A Day
IN THE Office
CASE STUDIES
IN PRIMARY
CARE

A Day IN THE Office
CASE STUDIES
IN PRIMARY CARE

JEFFREY A. EATON, MS, ARNP

JOYCE D. CAPPIELLO, MS, ARNP

Assistant Professors
Department of Nursing
University of New Hampshire
Durham, New Hampshire

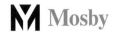 Mosby

St. Louis Baltimore Boston Carlsbad Chicago Naples New York Philadelphia Portland
London Madrid Mexico City Singapore Sydney Tokyo Toronto Wiesbaden

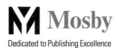
Mosby
Dedicated to Publishing Excellence

A Times Mirror
Company

Publisher **Sally Schrefer**
Developmental Editor **Michele D. Hayden**
Project Manager **Dana Peick**
Production Editor **Jeffrey Patterson**
Composition Specialist **Wendy Bellm**
Designer **Amy Buxton**
Manufacturing Manager **Don Carlisle**

A NOTE TO THE READER

The authors and publisher have made every attempt to check dosages and content for accuracy. Because the science of pharmacology is continually advancing, our knowledge base continues to expand. Therefore we recommend that the reader always check product information for changes in dosage or administration before prescribing or administering any medication. This is particularly important with new or rarely used drugs.

Printed in the United States of America
Composition by Mosby Electronic Production
Printing/binding by R.R. Donnelley

Mosby, Inc.
11830 Westline Industrial Drive
St. Louis, Missouri 63146

ISBN 0-8151-1559-8

98 99 00 01 02 / 9 8 7 6 5 4 3 2 1

ACKNOWLEDGEMENTS

Thanks to Sally Schrefer and Shelly Hayden from Mosby, who have seen us through this challenging process with the right mix of humor and persistence. Also thanks to our local Mosby representative Toni Fournier, who suggested this book in the first place in response to our lamentations about the lack of a case study book for nurse practitioners.

Thanks to the members and students of the Department of Nursing at UNH for their collegiality and direct and indirect contributions to this book.

We would also like to recognize Howard Barrows and Charlotte Paolini for opening us up to the world of Problem-Based Learning. Thanks also to Janet Anderson, Hannah Frank, and Dan Cappiello for editorial comments.

A special thanks to Gene Harkless for her vision in nurse practitioner education at UNH and for her mentorship and friendship.

Special thanks to my parents, David and Marjorie Eaton, my children Carla, Colin, and Cody, and of course my most special thanks to my wife Janet, without whom any contribution I have made would not have been possible.

Jeffrey A. Eaton

This is a special thank you to my health care colleagues and students for their encouragement and insightful comments. To my children, Nick, Lena, and Ben, thank you for your patience while I worked on this book. And a big thank you to my husband Dan for his encouragement.

Joyce D. Cappiello

REVIEWERS & CONSULTANTS

Jean Krajicek Bartek, PhD, ARNP
Associate Professor
University of Nebraska Medical Center
College of Nursing and Medicine/Pharmacology
Omaha, Nebraska

Bruce Bates, DO
Associate Dean for Clinical Affairs
University of New England
College of Osteopathic Medicine
Biddeford, Maine

Wendy Biddle, PhD, ARNP
Research Associate Professor
Dartmouth-Hitchcock Medical Center;
Assistant Professor
Department of Nursing
University of New Hampshire
Durham, New Hampshire

Theodore Chang, MD
Private Practice, Urology
Albany, New York

Joyce E. Dains, DrPH, JD, RN, CS, FNP
Assistant Professor
Department of Family Medicine
Baylor College of Medicine
Houston, Texas

Stefanie Diamond, PA-C
Emergency Department
Concord Hospital
Concord, New Hampshire

Trish Bagley Fairall, ARNP
Women's Health Care Specialist
The Clinic
Dover, New Hampshire

Colleen Grebus, MS, ARNP
Milford Family Practice
Milford, New Hampshire

Gene Elizabeth Harkless, DNSc, ARNP
Associate Professor
Department of Nursing
University of New Hampshire
Durham, New Hampshire

Susan Horton, MSN, RN
Cardiac Clinical Nurse
Optima Health
Manchester, New Hampshire

Gale Johnsen, PhD, FNP
Clinical Assistant Professor
Graduate Nursing
Simmons/Westbrook Partnership in Primary
   Healthcare at UNE
Simmons College
Boston, Massachusetts

Neil Korsen, MD
Medical Director
Sacopee Valley Health Center
Kezar Falls, Maine

Liza Little, PsyD, RN
Associate Professor
Department of Nursing
University of New Hampshire
Durham, New Hampshire

Charlotte Paolini, DO
Private Practice, Family Practice
Kennebunk, Maine

JoAnne Peach, MSN, RN, FNP-C
Assistant Professor
University of Virginia
School of Nursing
Charlottesville, Virginia

Stephanie Pluhar, MS, ARNP
Assistant Professor
Department of Nursing
University of New Hampshire
Durham, New Hampshire

Linda Robinson, MS, MA, RN
Assistant Professor
Department of Nursing
University of New Hampshire
Durham, New Hampshire

Michael Romanowsky, MD
Private Practice, Family Practice
Windham, New Hampshire

Victoria Scott, PA-C, MHS
Assistant Clinical Professor
Department of Community and Family Medicine;
Director of Preclinical Education
Physician Assistant Program
Duke University Medical Center
Durham, North Carolina

Amy Spearman, MSN, FNP, PNP, RN-CS
Clinical Assistant Professor
University of Alabama at Huntsville
Huntsville, Alabama

Susan F. Wilson, PhD, RN, FNP
Associate Professor
Harris College of Nursing
Texas Christian University
Fort Worth, Texas;
Family Nurse Practitioner
Medical Center at Riverside
Grand Prairie, Texas

INTRODUCTION

Case Studies in Primary Care: A Day in the Office is written with the objective of allowing a student or clinician to experience the clinical reasoning process just as it would occur in an office setting. We use "real" cases because they are ill-structured problems like those encountered in office practice. Textbook cases occur primarily in textbooks and not in clinical practice. Identifying information has, of course, been changed to protect the privacy of the individual.

These cases have been reviewed by experienced nurse practitioners, physician assistants, and physicians. Efforts have been made to ensure that the information presented is correct. It must, of course, be accepted that health care is a rapidly changing discipline and that new knowledge may be available that was not available when this book was written. Since the ultimate decision and responsibility belong to the individual clinician, cases in which the reader disagrees with what is written may actually provide a greater opportunity for discussion and learning. This book is not intended to be a textbook but an opportunity to exercise knowledge and abilities.

How to Use These Cases

SCHEDULE

You are encouraged to consider the time of day and length of visit for which each patient is scheduled. Time restraints and the appropriate strategies should be considered, such as scheduling a follow-up visit for further evaluation or intervention.

CASES

All of the cases that follow are "real." They are based on individuals, or composites of patients, who have been cared for by the clinicians who have contributed to this book. In the cases where composites have been used, it has been done to protect individual privacy rather than to create a case that reflects a certain pathology. In those cases in which a composite has been used, several clinicians have reviewed the case to ensure that it is a plausible scenario.

The formats of the cases are subtly different. This is in a deliberate effort to stimulate different portions of the clinical reasoning process. In some cases you will be asked to make decisions with limited information, and in others you will be given far more information than would actually be available in a clinical encounter. In each case the objective is to ask, "Do I need this information?" "How can I use this information?" "What does this information really mean?"

Once you have reviewed the case, you may want to investigate certain issues before completing the Assessment and Plan sections.

If you are perplexed about where to begin thinking through these problems, you can look at the inside front cover of the book. There are some general questions that may help start the process. The Learning Issues box in the Case Discussion may also provide some guidance. Each clinician will find a way of organizing the collection, evaluation, and synthesis of information that fits his or her individual style.

Prescription Blanks

Prescription blanks are provided for practice in writing out prescriptions. You are encouraged to review these with faculty or an experienced practitioner.

The number of prescription blanks appearing with each case varies. This is not intended to indicate that a certain number are required, however. You are encouraged to use discretion in writing prescriptions that you feel are necessary. Additional prescription blanks are included at the back of the book to be used as needed.

CASE DISCUSSION

After completing the Assessment and Plan or addressing the challenge offered, you may review the Case Discussion section for that case. Learning Issues and Discussions are intended to provide a basis for comparison with other clinicians' learning needs and approaches and are not intended to be interpreted as "right" answers. In primary care the right answer may depend on the resources of the client and practitioner and may vary greatly from instance to instance. Discussions are provided to show opinions from the literature as well as other anecdotal information when appropriate.

As noted, there is no single right answer in the vast majority of cases, but the range of options will be defined by a rational, evidence-based approach to clinical problems. Unfortunately there is not always research evidence available or research may be flawed or contradictory. These discussions reflect the synthesis of current information by experienced clinicians. We believe them to be, in all cases, a reasonable approach to the problem described. They may not, however, be the best approach for a given patient or a given clinician, or additional knowledge may now exist that would change the possible outcome of the case. You may create a more complete or elegant approach than those described in the case discussions.

Learning Issues

Often students have a difficult time deciding how to approach a problem, especially early in their education. By contrast, experienced clinicians may focus on one diagnosis or option without consciously considering all possibilities. In many cases this is not a defect in the clinical reasoning of the experienced clinician but a sign of an expert reasoning process. When an experienced clinician encounters an unfamiliar or otherwise "ill-structured" problem, however, the ability to think things through deliberately becomes important. Some references refer to this increased attention to the process of how to think through problems as being "metacognitive."

The Learning Issues box provides issues that have been generated by the authors and previous tutorial groups. This section is not meant to be exhaustive, and you will often have very different learning issues depending on your own level of development.

Initial Ideas

When a clinician sees a problem on a schedule book, ideas are quickly generated as to the etiology of that problem as well as possible treatments. Rather than deny that this process exists it is worthwhile to acknowledge this process and utilize it to achieve positive results while preventing or minimizing any negative results. Further, these initial ideas will drive the collection of data.

Interpretation of Cues, Patterns, and Information

Symptom analysis is the process by which most people begin collecting data. One mnemonic that may help in the collection of data is OPQRSTU:

- O: Are Other people sick?
- P2: Provocative and Palliative actions: What makes it better? What makes it worse?
- Q2: What are the Quality and Quantity of the pain?
- R3: Region, Radiation, Recurrence: Where is it? Does it go anywhere else? Have you ever had this before?

- S2: Severity, Symptoms: Similar to quantity but may have a somewhat more subjective flavor. Are you having any other symptoms?
- T3: Timing, Temporal, Treatment: When did it first come on? What time of day is it better or worse? What other treatments have you tried?
- U: What do *you* think is wrong?

Although OPQRSTU does not necessarily allow for a story to be told in its most logical form, it is a valuable mechanism to go back over a patient's story to ensure that the necessary information has been obtained.

Once data is collected, certain patterns may appear that support or dispute a particular etiology for the patient's problem. These patterns are interpreted based on the knowledge base and the experience of the clinician. These patterns may indicate the need for further investigation through history, physical examination, or other diagnostic testing, or they may lead to a specific theory of the cause of the problem or problems.

Revised Ideas

Once appropriate history and physical examination have been completed, there will be new thoughts about the most probable causes of the patients problem. Since the differential diagnosis will drive some of this data collection, this is often similar to the differential itself.

Differential Diagnosis[*]

A differential diagnosis is merely a "laundry list" of the possible causes for a particular symptom, sign, or syndrome. Most clinicians include about four to six possibilities in their working differential. Usually these are the possibilities that are the most common and/or the most dangerous causes of the signs or symptoms.

The differential diagnosis is an excellent guide to action since the objective is to rule in or rule out the possibilities. A symptom may have more than one cause, so it may be necessary to rule out problems on the differential even when another possibility has been ruled in. For example, even when history findings are conclusive that a viral illness is present in a patient with pharyngitis, it may be necessary to test for strep infection to eliminate the possibility of coexisting viral and bacterial infections.

---

[*]A word about Zebras. There is an old adage in clinical practice: "When you hear hoofbeats look for horses before you look for Zebras." Although there is great truth to this adage, you cannot forget that occasionally a Zebra will occur. Patients ask their health providers to provide the greatest assurance possible that they do not have a dangerous condition. Often, just by a few strategic history questions or physical assessment techniques, you can rule out potentially dangerous conditions. Laboratory and other diagnostic tests can then be used judiciously.

Diagnostic Options

Many times after a patient encounter is completed, the clinician has a "working" diagnosis but does not necessarily have a definite answer of what is wrong. A trial of therapy, referral to another provider, or laboratory or other diagnostic testing are all options at this point. The clinician must be able to make an appropriate choice based on efficacy and safety.

Therapeutic Options

Once a decision has been made to provide treatment to an individual, there are several other choices to be made. Will I prescribe a medication? If so which one? What other treatments can be used, such as physical therapy or environmental alteration? In addition, are there other treatments (such as those specific to a particular culture) that this patient will want to include as part of an overall approach?

Pharmacological When choosing a medication, there are many different factors to consider. What is the drug of choice for this problem? Are there other factors to consider (such as allergies, pregnancy, or drug interactions)? What is the best route and dosage for this patient?

Educational Are there educational needs of this patient and/or the family? When caring for an individual, there must be recognition that the individual and/or family are really the ones that determine what treatment will be carried out. Education about treatment options, reasons for treatment, and the treatment itself are essential.

Other Nonpharmacological options Included in this section are options such as physical therapy, culturally prescribed approaches, and alternative therapies.

Follow-Up

It is often a challenge for a fledgling clinician to decide when (and if) to ask a patient to return for a follow-up visit. Does this person only need to return if there is no improvement, or should a recheck be scheduled whether they feel that they have improved or not? Is phone follow-up appropriate? Research in this area is limited, so the individual clinician must often wrestle with this issue.

REFERENCES AND FURTHER READING

References are provided for two reasons. The first is to provide documentation of the accuracy of information. Those references are included with each case. The second reason is to allow an opportunity for additional investigation of a particular topic area.

References provided may be recent textbook or pocket references that are utilized by many clinicians in day-to-day practice as well as journal articles. This is a reflection of the pragmatic reality that often a general reference must be used for at least a portion of understanding an issue.

The book is intended to allow you to exercise your clinical reasoning abilities to the extent possible in this format. Our students have found these cases extremely helpful, and we hope that others will also.

Jeffrey A. Eaton
Joyce D. Cappiello

CONTENTS

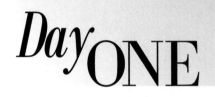

Day ONE

OPENING SCENARIO

Harold Baron is a 56-year-old male on your schedule for an annual physical examination because he wants to start an exercise program. He has been seen in your practice for the past 3 years.

HISTORY OF PRESENT ILLNESS

"I feel that I'm getting older and I've put on a few pounds, so I think I should start exercising. I'll probably just start out with brisk walking, but I'd like to get up to running a few miles a day. I've been in your practice for several years, but I have not taken your advice to come in for a complete physical. I feel very healthy."

MEDICAL HISTORY

Tonsillectomy and adenoidectomy as a child. No history of heart disease, hypertension, or diabetes. Usual childhood immunizations. Not immunized for hepatitis B. Unsure of last tetanus immunization.

FAMILY MEDICAL HISTORY

MGM: Died at 82 yr (breast cancer)
MGF: Died at 77 yr (myocardial infarction [MI])
PGM: Died at 80 yr (complications of Type II diabetes mellitus [DM])
PGF: Deceased at 74 yr (stroke)
Mother: 81 yr (A&W)
Father: Died at 80 yr (stroke 2 years ago)
Daughter: 32 yr (A&W)
Son: 30 yr (A&W)
Four grandchildren: None with health problems

SOCIAL HISTORY

Married for 34 years. Works in a post office. Active job of bending and lifting. No recreational exercise. Quit smoking 15 years ago. Alcohol occasionally (less than 2 ounces per week). Caffeine: 2 cups of coffee per day. Sleeps soundly 7 hours per night.

MEDICATIONS

One multivitamin with minerals daily
Vitamin E: 400 mg daily
Vitamin C: 1000 mg daily

ALLERGIES

None

REVIEW OF SYSTEMS

General: Good energy level
Skin: No itching or rashes
HEENT: No history of head injury; pupils equal and reactive to light; wears glasses for reading only; denies eye pain, excessive tearing, blurring, or change in vision; no tinnitus or vertigo; denies frequent colds, hay fever, or sinus problems; regular dental care
Neck: No lumps, goiters, or pain
Cardiac: Denies chest pain, shortness of breath, or elevated blood pressure
Respiratory: Denies shortness of breath, cough, dyspnea
Gastrointestinal: No nausea or vomiting, constipation, or diarrhea; denies heartburn, belching, bloating, stomach pain, black or clay colored stools
Genitourinary: No dysuria; no difficulty starting stream; sexually active (denies problems)
Extremities: Mild knee pain with significant activity
Neurological: No severe headaches, occasional mild headache relieved by acetaminophen; no history of seizures, weaknesses
Endocrine: No polyuria, polyphagia, polydipsia; temperature tolerances good
Hematological: No excessive bruising; no history of transfusions

PHYSICAL EXAMINATION

Vital signs: Temperature: 98.4° F; *Pulse:* 74 beats/min; *Respirations:* 20 breaths/min; *BP:* 126/82 mm Hg
Height: 5' 9"; *Weight:* 178 lb; *BMI:* 26-27
General: Well nourished, well developed; in no acute distress; appears younger than stated age
HEENT: Normocephalic without masses or lesions; pupils equal, round, and reactive to light; extraocular movements intact; fundi benign; nares patent and non-injected; throat without redness or lesions

Neck: Supple without thyromegaly, adenopathy, or carotid bruits

Heart: Regular rate and rhythm; no murmurs, rubs, or gallops

Lungs: Clear to auscultation

Gastrointestinal: No hepatosplenomegaly; abdomen soft, nontender; bowel sounds normoactive

Genitourinary: Normal male; circumcised; both testicles descended; prostate slightly enlarged symmetrically, smooth, firm

Extremities: Range of motion functionally intact; no cyanosis, clubbing, or edema; normal stance and gait; right and left knees: no bruising, swelling, erythema; no point tenderness; full range of motion without pain; no ballottement, negative bulge sign, negative drawer tests

Neuromuscular: Reflexes 2+ at Achilles, patellar, biceps, triceps, and brachioradialis; no Babinski sign present

ASSESSMENT   *Please indicate the problems or issues you have identified that will guide your care (preferably in list form):*

PLAN   *Please list your plans for addressing each of the problems or issues in your assessment:*

Community Clinic
Jeffrey A. Eaton, NP
Joyce D. Cappiello, NP

Name:_____ DOB_____
Address_____ Date_____

Rx

"label all unless indicated"
Refill:_____ times-- Do not refill ( )

Signed:_____
DO NOT TAKE THIS TO YOUR PHARMACIST

Community Clinic
Jeffrey A. Eaton, NP
Joyce D. Cappiello, NP

Name:_____ DOB_____
Address_____ Date_____

Rx

"label all unless indicated"
Refill:_____ times-- Do not refill ( )

Signed:_____
DO NOT TAKE THIS TO YOUR PHARMACIST

CASE
1 Discussion

INITIAL IDEAS

- Need for appropriate exercise plan
- Health maintenance issues

INTERPRETATION OF CUES, PATTERNS, AND INFORMATION

1. *Weight:* A quick way to approximate IBW for men is as follows:

$$(10 \text{ kg} \times \text{ft}) + (2.3 \text{ kg} \times \text{each additional inch}) =$$
$$(10 \text{ kg} \times 5 \text{ ft}) + (2.3 \text{ kg} \times 9 \text{ in}) =$$
an estimated IBW of 70.7 kg (155.54 lb)
or
$$(20 \text{ lb} \times \text{ft}) + (7 \text{ lb} \times \text{each additional inch}) =$$
$$(20 \text{ lb} \times 5 \text{ ft}) + (7 \text{ lb} \times 9 \text{ in}) =$$
an estimated IBW of 163 lb

The Metropolitan Life Insurance company has issued standard height and weight tables that reflect desirable weights, those at which people live the longest. These weights have long been interpreted as ideal. This became somewhat controversial when new standards were issued in 1983 that allowed an increase of 2 to 15 pounds for men and 2 to 12 pounds for women above the 1959 tables. Many health care providers feel this change is not in line with current research, which links obesity with cardiovascular disease. Mr. Baron is overweight using either the 1959 or the 1983 tables.

For body mass index (BMI), either use a BMI chart or compute weight (in kilograms) divided by height (in meters) squared. This would yield a BMI of 26.4. The criteria for obesity is 27. Based on any of these calculations of IBW, Mr. Baron is overweight but does not meet the criteria for obesity, which is >20% over IBW.

2. *Intake of vitamins C and E exceeding the recommended daily allowance (RDA):* His vitamin intake of C and E exceeds the RDA, although these are common supplement levels. Data exist that suggest that the antioxidant effect of vitamin C and E may decrease the risk of chronic diseases, although the optimal therapeutic dose is unclear.

3. *Increased risk for coronary artery disease (CAD):* An assessment of his coronary risk factors is necessary. Look at the following factors:

   a. He quit smoking 15 years ago. He probably had 20+ pack years (years smoked times average packs per day), but most of the effect has been "reversed" by his lack of smoking for 15 years. This will certainly have reduced his risk of hypertension and CAD.

   b. Although he has a family history of CAD and DM, the earliest death of a relative occurred at age 74. There does not appear to be a major risk of inherited premature death.

   c. He is a male over the age of 50 years. Gender and age are risk factors.

   d. He is more than 15% above IBW.

   e. He does not currently have a regular exercise program.

   f. In spite of his lack of a formal exercise program, his overall health so far seems reasonable. The fact that his blood pressure is normal is a very positive indicator of his health.

4. *Seeking medical clearance to begin an exercise program:* Consider what kind of a workup is necessary to clear him for increasing his activity and what specific recommendations you will suggest.

5. *Mild joint pain with significant activity:* You could suspect early osteoarthritis.

6. *Health maintenance:* All patients' annual physicals have health maintenance as an issue.

REVISED IDEAS

- Overweight
- Inactive lifestyle
- Mild joint pain with significant activity
- Family history of CAD
- Health maintenance issues

DIAGNOSTIC OPTIONS

1. First analyze the need for preexercise screening. The Guide to Clinical Preventive Services (1996) does not recommend preexercise screening for middle-age and older men and women who do not have symptoms of CAD with resting electrocardiography (ECG) or exercise ECG. This is based on the limited sensitivity and low predictive value of an abnormal resting ECG in asymptomatic persons and the high costs of screening and follow-up. Their recommendation is to focus on modifiable cardiac risk factors such as hypertension, smoking, elevated serum cholesterol level, diet, physical activity, and perhaps the daily intake of low dose aspirin.

The exercise ECG is more accurate than the resting ECG for detecting clinically important CAD, but most patients with asymptomatic CAD do not have a positive test, and most asymptomatic patients with an abnormal exercise ECG result do not have underlying disease (US Preventive Services Task Force, 1996). Because of Mr. Baron's history of joint pain, your recommendation might include a slow progression of exercise to avoid aggravating his joints, which will gradually increase his endurance, causing less stress on his cardiovascular system.

2. Based on his age, gender, and weight, an assessment of his cholesterol level is important. A fasting lipid profile seems reasonable. Since he has a relative with DM, a serum glucose test would be appropriate. You may also decide to order a limited chemistry profile for baseline data since it would include the glucose and is low cost; however, reimbursement may be a factor in this decision.

3. You consider doing thyroid testing, but based on his age, gender, and lack of symptoms, you decide that the cost/benefit analysis will not support doing this testing at this time.

THERAPEUTIC OPTIONS

1. Since Mr. Baron is overweight, encourage his idea of an activity program. It is also important to begin to look at his dietary intake. There are several options to consider regarding this:

a. Refer him to a dietitian.

b. Suggest a dietary intake of approximately 1800 calories.

c. Begin some brief diet teaching and provide him with some handouts. Plan for further assessment and intervention on later visits.

d. Weight loss may decrease stress on his knees.

2. Discuss with him that it probably is not essential that he continue his extra vitamin C and vitamin E intake, but the use of antioxidant vitamins seems reasonable. Some clinicians feel that there is a theoretical risk of kidney stones with excessive vitamin C intake. Although 1000 mg is not excessive, he could be warned of this. A 500 mg dose of vitamin C would give an antioxidant effect and would be well below a level that could cause side effects.

3. Consider low-dose daily acetylsalicylic acid (ASA) prophylaxis. A large randomized, controlled trial in the United States found a significant reduction in the incidence of MIs in the group receiving 325 mg of aspirin (Manson et al, 1991). A much smaller British study did not show a reduction in cardiovascular disease with 500 mg of aspirin (Pero et al, 1988). If considering aspirin use, keep in mind the potential adverse effects, especially on the gastrointestinal system. If you are convinced by the research, discuss it with Mr. Baron and make a joint decision based on risk/benefit analysis.

4. An exercise program is discussed and you recommend that he do the following:

a. Begin gradually with walking rather than running.

b. Monitor his pulse—initially in the 55% to 60% maximum range (about 90 to 100 beats/min).

$$\text{Maximum range} = 220 - \text{age}$$

c. Exercise at least three times per week.

d. Stretch before and after exercise.

e. Suggest a formal exercise program of muscle strengthening especially with his knees. Resistance work on machines at a gym or with free weights would be very helpful for him.

f. Suggest protective measures such as wearing reflectors if walking at night, wearing good quality athletic shoes with adequate cushioning, and calling his provider about any new or increased joint problems.

5. Regarding his joint pain you decide to do the following:

a. Further assess and monitor it as he begins his exercise program and/or recommend mild analgesics to help him manage this pain. Acetaminophen (Tylenol) has no gastrointestinal concerns but many clinicians use nonsteroidal anitinflammatory drugs (NSAIDs). Topical capsaicin products are pepper derivatives that are capable of stimulating nerve endings to release more than their usual amounts of substance P, a highly inflammatory vasoactive peptide. With recurrent use, these agents are capable of actually depleting the nerve endings of substance P, ultimately leading to less pain and inflammation (Peck, 1997). At first the cream will cause a prickly or burning feeling, but this will improve with repeated use of the cream.

b. If the joint pain worsens, consider a physical therapy referral for evaluation and recommendations of ways to increase the strength of the joints.

6. Health maintenance interventions

a. Colorectal cancer screening: The digital rectal examination (DRE) is of limited value as a screening test for cancer because the examining finger does not have access to the entire rectal mucosa. Consider three fecal occult blood tests (FOBT) for him to use at home. The U.S. Preventive Services Task Force recommends screening for colorectal cancer for all persons 50 years of age and older with annual FOBT, sigmoidoscopy, or both. The frequency for sigmoidoscopy screening varies from recommendations of every 3 to 5 years from the American Cancer Society, the American

Gastroenterological Association, and the American College of Obstetricians and Gynecologists to every 10 years by the American College of Physicians (US Preventive Services Task Force, 1996).

b. Prostate cancer screening: The sensitivity of the DRE is limited because the examining finger can palpate only the posterior and lateral aspects of the gland. The prostate-specific antigen (PSA) is a serum tumor marker available for screening. To date, the National Cancer Institute, the National Institutes of Health, and the U.S. Preventive Services Task Force have not yet endorsed PSA screening in asymptomatic patients. It has not been documented that early detection of prostate cancer leads to an increased survival rate (US Preventive Services Task Force, 1996). The American Cancer Society, the American Urological Association, and the Food and Drug Administration (FDA) have endorsed the use of PSA for the early detection of prostate cancer in men 50 years of age and older, in Black men, and in patients with a family history of prostate cancer at age 40. Discuss the pros and cons of testing with Mr. Baron.

c. Update his tetanus-diphtheria (Td) immunization if necessary.

d. Recommend an annual dental examination.

e. Recommend glaucoma screening. Mr. Baron would be at an increased risk for glaucoma if he is Black because glaucoma is the leading cause of blindness in Blacks. Effective screening for glaucoma is best performed by eye specialists who have access to specialized equipment to evaluate the optic disc and measure visual fields (US Preventive Services Task Force, 1996).

f. Discuss safety belt use, smoke detector use, and accident prevention.

g. Review any risk factors for hepatitis B and decide accordingly on his need for immunization.

FOLLOW-UP

When should the patient return? This is often a difficult decision-making area for new providers since there are few guidelines to follow. A return visit in 2 to 4 weeks to monitor his progress, review his laboratory work, and determine further plans seems reasonable.

References

Manson JE et al: Baseline characteristics of participants in the Physician's Health Study: a randomized trial of aspirin and beta-carotene in U.S. physicians, *Am J Prevent Med* 7:150, 1991.

Peck B: Osteoarthritis treatment, *Adv Nurs Pract* 4(7):32, 1977.

Pero R et al: Randomized trial of prophylactic daily aspirin in British male doctors, *Br Med J* 296:313, 1988.

US Preventive Services Task Force: *Guide to clinical preventive service,* Baltimore, 1996, Williams & Wilkins.

CASE
2

OPENING SCENARIO

Kate Smith is a 29-year-old female scheduled for an episodic visit with a complaint of painful urination. This is her first visit to your practice.

HISTORY OF PRESENT ILLNESS

"I'm having difficulty urinating. I had something like this 5 years ago and it was a urinary tract infection. I have been urinating more often, have burning with urination, and sometimes can't start the flow of urine for a while. This started yesterday, woke me during the night, and has made me very uncomfortable this morning. I am also having some sharp pain in the area of my bladder. I took one ibuprofen last night and this morning, but it didn't help all that much."

MEDICAL HISTORY

Urinary tract infection (UTI) 5 years ago that resolved with antibiotic use. No history of kidney infections or renal calculi. No history of major medical problems. Tonsillectomy and adenoidectomy as child. No other hospitalizations.

FAMILY MEDICAL HISTORY

Mother: 47 yr (A&W)
Father: 50 yr (hypertension)
Two brothers: 23 and 20 yr (A&W)

SOCIAL HISTORY

Moved here 3 months ago to begin graduate school. Single, lives with a female roommate. Two male sexual partners in the past 6 months.

MEDICATIONS

Occasional ibuprofen: 200 mg tabs
Triphasil-28

ALLERGIES

None

REVIEW OF SYSTEMS

General: Feels very healthy
Gastrointestinal: Occasional diarrhea with high stress; no diarrhea since symptoms began
Gynocological: G1P0Ab1 2 years ago; clear mucus discharge for 3 days; treated for monilia 2 years ago; using Triphasil-28 for $1^1/_2$ years; last menstrual period (LMP): 1 week ago, normal withdrawal bleeding; regular menstrual bleeding both on and off the pill; denies any missed pills; two male sexual partners in the past 6 months; partners use condoms most of the time; treated for chlamydia 3 years ago; Last Pap smear: 9 months ago; all Pap smears within normal limits; no dyspareunia or postcoital bleeding

PHYSICAL EXAMINATION

Vital signs: Temperature: 98.4° F; *Pulse:* 70 beats/min; *Respirations:* 16 breaths/min; *BP:* 110/60 mm Hg
General: Healthy-appearing female in no acute distress
Abdomen: Slight tenderness to palpation in suprapubic area; soft without masses; no costovertebral angle (CVA) tenderness
Genitourinary: Vulva without lesions, erythema, edema; vagina: moderate amount of clear, mucous discharge; cervix: os closed, Nabothian cyst, 11 o'clock, 3 mm; uterus: small, smooth, anteverted, midline, no cervical motion tenderness; adnexa: nonpalpable, nontender

Laboratory Results

Wet prep: occasional white blood cell (WBC), without monilia, clue cells, or motile trichomonas; ph: 4.1; Whiff test: negative; Urine dipstick test (Table 2-1)

Table **2-1** *Urine Dipstick Test for Kate Smith*

TEST	RESULT
Color	Yellow
Appearance	Cloudy
Glucose	Negative
Bile	Negative
Ketones	Negative
SG	1.025
Blood	Trace
ph	6.5
Protein	Trace
Urobilinogen	1.0
Leukocyctes	Moderate amount
Nitrites	Negative

ASSESSMENT   *Please indicate the problems or issues you have identified that will guide your care (preferably in list form):*

PLAN   *Please list your plans for addressing each of the problems or issues in your assessment:*

Community Clinic
Jeffrey A. Eaton, NP
Joyce D. Cappiello, NP

Name:_____ DOB_____
Address_____ Date_____

Rx

"label all unless indicated"
Refill:_____ times-- Do not refill ( )

Signed:_____
DO NOT TAKE THIS TO YOUR PHARMACIST

Community Clinic
Jeffrey A. Eaton, NP
Joyce D. Cappiello, NP

Name:_____ DOB_____
Address_____ Date_____

Rx

"label all unless indicated"
Refill:_____ times-- Do not refill ( )

Signed:_____
DO NOT TAKE THIS TO YOUR PHARMACIST

LEARNING ISSUES

In order to resolve this patient's problem, you will need to consider and address the following issues (you may generate additional issues as well):

- Analysis of the chief complaint in an episodic visit
- Differential diagnosis
- Useful physical examination techniques in a patient with dysuria
- Laboratory testing: How do the issues of cost, ease of testing, turnaround time for results, and accuracy of testing impact your decision making?
- Screening for vaginitis
- Choice of therapeutics: How do the issues of efficacy, cost, dosing, length of therapy, and side effects influence the choice? What is the current research on 1-, 3-, or 10-day therapy for UTI?
- Pain management
- Follow-up
- Preventive measures

INITIAL IDEAS

- UTI
- Sexually transmitted disease (STD)
- Vaginitis

INTERPRETATION OF CUES, PATTERNS, AND INFORMATION

The first decision to consider is whether this is an acute, uncomplicated UTI or a complicated UTI. An acute, uncomplicated UTI is a very common health concern in young women; it usually responds well to antibiotic therapy without sequelae. A complicated UTI includes recent antibiotic use, symptoms for more than 7 days, diabetes, immunosuppresion, hospital-acquired infection, pregnancy, recent urinary tract instrumentation, or known urological abnormality. The workup and treatment are very different for a complicated UTI, but fortunately for Ms. Smith, by history she does not appear to meet any of these criteria.

An important clue is that she has had symptoms similar to this in the past that were diagnosed as a UTI. Also, this past infection was 5 years ago, so there is no concern about a recurrent or resistant infection. Her temperature is not elevated, which is reassuring. A high fever and/or chills, especially with flank pain and positive CVA tenderness, would indicate a greater likelihood of a pyelonephritis. Fortunately, none of these findings are present.

Renal calculi usually present with severe pain. CVA tenderness may be present as well as changes in the urinalysis, which may show red blood cells (RBCs). The spun urine would typically show crystals and casts.

An STD is certainly a possibility given her history of two sexual partners in the past 6 months and lack of regular condom use.

A vaginitis such as a *monilia* or *trichomonas* infection can cause intense symptoms, although the onset may not be so rapid. It certainly belongs in your differential diagnosis since she is complaining of a vaginal discharge for 3 days.

DIAGNOSTIC OPTIONS

What is a cost-effective, timely test to evaluate the possibility of a UTI? The traditional testing has been to order a complete urinalysis followed by a culture, treatment, and a follow-up culture in 10 days. Using this recommendation, one episode of an uncomplicated UTI would cost approximately $200 (Barry, Ebell, and Hickner, 1997). Given that UTIs account for more than 7 million visits to health care offices each year, this is a significant contribution to escalating health care costs.

Using the above regimen, a urinalysis would provide information immediately if a dipstick is used in the office, but a spun urine is usually sent out to a laboratory with results available the next day. The culture report would not be available for 48 hours. The culture would essentially confirm your diagnosis and treatment but not help you establish them. The information would be helpful if the treatment was not working and an alternate medication had to be prescribed.

Microscopic examinations of unspun and spun urine can establish a presumptive diagnosis. Pyuria is defined as the presence of five or more leukocytes per high power field. These tests are Clinical Laboratory Improvement Act (CLIA) monitored tests that require quality control testing and skilled laboratory staff, which add to the cost of care.

A simple office-based test that would confirm the presence of a UTI seems necessary. The leukocyte esterase dipstick, common to most offices, has a reported sensitivity of 75% to 96% in detecting pyuria associated with infection. The nitrite portion of the test depends on the conversion of nitrates in the diet to nitrite by the action of gram-negative bacteria in the urine. The urine must be in the bladder for several hours for this to occur. If the patient is voiding every few minutes, the nitrite test may be negative only because the urine has not been in the bladder long enough for this breakdown to occur. The leukocyte portion of the test is more likely to be positive in the presence of frequent urination. A positive dipstick test is defined as one in which nitrites, leukocyte esterase, or both are present.

Some studies have focused on empiric treatment of acute, uncomplicated UTIs without any laboratory testing with good results (Barry, Ebell, and Hickner, 1997). Some providers have found telephone triage without an office visit adequate to successfully treat established patients.

STD testing: What should it focus on? A herpes infection could cause dysuria, but lesions are usually visible on physical examination. Chlamydia is more likely than gonorrhea to cause dysuria, but both can be tested for readily during the examination. Screening will add to the cost of the visit but may ultimately be cost effective if it detects chlamydia at an early stage.

The wet prep of the vaginal discharge performed in the office did not indicate the presence of monilia, trichomonas, or bacterial vaginitis. The pH of 4.1 (normal pH of the vagina is 3.8 to 4.2) and negative whiff test also help rule out vaginitis, particularly the very common bacterial vaginosis.

REVISED IDEAS

- UTI
- Chlamydia

THERAPEUTIC OPTIONS

Pharmacological

Stamn and Hooten (1993) outline the following approach to UTIs in women:

1. Since *E. coli* is implicated in 80% of acute, uncomplicated UTIs and is predictable in its antimicrobial susceptibility, an abbreviated laboratory workup can be used followed by empirical treatment.
2. An abbreviated laboratory workup is defined as leukocyte esterase testing or pyuria on microscopy.
3. No urine culture is performed.
4. A short course of antimicrobial therapy is given.
5. No follow-up visit or culture is recommended unless symptoms persist or recur.
6. If pyuria is absent or there are atypical clinical features that suggest a complicated infection, a culture should be performed before therapy is started.
7. This approach is efficacious, safe, and cost effective.

Numerous studies have focused on the optimal length of antibiotic therapy. Studies have focused on 1-, 3-, 7-, and 10-day therapy and have found that 3-day therapy is highly effective, inexpensive, and well tolerated. The 3-day therapy is more effective than the single dose therapy and is as effective as the longer course of medication in uncomplicated UTIs (Stamn and Hooten, 1993). The 3-day therapy also reduces the risk of *monilia* infections and drug induced rashes.

Various studies have compared antibiotics in 3-day therapy. A 3-day regimen of trimethoprim sulfamethoxazole (TMP/SMX [Bactrim or Septra]) DS tablets bid is more effective and less expensive than 3-day regimens of nitrofurantoin, cefadroxil, or amoxicillin for treatment of uncomplicated cystitis in women. The increased efficacy of TMP/SMX is likely related to its antimicrobial effects against *E. coli* in the rectum, urethra, and vagina (Hooten et al, 1995).

A cystitis pack of ciprofloxacin 100 mg bid is available, very effective, and well tolerated, but it is more expensive than TMP/SMX.

Educational

Several suggestions are given to women regarding the prevention of UTIs, but only a few of these have been supported by research. Studies have shown the most consistent factors associated with acute UTI to be sexual activity, the use of diaphragms with spermicides, and a history of recurrent UTIs (Hooten et al, 1996).

Some clinicians speculate that urethral trauma, decreased urge to void, and an increase in residual urine could serve as reasons why the diaphragm may be a risk factor. An association has also been found between diaphragm users and vaginal *E. coli* colonization, possibly because of the effect of the spermicide. Some studies have implicated the lack of postcoital voiding as a risk factor (Leiner, 1995).

To date, the literature has not supported the common advice given to women to prevent UTIs, such as direction of perineal wiping, bubble bath use, douching, tight pants or pantyhose, synthetic underwear, tampon use, and dietary factors (such as intake of coffee, alcohol, or carbonated beverages) (Leiner, 1995).

Recent studies have confirmed that cranberry or blueberry juice contain a substance with biological activity that can reduce bacterial adhesion to uroepithelial cells. Drinking 300 ml of cranberry juice each day may decrease the infection rate in some women.

FOLLOW-UP

There is no need for follow-up testing of the urine if the patient feels better. A resistant infection would indicate the need for a urine culture. The more common problem is the patient with recurrent infections (several per year). In the past, a urological workup was suggested for these patients, but the yield on this testing was very low. Rarely was a structural abnormality the cause of the frequent UTIs. Currently empiric management of recurrent UTIs is done with one TMP/SMX DS prophylactically postcoitus or low-dose, daily suppressive therapy of TMP/SMX (1 single strength tab po qd long term) (Sanford, Gilbert, and Sande, 1996). Some providers recommend patient-initiated therapy for those with only a few infections each year. Prescriptions are given in advance for a course of antibiotics to be started at the onset of symptoms (Stamn and Hooten, 1993).

References

Barry H, Ebell M, Hickner J: Evaluation of suspected urinary tract infection in ambulatory: a cost-utility analysis of office-based strategies, *J Fam Pract* 44(1):49, 1997.

Hooten TM et al: Randomized comparative trial and cost analysis of 3-day antimicrobial regimens for treatment of acute cystitis in women, *JAMA* 273(1):41, 1995.

Hooten TM et al: A prospective study of risk factors for symptomatic urinary tract infection in young women, *N Engl J Med* 335:468, 1996.

Leiner S: Recurrent urinary tract infections in otherwise healthy adult women, *Nurs Prac,* 20(2):48, 1995.

Sanford JP, Gilbert DN, Sande MA: *The Sanford guide to antimicrobial therapy,* Dallas, 1996, Antimicrobial Therapy.

Stamn WE, Hooten TM: Management of urinary tract infections in adults, *N Engl J Med* 329:1328, 1993.

CASE
3

OPENING SCENARIO

Francis Coulter is a 32-year-old male here for an episodic visit with a complaint of head congestion. He has been seen in your practice for the past 2 years.

HISTORY OF PRESENT ILLNESS

"I have had a cough and runny nose for over a week. About 3 days ago I developed a headache and started blowing thick, yellow-green mucus out of my nose. Bending over seems to make the headache worse. Acetaminophen improves the headache but doesn't take it away. I've also been using pseudoephedrine 30 mg, 2 tablets every 12 hours with little relief." The patient denies tooth pain or pain with mastication.

MEDICAL HISTORY

Seen here for a physical examination 1 year ago with no positive findings. No history of surgery, hospitalizations, coronary artery disease (CAD), hypertension, or diabetes.

MEDICATIONS

Pseudoephedrine HCl: 60 mg q12h for the past 3 days
Cough drops for sore throat
Acetaminophen: 1000 mg q4h for headache prn

REVIEW OF SYSTEMS

HEENT: Mild pain with swallowing; denies ear pain or discharge; no tinnitus or vertigo; describes purulent nasal discharge; has no history of allergies or allergic rhinitis; denies a history of frequent colds, hayfever, sinus problems; denies tooth pain
Cardiac: Denies chest pain
Respiratory: No shortness of breath or asthma; nonproductive cough
Gastrointestinal: No symptoms of nausea, vomiting, diarrhea
Neurological: Dull frontal headache, worse with bending over, for 3 days (4 on scale of 1 to 10)

PHYSICAL EXAMINATION

Vital signs: Temperature: 99.6° F; *Pulse:* 72 beats/min; *Respirations:* 16 breaths/min; *BP:* 126/82 mm Hg
HEENT: Tenderness to palpation over frontal area, no maxillary tenderness; tympanic membranes dull but not red, landmarks visible; nasal mucosa erythematous, boggy turbinates, no polyps noted; purulent yellow-greenish nasal discharge; pharynx: erythematous, cobbled appearance; no obvious dental disease; submaxillary nodes enlarged; no cervical adenopathy
Heart: Regular rate and rhythm; no murmurs, rubs, or gallops
Lungs: Clear to auscultation

ASSESSMENT   *Please indicate the problems or issues you have identified that will guide your care (preferably in list form):*

PLAN   *Please list your plans for addressing each of the problems or issues in your assessment:*

Community Clinic
Jeffrey A. Eaton, NP
Joyce D. Cappiello, NP

Name:_____ DOB_____
Address_____ Date_____

Rx

"label all unless indicated"
Refill:_____ times-- Do not refill ( )

Signed:_____
DO NOT TAKE THIS TO YOUR PHARMACIST

Community Clinic
Jeffrey A. Eaton, NP
Joyce D. Cappiello, NP

Name:_____ DOB_____
Address_____ Date_____

Rx

"label all unless indicated"
Refill:_____ times-- Do not refill ( )

Signed:_____
DO NOT TAKE THIS TO YOUR PHARMACIST

Community Clinic
Jeffrey A. Eaton, NP
Joyce D. Cappiello, NP

Name:_____ DOB_____
Address_____ Date_____

Rx

"label all unless indicated"
Refill:_____ times-- Do not refill ( )

Signed:_____
DO NOT TAKE THIS TO YOUR PHARMACIST

Community Clinic
Jeffrey A. Eaton, NP
Joyce D. Cappiello, NP

Name:_____ DOB_____
Address_____ Date_____

Rx

"label all unless indicated"
Refill:_____ times-- Do not refill ( )

Signed:_____
DO NOT TAKE THIS TO YOUR PHARMACIST

CASE
3 Discussion

LEARNING ISSUES

In order to resolve this patient's problem, you will need to consider and address the following issues (you may generate additional issues as well):

- **Pertinent physical examination techniques**
- **Choosing therapeutics: issues of efficacy, cost, dosing, and side effects. What resources are helpful?**
- **Length of course of antibiotics**
- **Pain management**
- **Role of decongestants**
- **Follow-up**

INITIAL IDEAS

- Upper respiratory infection (URI) possibly complicated by a concurrent sinusitis

INTERPRETATION OF CUES, PATTERNS, AND INFORMATION

Before a decision can be made on the final diagnosis in this case, the symptoms must be analyzed. With sinusitis, you typically think of headache, purulent nasal discharge, facial and/or dental pain, facial or head pain with bending over, and a URI.

A study by Williams and Simel (1993) showed poor accuracy of the diagnosis when based on any individual symptom (e.g., green nasal discharge), but symptoms in combination could be diagnostic. They identified three subjective complaints of maxillary toothache, poor response to nasal decongestants, and history of colored nasal discharge. Two objective signs as the best predictors of sinusitis are purulent nasal secretion and abnormal transillumination.

When none of these findings were present, sinusitis could be ruled out. When four or five were present, the likelihood of sinusitis was high. The common symptom of headache when leaning over was not studied.

Accurate transillumination in this study required a completely darkened room, adequate time for dark adaptation, and practice. The otolaryngologists were better with this skill than the primary care providers, which points to the value of practice with this technique (Williams and Simel, 1993).

In this case study, Mr. Coulter presented with two of the symptoms and one of the physical examination findings, which gives him a lower likelihood of sinusitis according to this research. Transillumination was not performed, which confounds the assessment. However, this man is symptomatic enough to seek health care and has a low-grade fever. The clinician must take all of this information and create an overall impression.

Are there other possible causes of his symptoms? Allergic rhinitis sufferers usually present with sneezing; pruritis; clear, watery discharge; and congestion. On physical examination the nasal mucosa is often pale and boggy. None of these clues were present.

Mr. Coulter is not taking any medications, so drug-induced rhinitis can be eliminated. Pregnancy (easily eliminated from your differential diagnosis) and hyperthyroidism both produce nasal congestion and nasal discharge. Hyperthyroidism was not specifically screened for, but his symptoms point to other causes.

Nasal polyps can contribute to nasal and/or sinus complaints and need to be considered if this becomes a chronic problem or if noted on examination.

DIAGNOSTIC OPTIONS

Are diagnostics such as x-ray examination or computerized tomography (CT) scan of the sinuses helpful or necessary with Mr. Coulter? Usually these tests are more useful if the patient is very ill, is immunocompromised such as with a malignancy or human immunodeficiency virus (HIV), has failed to respond to treatment, is developing potential complications (such as subperiosteal abscess, orbital cellulitis, or abscess), or is soon to have sinus surgery.

X-ray examinations are less costly, but CT scans have superior diagnostic ability to evaluate all sinus cavities in ill patients. CT scans in patients with a low clinical suspicion for sinusitis must be interpreted cautiously since 15% to 40% of abnormalities, such as mucosal thickening, are seen in patients without sinusitis. Magnetic resonance imaging (MRI) evaluations are only useful in evaluating fungal or neoplastic disease in chronic sinusitis (Lorenz, 1996). The exact role of ultrasound as a diagnostic test for sinusitis remains unclear (Schwartz, 1994). Usually imaging is not necessary to make the diagnosis for acute sinusitis nor is it cost effective.

Since diagnostic testing is unlikely to be helpful, the clinician's overall impression of symptoms and physical examination findings will make this a diagnosis of sinusitis. Although the diagnostic criteria for acute sinusitis is somewhat controversial, most clinicians would agree that this man has some sinus involvement and needs treatment.

THERAPEUTIC OPTIONS

Antibiotic Therapy

The importance of antibiotic therapy in acute and chronic sinusitis has not been well tested. It is not clear when viral or allergic sinusitis is superseded by bacterial infection. As demonstrated in a CT study of the common cold and in the few placebo-controlled trials of antibiotic therapy in sinusitis, many patients with acute sinusitis have spontaneous resolution of their symptoms (Lorenz, 1996).

A decision needs to be made whether to use antibiotic therapy on Mr. Coulter. Many clinicians would do so based on his complaints of headache, green nasal discharge, and pain with bending over.

The most commonly used antibiotics have been amoxicillin, ampicillin, augmentin, or trimethroprim sulfamethoxazole (TMP/SMX). Amoxicillin or TMP/SMX has traditionally been the first choice of many providers because they are generally well tolerated, low cost, and effective against *Streptococcus pneumoniae.* Augmentin (AM/CL 500/125 mg tid or 875/125 bid) is now listed as first-line therapy by the Sanford Guide because of the high incidence of penicillin-resistant pneumococci (Sanford et al, 1997).

Other drugs active against *Staphylococcus aureus* plus the beta-lactamase—producing strains of *H. influenzae, Moraxella catarrhalis,* some anaerobes, and many gram-negative aerobic bacilli include oral cephalosporins, macrolides, and azolides (Lorenz, 1996). Although these medications are more costly, some offer the advantage of once-a-day dosing.

Treatment for 10 to 14 days has been advised based on numerous studies. To date, only one study has shown efficacy with a short course (3-day) of therapy (Williams, Holleman, and Samsa et al, 1995).

Decongestant Use

Decongestants can help in meeting the management goals of reduction of tissue edema, facilitation of drainage, and maintenance of patency of the sinus ostia (Schwartz, 1994). Mr. Coulter describes a 3-day history of oral decongestant use with presumably no relief. With the addition of the antibiotic, the decongestant may be more successful.

Adrenergic nasal sprays (such as oxymetazoline) may shrink the nasal mucosa membrane and provide symptomatic relief but should only be used for 2 to 3 days because of the rebound phenomena. This could be used for 3 days assuming that by then the antibiotics would have taken effect in improving his clinical symptoms and should be discontinued.

Topical saline sprays may be given to liquefy and clear secretions without concern of rebound effect. Oral guaifenesin or nasal saline irrigation may also promote clearance of secretions.

Topical steroid sprays would take 3 to 4 days to take effect, and their use has not been shown to be definitely helpful in this situation. In acute sinusitis, antihistamines may cause impairment of mucociliary clearance because of their drying effect on nasal secretions. They may, however, have a use in chronic sinusitis related to allergic rhinitis.

Pain Relief

Continuing acetaminophen use or switching to any of the over-the-counter (OTC) nonsteroidal antiinflammatory drugs (NSAIDs) may help with the headache pain. Symptomatic relief with showers, warm compresses to the forehead, and increasing fluids may also help with the discomfort.

FOLLOW-UP

A safe course of action is to instruct Mr. Coulter to call for further evaluation if he worsens or if symptoms are not improving in 48 to 72 hours. What you do not want to miss is the rare complication of a facial cellulitis and its risk of intracranial infection.

If he is feeling better and symptoms are cleared, a follow-up visit is not necessary. It is always good practice to tell patients to call if they have any concerns.

A referral to an otolaryngologist may be necessary if Mr. Coulter develops a complication of sinusitis, all medical therapy fails, or he has frequent recurrent sinusitis. Referrals are also indicated if a patient has severe, acute sinusitis, has an anatomical nasal obstruction such as polyps or septal deviation, or is immunocompromised (Lorenz, 1996).

References

Lorenz K: Community-acquired bacterial sinusitis, *Prim Care* 2(24):217, 1996.

Sanford J et al: *The Sanford guide to microbial therapy,* Dallas, 1996, Antimicrobial Therapy.

Schwartz R: The diagnosis and management of sinusitis, *Nurs Pract* 19(12):58, 1994.

Williams J, Holleman D, Samsa G et al: Randomized controlled trial of 3 vs 10 days of trimethoprim/sulfamethoxazole for acute maxillary sinusitis, *JAMA* 272:1015, 1995.

Williams J, Simel D: Does this patient have sinusitis? diagnosing acute sinusitis by history and physical examination, *JAMA* 270:1242, 1993.

CASE
4

9:45 AM
Lianne Pierce
Age 6 years

OPENING SCENARIO

Lianne Pierce is a 6-year-old female on your schedule for rash with sore throat and fever. Her mother is present and appears to be in her late twenties. Lianne is sitting quietly on the examination table.

HISTORY OF PRESENT ILLNESS

(Obtained from mother)

"Lianne has been sick for about 4 days. It started with a headache, but she has been complaining of headaches lately anyway, so I didn't think much of it. Then she got a sore throat and runny nose. Now she feels like she has a fever (but I couldn't find my thermometer since we just moved) and this rash, so I thought I should bring her in. The rash came on about this time yesterday, and it has not really changed since it started. She says the rash is just a little itchy." Lianne's mother has made no changes in laundry detergent. Lianne has not eaten any new foods recently; no seafood in the past week. No new clothing recently. Denies known exposure to anyone with chicken pox or any other rash. You have not seen any similar cases recently in your practice. Lianne has no history of similar rashes or upper respiratory infections (URIs).

MEDICAL HISTORY

Growth percentiles within normal limits on previous visits. Milestones all within normal limits on previous visit. Has not had chicken pox. Immunization record is shown in Table 4-1.

FAMILY MEDICAL HISTORY

MGM: 51 yr (A&W)
MGF: 50 yr (high cholesterol)
PGM: 48 yr (breast cancer)
PGF: 50 yr (A&W)
Mother: 27 yr (A&W)
Father: 27 yr (A&W)
One brother: 8 yr (A&W)

SOCIAL HISTORY

Lives with mother. Spends every other weekend with father in a city with a population of 30,000 about one half hour away. Mother is an accountant. Father is an administrator of a public social service agency. Parents have been divorced about 2 years. In first grade; doing well. Sleeps well. No behavioral problems.

MEDICATIONS

None

ALLERGIES

None

REVIEW OF SYSTEMS

General: Good energy level
Skin: No itching or chronic or recurrent rashes
HEENT: Denies colds more frequent than normal; gets about three a year
Neck: No lumps, goiters, or pain
Thorax: Denies shortness of breath
Cardiac: No changes in color
Gastrointestinal: No vomiting, constipation, or diarrhea

Table **4-1** *Immunization Record for Lianne Pierce*

Vaccine	Date	Initials	Notes
DPT	2 mo	MDO	Tetramune
DPT	4 mo	KJ	Tetramune
DPT	6 mo	MDO	Tetramune
DPT	18 mo	MDO	Tetramune
DPT	5 yr	KJ	Acellular
Td			
OPV	2 mo	MDO	
OPV	4 mo	KJ	
OPV	18 mo	MDO	
OPV	5 yr	KJ	
MMR	13 mo	KJ	
MMR	5 yr	KJ	
HBV			
HBV			
HBV			
Hib	2 mo	MDO	Tetramune
Hib	4 mo	KJ	Tetramune
Hib	6 mo	MDO	Tetramune
Hib	18 mo	MDO	Tetramune

Genitourinary: No odor to urine
Extremities: No joint swelling
Neurological: No seizures
Nutritional: No problems

PHYSICAL EXAMINATION

Vital signs: Temperature: 100.8° F (oral); *Pulse:* 96 beats/min; *Respirations:* 26 breaths/min
Height: 46" (at 6-year check-up); *Weight:* 42 lbs
General: Well nourished, well developed; in no acute distress
Skin: Confluent maculopapular rash; no pustules; no desquamation; rash is predominantly over trunk, but there are a few (about 3) vesicles located on the lateral aspect of the upper trunk; vesicles are nonlinear in distribution and are about 6 to 8 cm apart
HEENT: Normocephalic without masses or lesions; conjunctiva noninjected; pupils equal, round, and reactive to light; extraocular movements intact; nares patent and non-injected; throat with redness and a moderate number of vesicles; tonsils 1+ with no apparent exudate; no petechiae on palate or uvula; teeth in good repair; tongue pink and in the midline; tympanic membranes (TMs) slightly dull and retracted, cone of light slightly diffused, TMs mobile
Neck: Supple without thyromegaly; a few mildly tender, minimally enlarged, anterior cervical nodes palpable; no posterior nodes palpable
Thorax: Clear to auscultation and percussion
Heart: Regular rate and rhythm; no murmurs, rubs, or gallops
Gastrointestinal: No hepatosplenomegaly; abdomen soft, nontender; bowel sounds normoactive
Extremities: Femoral pulses 2+; full range of motion of hips
Neurological: No Babinski signs present

Diagnostics

- Streptococci screen: Negative
- Throat culture: Positive for non-group A β-hemolytic streptococci

---

ASSESSMENT *Please indicate the problems or issues you have identified that will guide your care (preferably in list form):*

PLAN   *Please list your plans for addressing each of the problems or issues in your assessment:*

Community Clinic
Jeffrey A. Eaton, NP
Joyce D. Cappiello, NP

Name:_____ DOB_____
Address_____ Date_____

Rx

"label all unless indicated"
Refill:_____ times-- Do not refill ( )

Signed:_____
DO NOT TAKE THIS TO YOUR PHARMACIST

Community Clinic
Jeffrey A. Eaton, NP
Joyce D. Cappiello, NP

Name:_____ DOB_____
Address_____ Date_____

Rx

"label all unless indicated"
Refill:_____ times-- Do not refill ( )

Signed:_____
DO NOT TAKE THIS TO YOUR PHARMACIST

CASE
4 Discussion

LEARNING ISSUES

In order to resolve this patient's problem, you will need to consider and address the following issues (you may generate additional issues as well):

- **Differential diagnosis of rash**
- **Rashes that cause vesicles**
- **Presentation of scarlet fever (scarlatina)**
- **Causes of sore throat**
- **Symptom management of pruritic rashes**
- **Throat cultures and rapid strep testing**

INITIAL IDEAS

- Viral exanthem
- Chicken pox
- Scarlet fever (scarlatina)
- Allergic reaction: topical, food, or medication
- Mononucleosis

INTERPRETATION OF CUES, PATTERNS, AND INFORMATION

Lianne has been sick for about 4 days, and her illness came on with a presentation similar to a viral syndrome. Two things that might be causing her rash and fever are chicken pox and a vesicle-causing viral exanthem. Is this rash consistent with chicken pox? A varicella rash usually begins with macules and papules that become vesicles within a few hours; these vesicles then burst and create a crust within 1 or 2 days. Characteristically, the child that presents with chicken pox will have lesions in all stages. Lianne's rash has been present for 24 hours, so you would expect to see many more vesicles than you see. You probably cannot rule out chicken pox at this point, but this would not be a classic presentation.

What kinds of viral exanthems cause vesicular rashes? The most common would be the Coxsackie viruses, but the classic presentation is hand-foot-and-mouth disease, in which the child gets vesicles on the hands and feet as well as in the mouth. Lianne has vesicles or her trunk and in her throat. You cannot rule out a Coxsackie virus, and although this would not be the classic presentation, there are other subtypes of the Coxsackie virus that can cause a rash such as this. Echoviruses and enteroviruses also occasionally cause vesicular rashes.

You may also have thought of scarlet fever (also known as scarlatina) because Lianne had a sore throat. Scarlet fever does not commonly present with vesicles, but missing it can have potentially serious consequences (such as rheumatic fever), so it is worth consideration. The negative throat culture, the lack of changes in the tongue, and the distribution of this rash essentially rule this out.

Allergic reaction is a possibility, but the lack of any contact or dietary changes makes it less probable. The symptomatic treatment will probably be similar to the treatment given for a pruritic viral exanthem, so it may not be essential to detect an allergic reaction at this point. If the symptoms fail to improve with the symptomatic treatment and time, then further investigation would be appropriate.

Another viral illness that can cause sore throat and rash is mononucleosis (mono). Many clinicians think of mono as a condition of adolescents, but at least 50% of children have had mono by age 5 (Berkow, 1992). The rash of mono is usually maculopapular and affects primarily the trunk area. The lack of palpable posterior cervical nodes makes this less probable, but again you cannot completely rule it out. A mono infection would not be unusual in a child this age.

Another piece of information to be considered in any plan is that Lianne's parents are divorced. This may be a factor in weekend travel to her father's house if there is concern regarding exposure to the least number of people or if you feel that the distance travelled might add to Lianne's fatigue.

DIFFERENTIAL DIAGNOSIS

1. *Kawasaki syndrome:* Lianne is at an age where this is a possibility. You do not know Lianne's heritage, but this will be a factor in considering the probability of Kawasaki syndrome since it is six times more common in Asian-Americans and three times more common in Black Americans as compared with White European-Americans. The ratio of its effect on males to females is 3:2, so that makes it somewhat less probable in Lianne. On reviewing the diagnostic criteria for Kawasaki syndrome, you can pretty much rule it out (she lacks the conjunctivitis and the fever for 5 days). If she develops desquamation, evidence of cardiac involvement, or a fever that does not respond to antipyretics, you may want to consider Kawasaki syndrome.

2. *Lupus:* A systemic problem like lupus could also present with fever and a rash, although a vesicular rash would be unusual. Since there are other things that have a much higher probability, and the long-term course of these problems would not be affected by earlier diagnosis, a trial of therapy may be appropriate. If the problem resolves without recurrence, then systemic causes can essentially be ruled out. If it does recur, or other symptoms of a systemic disease occur, then further investigation can be carried out.

3. *Bacterial infection:* Another possibility that exists is that the vesicles represent bullae, and that they may be indicative of bacterial infection. If that is the case, culture and or antibiotic therapy could be considered.

4. *Pityriasis rosea:* This is more common in the 10 to 35 age range and would not usually include vesicles. The accompanying URI symptoms also make this less probable.

DIAGNOSTIC OPTIONS

Group A β-hemolytic streptococci (GABHS) infection has already been ruled out using a throat culture, so the most probable causes of her fever and rash at this point are some sort of viral exanthem (including those that would be caused by mononucleosis and varicella zoster virus [VZV]). Group C streptococci can cause a sore throat, and her throat culture may be consistent with a GABHS infection, but since it does not cause the long-term problems of GABHS, it is often not treated with antibiotics. Thus a "trial of therapy" may be appropriate, although in this case the therapy will be primarily supportive and symptomatic. If antibiotics were chosen, Group C streptococci should be sensitive to penicillin.

THERAPEUTIC OPTIONS

Pharmacological

Symptomatic drug therapy will depend on how much the itchiness of the rash is bothering Lianne. Diphenhydramine (Benadryl) may provide symptomatic relief for the itching. The dosage would be 5 mg/kg/day, or about 100 mg/day since Lianne weighs almost 20 kg. There are several options in prescribing. One would be 1.5 tsp (12.5 mg/5 ml or 18.75 mg/dose) every 4 hours prn.

Atarax syrup would also be an option (a sample prescription might be 1 $\frac{1}{4}$ tsp qid prn: 10 mg/5 ml→50 mg per day→12.5 mg per dose). Aveeno baths are also used for itching, although Lianne's does not seem severe. Calamine lotion or a comparable preparation may also provide topical relief.

Educational

Since the diagnosis of Lianne's problem is far from certain, the most important educational intervention is to let Ms. Pierce know what problems to look for and how not to expose anyone else to potential illness. She should be instructed to limit Lianne's exposure to anyone who has not had chicken pox on the outside chance that this rash will develop into a rash more like chicken pox. She should also be informed that a varicella vaccine now exists, and that it should be considered for Lianne at some point if this turns out to be something other than VZV. Lianne should probably be kept home from school for a few days until the rash improves and she has been without a fever for at least 24 hours. Ms. Pierce should also be given instructions to call back in a couple of days if Lianne's fever is not gone. Having the office staff call Ms. Pierce in 1 or 2 days for an update may provide reassurance to both the family and the clinician. Traveling to the father's house should probably be avoided until Lianne is better, although a provider must be aware that issues such as this can cause friction in a relationship that may already be adversarial. A delicate exploration of the issue with the mother and an offer to discuss the issue with the father if he has concerns may defuse any potential controversy.

Other Nonpharmacological Options

As noted, Aveeno baths may be helpful. If the weather is warm, ultraviolet light may decrease the itching, although sunlight that causes sweating may actually make Lianne more uncomfortable.

HEALTH PROMOTION/HEALTH MAINTENANCE

Lianne is 6 years old, and her immunizations are up-to-date. She has not had VZV or hepatitis B vaccinations, so those can be discussed. Currently, if a child has not had a hepatitis B vaccination, the recommendation is to begin the series at the entry into secondary school.

FOLLOW-UP

As noted, telephone follow-up is an option; otherwise Lianne probably does not need to return until she has a need for other treatment or a health maintenance visit per your usual protocol.

References

Berkow R, editor: *Merck manual*, ed 16, Rahway, NJ, 1992, Merck.

CASE
5

OPENING SCENARIO

Wendy Raymond is a 38-year-old female who is new to this practice. Her primary complaint today is of problems with migraine headaches.

HISTORY OF PRESENT ILLNESS

"I have had migraines for about 10 years. I have about 4 to 5 per month, and they are very severe. I have nausea and occasional vomiting. I have the sensation of flashing lights in my eyes before I get the headache. The headaches are more often on the right than left. They seem to come most frequently on weekends and when I am due for my period. They last about 6 to 8 hours, and they are improved by going into a dark room and lying down with a cool cloth on my forehead. I haven't sought treatment before because I hate doctors and I've just been too busy. I finally decided that I needed to do something now because I've been missing work, and they seem to be getting more frequent. I have tried acetaminophen 1000 mg every 4 hours when I get a headache, but it has minimal effect. I have not noticed particular foods or activities that cause my headaches. I have no history of head trauma."

MEDICAL HISTORY

Tonsillectomy and adenoidectomy as a child and endometriosis

FAMILY MEDICAL HISTORY

MGM: 82 yr (mild arthritis)
MGF: Died at 71 yr (heart attack)
PGM: Died at 64 yr (Alzheimer's disease)
PGF: Died at 79 yr (stroke)
Mother: 63 yr (mild hypertension)
Father: 65 yr (chronic obstructive pulmonary disease; occasionally has problems with his eyes "going out of focus")
Two sisters: 35, 41 (A&W)

SOCIAL HISTORY

Married for 17 years. Works as a fourth grade teacher. Never smoked. Alcohol very rarely (only for a toast at a wedding). Has 1 cup of regular coffee each morning. Denies other caffeine intake.

MEDICATIONS

Acetaminophen: 1000 mg q4h (when she gets a headache)

ALLERGIES

None

REVIEW OF SYSTEMS

General: Good energy level
Skin: No itching or rashes
HEENT: No history of head injury; no corrective lenses; denies eye pain, excessive tearing, blurring, or change in vision; no tinnitus or vertigo; denies frequent colds, hay fever, or sinus problems; headaches as noted under History of Present Illness
Neck: No lumps, goiters, or pain
Thorax: Denies shortness of breath, paroxysmal nocturnal dyspnea
Cardiac: No chest pain, no shortness of breath with normal activity
Gastrointestinal: No nausea, vomiting, constipation, or diarrhea; denies belching, bloating, and black or clay colored stools
Genitourinary: No dysuria; no difficulty starting stream; current contraception: diaphragm; her endometriosis has been followed by her gynecologist, and she does not currently perceive it to be a problem
Extremities: No joint pains or swelling
Neurological: No seizures
Endocrine: No polyuria, polyphagia, polydipsia; temperature tolerances good
Hematological: No excessive bruising; no history of transfusions

PHYSICAL EXAMINATION

Vital signs: Temperature: 98.0° F; *Pulse:* 76 beats/min; *Respirations:* 18 breaths/min; *BP:* 120/74 mm Hg
Height: 5' 6"; *Weight:* 127 lb
General: Well nourished, well developed; in no acute distress; appears stated age

HEENT: Normocephalic without masses or lesions; pupils equal, round, and reactive to light; extraocular movements intact; fundi benign; nares patent and noninjected; throat without redness or lesions; no tenderness on temporal palpation or on sinus percussion or palpation; no deviation or clicks on mandibular opening; teeth in good repair

Neck: Supple without thyromegaly or adenopathy

Heart: Regular rate and rhythm; no murmurs, rubs, or gallops

Lungs: Clear to auscultation and percussion

Abdomen: No hepatosplenomegaly; abdomen soft, nontender; bowel sounds normoactive; rectal without masses; stool brown; guaiac negative

Extremities: Range of motion functionally intact; no cyanosis, clubbing, or edema

Neurological: Reflexes 2+ at Achilles, patellar, biceps, triceps, and brachioradialis; no Babinski signs present; cranial nerves 2 to 12 intact; negative Romberg; heel-to-shin and finger-to-nose movements intact; motor and sensory findings normal and symmetrical

ASSESSMENT   *Please indicate the problems or issues you have identified that will guide your care (preferably in list form):*

PLAN   *Please list your plans for addressing each of the problems or issues in your assessment:*

Community Clinic
Jeffrey A. Eaton, NP
Joyce D. Cappiello, NP

Name:_____ DOB_____
Address_____ Date_____

Rx

"label all unless indicated"
Refill:_____ times-- Do not refill ( )

Signed:_____
DO NOT TAKE THIS TO YOUR PHARMACIST

Community Clinic
Jeffrey A. Eaton, NP
Joyce D. Cappiello, NP

Name:_____ DOB_____
Address_____ Date_____

Rx

"label all unless indicated"
Refill:_____ times-- Do not refill ( )

Signed:_____
DO NOT TAKE THIS TO YOUR PHARMACIST

Community Clinic
Jeffrey A. Eaton, NP
Joyce D. Cappiello, NP

Name:_____ DOB_____
Address_____ Date_____

Rx

"label all unless indicated"
Refill:_____ times-- Do not refill ( )

Signed:_____
DO NOT TAKE THIS TO YOUR PHARMACIST

Community Clinic
Jeffrey A. Eaton, NP
Joyce D. Cappiello, NP

Name:_____ DOB_____
Address_____ Date_____

Rx

"label all unless indicated"
Refill:_____ times-- Do not refill ( )

Signed:_____
DO NOT TAKE THIS TO YOUR PHARMACIST

CASE
5 Discussion

INITIAL IDEAS

When a patient comes in and tells you what the diagnosis is, the clinical reasoning process becomes subtly different. In this case, most clinicians will ask themselves the following questions:
- Does she really have migraine headaches? Are there other things I need to consider?
- If she does have migraines, what type of migraines does she have?

INTERPRETATION OF CUES, PATTERNS, AND INFORMATION

The most recent classification of migraine headaches (Stewart and Lipton, 1992) requires at least two of the following to be present:
1. Unilateral location
2. Pulsating quality
3. Moderate to severe intensity
4. Exacerbation by physical activity

Ms. Raymond clearly meets criteria 1 and 2 and probably 4.

The headache must also be accompanied by nausea or vomiting, photophobia, or phonophobia. Ms. Raymond meets at least two of these criteria and would probably meet the third if questioned. Her complaints of flashing lights before the onset of the headache define her headaches as migraine with aura (classic migraine).

32

A family history of migraines also makes you more suspicious of migraines, and her father's history of "eyes going out of focus" may actually represent a migraine. Migraines also often occur during or just after a stressful time. Many people experience a migraine after they have started to relax after stress. The presentation on weekends with Ms. Raymond may be consistent with this. Caffeine and certain other substances may trigger migraines. Ms. Raymond's one cup of coffee in the morning is not a problem since it is consistent; however, she may change this pattern on weekends, and that may also help to explain why her headaches are occurring on weekends.

Is her endometriosis an issue? You need to know the level to which this is an issue for her. Are there fertility issues? Is it causing her much pain? What has been told about it so far? This is probably an issue that can be fully dealt with on a follow-up visit to her gynecologist, but you will need to define and negotiate your role as the primary care provider.

DIFFERENTIAL DIAGNOSIS

1. *Space occupying lesion:* This is very improbable because of the timing and temporal aspects of these headaches. A lesion is not often present for 10 years without a progression of symptoms, and symptoms would not usually increase and abate. Therefore no need for any imaging is seen in this case.
2. *Sinusitis:* Sinusitis could be considered, but there is not a lot of evidence here either. There is no noted history of a upper respiratory infection (URI) or allergies, and the timing of symptoms again argues against it. The aura essentially rules this out.
3. *Cluster headache:* Cluster headaches are more common in men and often include symptoms of nasal stuffiness, lacrimation, and facial flushing on the affected side. That pain is often a stabbing pain. Cluster headaches are usually not throbbing and lack the other characteristics of migraines.

DIAGNOSTIC OPTIONS

A computerized tomography (CT) scan would be ordered by some clinicians, but most would reserve this for patients with signs or symptoms of a space-occupying lesion, such as papilledema, or widening pulse pressure. Other indications might be a complaint of "the worst headache I've ever had," which may be the complaint in a subarachnoid hemorrhage. In a patient with a history of more than 1 year of a similar type of headache, the probability of a bleed or tumor goes down dramatically.

A *headache diary* will be very helpful no matter which treatment approach is chosen. Perhaps this will identify "triggers." She has more headaches on weekends. Is this a let-down period from stress? A headache diary will also either verify a reduction in frequency or will substantiate a lack of efficacy of treatments.

The database could also be more complete. Family history can often be helpful in patients with migraines both to establish the diagnosis and to help them find out coping strategies that other family members have used. Some clinicians would have done a more extensive neurological examination, and this would have been very reasonable. Think about what exactly you are looking for to plan that examination. Temporomandibular joint dysfunction could be possible, and history should focus as much on behaviors such as gum chewing, playing of musical instruments, grinding and clenching of teeeth, as well as on any physical symptoms.

Her caffeine intake could be a factor both as a trigger and also from caffeine "withdrawal," such as having less coffee on weekends.

THERAPEUTIC OPTIONS

Pharmacological

There are many options for dealing with her migraines. The first thing you must decide about pharmacological treatment is whether to focus on abortive or prophylactic treatment. Criteria for preventive therapy would be two to three incapacitating headaches per month or one prolonged severe attack, abortive therapy that does not work, a situation in which abortive therapy is contraindicated, medically significant side effects expected from abortive therapy, or a patient with a psychological inability to deal with headaches. Since her headaches are occurring more than two to three times per month, the case for prophylactic as well as abortive therapy could be made. Alternatively, if she is willing, it may be reasonable to try a better approach to abortive therapy and see if long-term, ongoing medication can be avoided. This is a decision that could only be made in collaboration with the patient.

1. *Prophylaxis* could include beta blockers or Depakote. Blocadren and propranolol (Inderal) are beta blockers currently approved by the Food and Drug Administration (FDA) for use with migraines. Depakote is best known as an anticonvulsant but is also approved for migraine prophylaxis. Other drugs commonly used but without an approved indication are tricyclic antidepressants (TCAs), selective serotonin reuptake inhibitors (SSRIs), and calcium channel blockers. Nonapproved drugs are of course used for various conditions, but this is a factor that should be taken into consideration when prescribing. Side-effect profiles are of course a major factor in drug choice. It should be remembered with beta blockers that many are antagonized by nonsteroidal antiinflammatory drugs (NSAIDs).

2. *Abortive therapy* options include the following:

   a. *NSAIDs:* They are particularly useful when used for premenstrual headaches when given on a scheduled basis for a couple of days before the onset of the menstrual period. Ibuprofen 800 mg tid-qid or Naproxen 500 mg bid would be reasonable approaches. Ms. Raymond may have tried these drugs at home but probably has not tried them in these dosages.

   b. *Cafergot or Wigraine:* Low-dose ergot with caffeine added. It may be better tolerated in some patients.

   c. *Midrin:* A caffeinelike drug; a mild sedative and acetaminophen make up this drug. Many migraine suffers get good relief from Midrin.

   d. *Methysergide (Sansert):* Another ergot that can be useful for severe, frequent, vascular headaches refractory to other drugs. It has fibrotic complications and a complicated dosing regimen, so it is used with great caution.

   e. *Opiates, Fiorinal (acetylsalicylic acid [ASA] and a mild barbiturate), Fioricet, or Esgic (acetaminophen with the barbiturate):* Fiorinal is a controlled ("scheduled") drug, but Fioricet and Esgic are not.

   f. *Opioids:* Opioids are usually avoided but may be useful in the acute phase. An injection of meperidine (often accompanied by an antiemetic) is what some migraine sufferers rely upon during their worst episodes. Alternatively, some clinicians are now using injectable ketorolac (Toradol) in this most acute phase. Ms. Raymond's pain currently does not require an injectable approach.

   g. *Narcotic agonist-antagonist drugs (Stadol nasal spray [butorphanol tartrate]):* These are also used for migraines. Stadol nasal spray absorbs in 15 to 60 seconds and can be used in the presence of nausea and vomiting. It is not a scheduled substance and seems to have a lower potential for abuse, although abuse does occur.

   h. *Imitrex (sumatriptan):* This is a tablet or subcutaneous injection that quickly relieves signs and symptoms of headache. It is a fairly selective cranial vasoconstrictor, but it can affect cardiac vessels. There have been a few deaths in young healthy women with this drug. The first dose should be given in the office because of its effect on coronary vessels. Some clinicians will not do this if the individual is low risk for unrecognized coronary artery disease, but the manufacturers recommendations are that the first dose be supervised. If Ms. Raymond does not have problems with the first dose, it is thought that she will do okay with future doses. Imitrex's effect on the headaches can be dramatic.

   i. *Dihydroergotamine (DHE):* A new nasal form of DHE may be on the market soon. DHE is currently only available in parenteral form but has a long history of being well tolerated, having a low incidence of side effects, being less prone to cause nausea and vomiting, and having little or no potential for addiction or rebound headaches.

j. *Propranolol:* Propranolol 20 mg bid for 3 days before menses may also be a middle-range approach between abortive therapy and prophylaxis.

A prescription for an antiemetic could also be included.

Nonpharmacological

Certain foods such as aged cheeses, chocolate, caffeine, pink lunch meats, certain nuts, and alcohol (especially red wine) have been identified as triggers for migraine headaches. A headache diary will allow a patient to correlate dietary issues with the onset of headache. Sleep patterns and stress level have also been correlated, and monitoring these should be included in instructions to patients when trying to identify triggers and subsequently avoid them.

You must be alert for an increase in headaches caused by a rebound effect from abortive therapy in some patients.

Further history about her endometriosis and child-bearing plans is necessary. It could even be considered in the development of a migraine management plan, since if she is planning on becoming pregnant in the foreseeable future, an appropriate migraine management plan could be chosen.

What other nonpharmacological measures has she tried? A combination of stress management and biofeedback therapy can be very effective.

HEALTH PROMOTION/HEALTH MAINTENANCE

There is little if any time for health maintenance concerns at this visit, but at subsequent visits you need to ascertain risk factors further, intervene with appropriate preventive activities, and provide anticipatory guidance.

1. Although she is probably young for getting a mammogram covered by insurance, she may be given the option of having one.
2. Update her tetanus-diphtheria (Td) immunization.
3. She should have a Pap smear now and every year for 3 years. If those are all negative, she could go to every 3 years. In utero exposure to diethylstilbestrol (DES) could also be assessed.
4. A risk assessment for human immmunodeficiency virus (HIV) behaviors could be done with very few strategic questions.
5. If tuberculosis (TB) is an issue in this community or has the potential, a purified protein derivative (PPD) could be considered. The population in her school would be a factor.
6. A clinical breast examination is indicated. There are controversies around teaching self breast examination, so you need to weigh the available information and make a recommendation.
7. A discussion of contraceptive issues may be helpful.
8. If she has fear of hepatitis B from kids getting hurt at school, she could be offered the hepatitis B vaccine. She will have to make the cost/benefit decision. Some schools cover the cost and she should explore this.
9. Titers or vaccine could be considered if she is considering pregnancy or is worried about her measles, mumps, or rubella (MMR) status. If she does receive the vaccine, the manufacturers' recommendations are that she avoid pregnancy for 3 months.
10. Use of seatbelts, smoke detectors, dental and vision care, and carbon dioxide detectors is recommended (some oil companies will lend these if cost is an issue).
11. Routine laboratory tests including nonfasting total cholesterol (+/- high-density lipoproteins [HDLs]) should be done.
12. The U.S. Public Health Service has a specific recommendation around folate intake for women of childbearing years, and you would have to decide whether to make specific recommendations in this case.
13. She should be encouraged to develop a program of regular activity; this could actually help with her migraines as well.
14. Teaching about skin changes and sun exposure may be appropriate.

FOLLOW-UP

Ms. Raymond should probably try whatever approach is decided upon for a month or so and then return for further discussion. A screening examination to address the above health-maintenance issues could also be scheduled at that time if appropriate.

References

Stewart WF, Lipton RB: Migraine headache: epidemiology and health care utilization, *Cephalalgia* 13(suppl 12):41, 1992.

OPENING SCENARIO

Liu Lee is a 24-year-old female scheduled for an episodic visit for unprotected coitus. Her last visit with you was 9 months ago for an annual gynecological examination.

HISTORY OF PRESENT ILLNESS

"My boyfriend and I have been using condoms for birth control. The condom broke last night, and my period was 2 weeks ago. I don't want to be pregnant because I am a graduate student in a doctoral program. I have at least 3 years of school ahead of me. Is there anything I can do at this point to prevent a pregnancy?"

MEDICAL HISTORY

A review of her records shows that her last gynecological examination was 9 months ago with a negative examination and negative Pap smear; G0P0; healthy female with regular 27- to 28-day cycles. No history of hospitalizations or surgeries. All immunizations up-to-date, including hepatitis B. Seen 3 months ago for an uncomplicated upper respiratory infection (URI).

FAMILY MEDICAL HISTORY

MGM: 70s (A&W)
MGF: 70s (A&W)
PGM: 73 yr (Type II diabetes mellitus [DM])
PGF: Died at 35 yr (accident)
Mother: 44 yr (A&W)
Father: 48 yr (high cholesterol)
One sister: 18 yr (A&W)

SOCIAL HISTORY

Has a steady boyfriend for the past 2 years whom she plans to marry in the future. At some point they would like to have a family. Smokes $1/2$ pack per day. Denies drug use. States consumption of one glass of wine with dinner 3 times a week. Denies domestic violence.

MEDICATIONS

None

ALLERGIES

None

REVIEW OF SYSTEMS

General: Feels healthy but often fatigued and stressed from demands of school; sleeps 5 to 6 hours per night; states she requires more sleep than this but needs the time for studying

HEENT: States no further upper respiratory symptoms since her visit 3 months ago; has not made any progress in decreasing smoking; states that the stress of graduate school makes smoking cessation difficult; wants to work on quitting in the summer since she will not attend summer school this year; thinks her stress level will be lower with just working; in addition, the restaurant where she will work as a waitress is a smoke-free environment; currently the cafe where she is employed has a smoking section, and that makes her want to smoke more

Thorax: Denies chest pain, shortness of breath, asthma, or any breathing difficulties

Breasts: No history of masses, skin changes, nipple discharge

Gastrointestinal: Denies heartburn, nausea and vomiting, abdominal pain, constipation, diarrhea, rectal bleeding; no history of hepatitis or liver disease

Genitourinary: No complaints of pelvic pain or unusual bleeding; no history of kidney disease, urinary tract infections (UTIs)

PHYSICAL EXAMINATION

Vital signs: Temperature: 98.0° F; *Pulse:* 68 beats/min; *Respirations:* 16 breaths/min; *BP:* 110/70 mm Hg
Height: 5' 2"; *Weight:* 100 lb
Physical examination not performed today.

ASSESSMENT   *Please indicate the problems or issues you have identified that will guide your care (preferably in list form):*

PLAN   *Please list your plans for addressing each of the problems or issues in your assessment:*

Community Clinic
Jeffrey A. Eaton, NP
Joyce D. Cappiello, NP

Name:_____ DOB_____
Address_____ Date_____

Rx

"label all unless indicated"
Refill:_____ times-- Do not refill ( )

Signed:_____
DO NOT TAKE THIS TO YOUR PHARMACIST

Community Clinic
Jeffrey A. Eaton, NP
Joyce D. Cappiello, NP

Name:_____ DOB_____
Address_____ Date_____

Rx

"label all unless indicated"
Refill:_____ times-- Do not refill ( )

Signed:_____
DO NOT TAKE THIS TO YOUR PHARMACIST

LEARNING ISSUES

In order to resolve this patient's problem, you will need to consider and address the following issues (you may generate additional issues as well):

- Use of medications "off label"
- Prevention of unplanned pregnancy
- Personal feelings regarding provision of emergency contraception
- Screening for risk factors
- Choice of medications
- Medication side effects
- Appropriate follow-up

INITIAL IDEAS

Before entering the room, you are reviewing this case in your mind. Ms. Lee is a healthy young woman with an essentially negative medical history. The chief complaint or concern is the desire to prevent pregnancy from the recent act of unprotected coitus. Think through what you need to assess (how to effectively present the available information on emergency contraception), decide if it is appropriate for Ms. Lee, and determine if both you and she are comfortable with the method.

INTERPRETATION OF CUES, PATTERNS, AND INFORMATION

As you review her history, you realize that she is at risk for pregnancy because she had unprotected coitus (condom broke) 13 days after the onset of menses in a regular 27- to 28-day cycles. She clearly states that she does not want a pregnancy nor does she want to be in the difficult situation of considering an abortion.

What is her actual risk of pregnancy? Depending on the study, theoretical conception rates vary from 20% to 60% per cycle. Whatever the actual risk, it is probably higher than this individual wants. Her maximum fertility is the 5 days before and the day of ovulation. Most women ovulate 14 days before the onset of menses. For example, if a woman has a 56-day cycle, she will still usually ovulate 14 days before the onset of her menses. The part of the cycle from the beginning of the menses to ovulation (the follicular stage) is the part of the cycle that varies. With Ms. Lee, who has a 27- to 28-day cycle, ovulation will occur approximately midcycle, which is 14 days before her menses is due. Since the unprotected coitus occurred at day 13, she is at the most risky time of her cycle.

Is there an effective emergency contraception method to offer her? The most commonly used emergency contraception is 2 doses of combination oral contraceptives (OCs) taken 12 hours apart within 72 hours of the unprotected coitus. The analysis of several studies indicates an approximate efficacy rate of 75% (Trussell, Ellertson, and Stewart, 1996). A copper T380A intrauterine device

(IUD) inserted within 5 days after unprotected intercourse is effective for emergency contraception. Since Ms. Lee is a nulliparous woman, this is not the best choice.

How does emergency contraception work? The mechanism of action of emergency contraceptive pills (ECPs) has not been clearly established. Several studies have shown that ECPs can inhibit or delay ovulation. It has also been suggested that ECPs may prevent implantation by altering the endometrium. However, the evidence for endometrial effects of ECP is mixed, and whether the endometrial changes that are observed in some studies would be sufficient to prevent implantation is not known. ECPs may also prevent fertilization or transport of sperm or ova, but no data exist regarding these possible mechanisms. ECPs do not interrupt an established pregnancy (Wells, Crook, and Muller, 1997).

Is the method safe for her? Are there any medical contraindications? Because this regimen consists of using combined OCs already on the market and because it has never been specifically regulated by the Food and Drug Administration (FDA) until very recently, the contraindications for its use have simply been adopted from those stated on the package insert for OCs:
- Current or past thromboembolic disorders
- Cerebrovascular disease
- Coronary artery disease
- Known or suspected carcinoma of the breast or endometrium
- Jaundice
- Hepatic adenoma or carcinoma
- Women older than 35 who smoke heavily

Some sources define smoking heavily as 1 pack per day or more. There is no specific data to state, for instance, that a woman over 35 years of age who smokes 1 pack per day is at risk for cardiovascular events if she takes 2 doses of OCs. It may well be that the risk of a pregnancy with any of the above conditions by far outweighs any risk from using a short dose of OCs. The general medical consensus based on many years of clinical use is that this regimen has no contraindications (International Medical Advisory Panel, 1994).

It is important to rule out the possibility of a preexisting pregnancy. This can be done with a thorough history: Was the last menstrual period (LMP) normal and was there any unprotected coitus since the LMP? If either response raises concern, then emergency contraception might be less effective than expected. Ms. Lee is quite clear about the normalcy of her LMP and the lack of unprotected coitus earlier in her cycle. In situations like this it is often difficult to confirm or rule out a preexisting pregnancy with a pregnancy test since current tests (blood or urine) can only show a positive result 8 to 10 days after conception.

What if you provided emergency contraception, it was not effective, and Ms. Lee chose to continue the pregnancy? Every provider fears prescribing a medicine that might cause a fetal malformation, but there is no evidence to support this concern with this regimen. A metaanalysis of 12 prospective studies failed to detect any statistically significant association between OC use early in the pregnancy and the risk of fetal malformation (Bracken, 1990) or specifically with the use of postcoital contraception (Cardy, 1995). According to the FDA (1997), "There is no evidence that these drugs (oral contraceptives), taken in smaller total doses for a short period of time for emergency contraception, will have an adverse effect on an established pregnancy"

What about side effects? Nausea and vomiting are the most common, with nausea occurring in 50% to 70% of those treated. As many as 25% experience vomiting. Most providers instruct clients to take the pills with food to reduce nausea, and if vomiting occurs, then to use an antiemetic. A study by Bagshaw, Edwards, and Tucker (1988) suggests that providers should routinely prescribe antiemetics prophylactically because nausea was reduced to 28% and vomiting to 10% among users of emergency contraception. Nonprescription dimenhydrinate (Dramamine) or prescription trimethobenzamide hydrochloride (Tigan) or promethazine hydrochloride (Phenergan) can be used.

Is this method cost effective? In the United States, pills are not specifically marketed for this purpose. You must either prescribe a month of pills at an approximate cost of $25 to $35 or simply cut up a sample package of appropriate pills and provide the number of pills needed. In European countries, tablets equivalent to 50 µg of ethinyl estradiol and 0.5 mg of norgestrel (Ovral) are available in four strips labeled explicitly for emergency use. Even at $35, this is still a cost-effective regimen. Providing a single ECP treatment in a managed care setting saves $142 in pregnancy care costs. Providing ECPs ahead of time to women using barrier contraceptives, spermicides, withdrawal, or periodic abstinence results in annual cost savings ranging from $263 to $498 in a managed care setting (Trussell et al, 1997).

Now that you have thought through the medical implications, what about the legal issues involved? Until recently this treatment involved use of an FDA-approved drug for a use that was not specifically approved. Would this have put the provider at risk? The 1982 FDA Drug Bulletin shown in Box 6-1 clarifies this.

Medications are commonly used off label (e.g., hormone replacement therapy [HRT] is approved only for treatment of menopausal symptoms, atrophic vaginitis, and osteoporosis). However, numerous studies have documented the role of HRT in prevention of heart disease, and it is widely prescribed for this reason. In spite of familiarity with the concept of off-label uses, emergency contraception remains an underutilized treatment.

As of February 1997, emergency contraception is an FDA-endorsed use of OCs. This came about through a very unusual set of circumstances. Usually, drug manufacturers submit such proposals to the FDA, but in this case they had little to gain financially since the medication is already on the market and thus were not interested in pursuing this. The Center for Reproductive Law and Policy filed a citizen petition asking the FDA to require manufacturers to amend their labeling and patient package inserts to include information regarding the use of OCs for emergency contraception. In

---

Box 6-1 Use of Approved Drugs for Unlabeled Indications

The appropriateness or the legality of prescribing approved drugs for uses not included in their official labeling is sometimes a cause of concern and confusion among practitioners. Under the federal Food, Drug, and Cosmetic (FD&C) Act, a drug approved for marketing may be labeled, promoted, and advertised by the manufacturer only for those uses for which the drug's safety and effectiveness have been established and which the FDA has approved. These are commonly referred to as *approved uses*. This means that adequate and well-controlled clinical trials have documented these uses, and the results of the trials have been reviewed and approved by the FDA. The FD&C Act does not, however, limit the manner in which a physician may use an approved drug. Once a product has been approved for marketing, a physician may prescribe it for uses or in treatment regimens or patient populations that are not included in approved labeling. Such "unapproved," or more precisely, "unlabeled" uses, may be appropriate and rational in certain circumstances and may in fact reflect approaches to drug therapy that have been extensively reported in medical literature. The term *unapproved* uses is to some extent misleading. It includes a variety of situations ranging from unstudied to thoroughly investigated drug uses. Valid new uses for drugs already on the market are often first discovered by serendipitous observations and therapeutic innovations, subsequently confirmed by well-planned and well-executed clinical investigations. Before such advances can be added to the approved labeling, however, data substantiating the effectiveness of a new use or regimen must be submitted by the manufacturer to the FDA for evaluation. This may take time and may never occur without the initiative of the drug manufacturer whose product is involved. For that reason, accepted medical practice often includes drug use that is not reflected in approved drug labeling. With respect to its role in medical practice, the package insert is informational only. The FDA tries to assure that prescription drug information in the package insert accurately and fully reflects the data on safety and effectiveness on which drug approval is based.

From Food and Drug Administration: Use of approved drugs for unlabeled indications, *FDA Drug Bulletin* 12:1, 1982.

February 1997, the FDA published a notice in the Federal Register concluding that the use of certain combined OCs for emergency contraception is safe and effective. Although the FDA cannot approve a drug for a new indication without an application from the drug's manufacturer, the publication of a notice in the Federal Register represents a strong FDA endorsement of off-label use of birth control pills currently on the market for emergency contraception.

DIAGNOSTIC IMPRESSION

Ms. Lee is at risk for unintended pregnancy.

THERAPEUTIC OPTIONS

Now you must decide if you will provide emergency contraception to this woman. If you are not comfortable doing so after this discussion, perhaps you can refer her to a colleague who will provide this service.

Is any diagnostic testing indicated? What physical examination techniques, if any, are appropriate? The medical problems that make emergency contraceptives contraindicated can be assessed with a careful history. A physical examination is not necessary unless the history indicates a problem or if the woman suspects she may already be pregnant since she is already a patient in your office with a database (Hatcher et al, 1994). There are no routine diagnostic tests indicated.

What OCs can be used? Ovral has traditionally been used, but it is not always readily available since it has been replaced by lower-dose pills. Other levonorgestrel-containing pills can be used. It may well be that any OC could be used, but the studies have only examined pills containing the progestin levonorgestrel. Ethinyl estradiol is the estrogen component in all levonorgestrel pills. The current cost of Ovral is approximately $40, while the cost of Triphasil is $26.

Dosage

- Ovral: 2 tabs (2 doses, 12 hours apart); total of 4 pills
- LoOvral, Nordette, Levlen: 4 tabs (2 doses, 12 hours apart); total of 8 pills
- Triphasil, Tri-Levlen (yellow pills only): 4 tabs (2 doses, 12 hours apart); total of 8 pills
- Allesse: 5 tabs (2 doses, 12 hours apart); total of 10 pills

FOLLOW-UP

Do you need to see her back? A routine follow-up visit is not necessary if she has withdrawal bleeding in the next 3 weeks. If she does not have bleeding within this time, she needs to return for a pregnancy test.

A major concern for Ms. Lee is the need to start a reliable method of contraception. This visit will need to include a discussion of birth control options acceptable to Ms. Lee. Emergency contraception is just that: meant for emergencies.

Since she had a gynecological examination 9 months ago, we can assume other health-maintenance issues such as immunizations were addressed at that time. A yearly examination, due in 3 months, would be an ideal time for follow-up on whatever contraceptive method she chooses today and to address health-maintenance issues.

Reenforce her plan to work on smoking cessation this summer.

A brief comment on the need to increase the amount of sleep at night and encouraging stress-reduction measures could be helpful.

References

Bagshaw SN, Edwards D, Tucker AK: Ethinyl estradial and D-norgestrel is an effective emergency postcoital contraceptive: a report of its use in 1200 patients in a family planning clinic, *Aust N Z J Obstet Gynaecol* 28:137, 1988.

Bracken MB: Oral contraceptives and congenital malformations in offspring: a review and meta-analysis of the prospective studies, *Obstet Gynecol* 76:552, 1990.

Cardy GC: Outcome of pregnancies after failed hormonal postcoital contraception: an interim report, *Br J Fam Plann* 21:112, 1995.

Food and Drug Administration: Prescription drug products: certain combined oral contraceptives for use as postcoital emergency contraception, *The Federal Register* 62:8610, 1997.

Food and Drug Administration: Use of approved drugs for unlabeled indications, *FDA Drug Bulletin* 12:1, 1982.

Hatcher R et al: *Contraceptive technology* New York, 1994, Irvington.

International Medical Advisory Panel of the International Planned Parenthood Federation: Statement on emergency contraception, *IPPF Medical Bulletin* 26(6):1, 1994.

Trussell J et al: Emergency contraception: a cost-effective approach to preventing unintended pregnancy, *Am J Public Health* 87:6, 1997.

Trussell J, Ellertson C, Stewart F: The effectiveness of the Yuzpe regimen of emergency contraception, *Fam Plann Perspect* 28(2):58, 1996.

Wells E, Crook B, Muller N: Emergency contraception: a resource manual for providers, *Program for Appropriate Technology (PATH)* i-24, 1997.

11:00 AM
Amber Jackson
Age 20 weeks

OPENING SCENARIO

Amber Jackson is a 20-week-old female in your office for a 4-month well child check (WCC). Both parents are present. The father is thin and appears to be in his late thirties. The mother looks younger, possibly in her twenties. She is Filipino, about 4'10", and less than 100 lbs.

HISTORY OF PRESENT ILLNESS

(Obtained from mother)

"Amber is just here for her shots. We do have some concerns. What should we be giving her for formula? She was getting constipated, so I put some Karo syrup in her formula (1 tsp per bottle) and switched her to Low-iron Similac. Is that okay? Also, she is still up twice a night. How much longer is that going to last?" The mother also expresses concern about her dose of inactivated poliovirus vaccine (IPV). "I was told that I had to have that before Amber could get hers."

MEDICAL HISTORY

Normal spontaneous vaginal delivery (NSVD) at term. Milestones all within normal limits on previous visit. Has just started to try to turn over. Immunization record is shown in Table 7-1. Growth is shown in Table 7-2.

FAMILY MEDICAL HISTORY

MGM: 44 yr (A&W)
MGF: 46 yr (A&W)
PGM: 53 yr (hypertension, diabetes mellitus [DM])
PGF: 58 yr (prostate cancer)
Mother: 27 yr (A&W)
Father: 37 yr (A&W)

SOCIAL HISTORY

Lives with both parents. Father works as a truck driver. Mother stays at home. Mother has been in this country for about 5 years. Mother describes Amber as a good baby who does not cry much.

Table **7-1** *Immunization Record for Amber Jackson*

VACCINE	DATE	INITIALS	NOTES
DPT	2 mo	MDO	Acellular
DPT			
DPT			
DPT			
DPT			
Td			
Td			
OPV	Held		
OPV			
OPV			
OPV			
MMR			
MMR			
HBV	2 mo	MDO	
HBV			
HBV			
Hib	2 mo	MDO	
Hib			
Hib			
Hib			

Table **7-2** *Growth of Amber Jackson*

MEASURE	AGE	RESULT	PERCENTILE
Length	2 wk	20"	45%
	2 mo	21 3/4"	45%
	4 mo	23 1/2"	40%
Weight	Birth	6 lb, 15 oz	
	2 wk	6 lb, 14 oz	25%
	2 mo	8 lb, 8 oz	20%
	4 mo	11 lb, 1 oz	15%
Head circumference	2 wk	34 cm	25%
	2 mo	37 cm	30%
	4 mo	39 cm	25%

MEDICATIONS

None

ALLERGIES

None

REVIEW OF SYSTEMS

(Obtained from mother)

General: Good energy level

Skin: No itching or rashes

HEENT: Denies colds

Neck: No lumps, goiters, or pain

Thorax: Denies appearance of shortness of breath

Cardiac: Color good

Gastrointestinal: No vomiting, constipation, or diarrhea; usually two soft, brown bowel movements per day until 2 weeks ago, then had 2 days without BM for which formula was still changed; strains with BMs at times

Genitourinary: No odor to urine; six to seven wet diapers per day

Extremities: No joint swelling

Neurological: No seizures

Nutrition: Was nursing until about 2 to 3 weeks ago; started on Similac but became very constipated so added 1 tsp of Karo syrup and switched to Low-iron Similac; taking 24 to 32 oz of formula per day; has not yet had cereal or other solid food

PHYSICAL EXAMINATION

Vital signs: Temperature: 98.0° F; *Pulse:* 106 beats/min; *Respirations:* 24 breaths/min

General: Well nourished, well developed; in no acute distress

HEENT: Normocephalic without masses or lesions; pupils equal, round, and reactive to light; extraocular movements intact; nares patent and noninjected; throat without redness or lesions; tympanic membranes (TMs) noninjected, cone of light crisp, TMs mobile; fontanels palpable, soft, and flat

Neck: Supple without thyromegaly or adenopathy

Thorax: Clear to auscultation and percussion

Heart: Regular rate and rhythm; no murmurs, rubs, or gallops

Gastrointestinal: No hepatosplenomegaly; abdomen soft, nontender; bowel sounds normoactive

Extremities: Femoral pulses 2+; full range of motion of hips; no Ortolani's sign; no cyanosis, clubbing, or edema

Neurological: Babinski signs equivocal

ASSESSMENT   *Please indicate the problems or issues you have identified that will guide your care (preferably in list form):*

PLAN   *Please list your plans for addressing each of the problems or issues in your assessment:*

Community Clinic
Jeffrey A. Eaton, NP
Joyce D. Cappiello, NP

Name:_____ DOB_____
Address_____ Date_____

Rx

"label all unless indicated"
Refill:_____ times-- Do not refill ( )

Signed:_____
DO NOT TAKE THIS TO YOUR PHARMACIST

Community Clinic
Jeffrey A. Eaton, NP
Joyce D. Cappiello, NP

Name:_____ DOB_____
Address_____ Date_____

Rx

"label all unless indicated"
Refill:_____ times-- Do not refill ( )

Signed:_____
DO NOT TAKE THIS TO YOUR PHARMACIST

LEARNING ISSUES

In order to resolve this patient's problem, you will need to consider and address the following issues (you may generate additional issues as well):

- **Procedure for a WCC**
- **Information included in a 4-month WCC**
- **Immunization schedules**
- **Criteria for constipation in a 4 month old**
- **Treatment of constipation in a 4 month old**
- **Bottle feeding (nutritional needs)**
- **Sleep issues**
- **Anticipatory guidance in a 4 month old**
- **Oral poliovirus vaccine (OPV) versus IPV**
- **Karo syrup and other conventional, but nonmedical, treatments**
- **Cultural issues in child rearing**
- **Weight patterns and flags for concern**
- **Age-appropriate vital signs**
- **Vaccine preparations for diphtheria-pertussis-tetanus (DPT) and *Haemophilus influenzae* type b (Hib)**
- **Physical examination of a 4 month old**
- **Hepatitis B vaccine (and level of risk for a 4 month old)**

INITIAL IDEAS

- You are optimistically hoping that this will be a routine WCC.
- You expect that you will review some history regarding development, diet, and sleep.
- You hope to check a quick physical examination to screen for gross abnormalities including abnormal patterns of growth.
- You will give some anticipatory guidance, and the staff can give Amber her immunizations.

INTERPRETATION OF CUES, PATTERNS, AND INFORMATION

After reviewing Amber's chart, you see that she did not receive her OPV at her last appointment because her mother was not immunized. This decision was already made, so there is nothing you can do about it now, but many clinicians would have gone ahead with OPV or IPV on the last visit. You should never miss an opportunity to immunize, but the Centers for Disease Control and Prevention

(CDC) give the option of delaying polio vaccine as long as you are confident that the child will be vaccinated as soon as the family contact has completed two doses of IPV (Atkinson et al, 1996).

Now you will have to decide whether to give the OPV or possibly IPV this time. Recommendations from the CDC Advisory Committee on Immunization Practices (ACIP) and the American Academy of Pediatrics have recently changed (MMWR, 1997) to include IPV for the 2- and 4-month doses of poliovaccine because of the risks of a live vaccine. Many practices are still in the process of dealing with these changes.

You also reviewed the growth patterns (see Table 7-2) and noticed that Amber had gone from the 25th percentile for weight to the 15th. Should this worry you? Baker (1996) suggests the crossing of two dark percentile lines as an index of concern.

Does the fact that the mother is of Filipino (Tagalog) heritage make a difference in how you will approach this family?

What do you need to assess further regarding Amber's constipation? Do you think the parents acted appropriately by adding the Karo syrup and changing the formula to low iron? Is Amber getting enough iron?

REVISED IDEAS

- Behind schedule on polio vaccine
- Constipation
- Weight measures indicating weight gain slowing; possible causes versus measurement issues
- Iron deficiency
- Knowledge deficit regarding normal sleep patterns and the promotion of good sleeping habits

DIFFERENTIAL DIAGNOSIS

1. *Constipation:* What can cause constipation in a 4 month old? Can this be considered a normal occurrence in this age group? Constipation is defined differently by different sources, but it usually involves some element of painful or difficult defecation. If after obtaining more history on Amber you believe that she is in fact having difficulty, then you will need to consider the possible causes. In many cases there is no organic cause detectable, and hence it may be defined as functional constipation. This should not interfere with growth and development, so symptomatic treatment is appropriate. Other possible causes would be hypothyroidism, Hirschsprung's disease, celiac disease, lead toxicity, or some sort of myelodysplasia. All of these are unlikely in Amber, although Hirshsprung's disease is common enough to merit a reasonably high level of vigilance. Hypothyroidism is rare in general, but if she was lethargic or had other evidence, it could be considered. Hirschsprung's disease is often diagnosed earlier than this, but as many as $1/3$ of cases are undiagnosed at 3 months of age (Dershewitz, 1993). Hirschsprung's disease is a problem with a lack of ganglia in the colon so that if only a small segment were affected, then symptoms could be relatively mild. If Amber's problems persist, then referral for rectal manometry could be considered. Celiac disease would be very improbable since it does not appear that Amber has had any gluten-containing foods introduced into her diet yet. Lead toxicity would only be of concern if there was an airborne source of lead or there was a contamination of the water source since Amber is probably too young to be putting lead-containing items in her mouth. Gross myelodysplasia can essentially be ruled out by examining Amber's lower extremities and checking urinary function by history and checking for bladder distention. Again if the constipation is very persistent, a mild case could be present.

Another thing to consider is that Amber had been constipated, but it may have been related to a self-limiting minor illness. If she had been mildly dehydrated, then she could have been constipated but would not be now even with a normal diet.

It is necessary to address the issue of iron as a cause of constipation. There is not currently any evidence that formulas with iron are constipating, although there are many people (including professionals) who believe that they are. This may be a challenge to balance iron needs with this belief in some individuals.

Should you do a rectal examination? This will be based on your index of concern regarding the more serious causes of her constipation. Even with a gentle approach using a lot of lubricant and your little finger, this is apt to be an uncomfortable experience for Amber.

2. *Weight gain slowing:* Do you even believe that Amber's weight gain has slowed? Unfortunately, between scale error and human error the certainty of weights is often an issue. You would want to trend her weight and continue to evaluate. Any metabolic or even functional issues such as constipation can cause slower gain of weight.

Genetics is also a factor, and Amber may be destined to be small like her mother. However, you should be vigilant for a problem that is amenable to intervention.

One red flag is usually crossing two dark percentile lines, which Amber has not done. Inadequate dietary intake is something else that you will want to consider as a cause of Amber's slowed weight gain. You probably want Amber to be having about 32 ounces of feedings per day, and she seems to be getting close to this, although an intake diary might give us a more accurate assessment.

3. *Iron deficiency:* The newborn has iron stores adequate for the first 3 to 4 months of life. This is a point in Amber's life where these stores will be running out. Thus she needs adequate iron intake. Formulas without iron are not recommended unless there is specific need, and some clinicians are now saying that they should only be available by prescription. What should you do to decide if Amber has iron deficiency? Checking a hemoglobin or hematocrit might tell you, but you need to ask yourself how that will change your treatment. If you are already committed to increasing Amber's iron intake, it may not add anything at this point unless you had concerns that the iron deficiency was significant and had caused an anemia that would require other intervention.

DIAGNOSTIC OPTIONS

Since most of the problems identified are either already better (the constipation) or are potential problems rather than current active problems, the most appropriate intervention may be to go ahead with the current plan and monitor its effect rather than doing any particular diagnostics at this point. A hematocrit might be a reasonable thing to do to assess whether the iron deficiency anemia was a real or potential problem.

THERAPEUTIC OPTIONS

Pharmacological

The parents have already used an osmotic laxative to address the constipation. It is probably reasonable to continue this, although a gradual decrease in the amount of the Karo syrup would be appropriate. You could ask the parents to call you if the constipation recurs, and then you could consider other options at that point.

Another pharmacological issue that you will need to address is what vaccines to give at this visit. Most difficult is the issue of the polio vaccine. You have three options:

1. Do not give the polio vaccine today, and give her mother the chance to have one more dose of IPV to provide her with increased protection.
2. Give Amber an OPV as soon as her mother has had her second dose of IPV.
3. Give Amber IPV today. Based on the most current recommendations, this may be the most appropriate approach, although it means giving Amber another injection. IPV may not be available at all sites as well.

Educational

Elements that would normally be included in a 4-month WCC (and basically all WCCs) are an interval history (including nutrition, sleep, elimination, growth and development, and parenting) and an assessment of development, a physical examination, and anticipatory guidance. At 4 months old, Amber should be holding her head well, she should have no head lag when pulled to sit, she should follow 180 degrees, her primitive reflexes should be diminished or gone, and she may be starting to roll from front to back. Anticipatory guidance at this age could include injury prevention, continued use of a car seat, discouraging the use of walkers, continued playing of games, and talking to Amber. The only laboratory test that is common is screening for sickle cell anemia if there is a family history.

It is very important to spend some time emphasizing the importance of adequate iron intake in this age group. Returning to an iron-fortified formula is the most logical approach. Addition of an iron-fortified cereal would also provide additional iron in the diet.

The usual educational approach for a 4-month WCC includes a review of the skills that the child can be expected to develop in the next 2 months, including sitting with support, rolling over, and increased vocalization. A discussion of the usual introduction of foods and the ages that they will be introduced would be a usual thing to cover at this visit. Use of car seats should be encouraged. A brief review of those things that require a call to the primary care provider including fevers or any health problems can give parents a sense that the provider is available.

HEALTH PROMOTION/HEALTH MAINTENANCE

Immunizations today would include DPT, Hib, and polio vaccine as discussed above. Injury prevention such as the use of car seats, setting the water heater temperature below 130° F, and cardiopulmonary resuscitation (CPR) training should be discussed. Lead-risk screening will be done at the next visit.

It is recommended to start supplementation of fluoride between 2 weeks and 6 months of age. The family can be assessing their water supply for fluoride (which will involve testing if it is well water) even if you do not recommend supplementation until 6 months of age.

FOLLOW-UP

The next scheduled visit for the 6-month WCC will be the next time Amber is seen unless she has problems.

References

Atkinson W et al, editors: *Epidemiology and prevention of vaccine preventable diseases*, Atlanta, 1996, CDC.

Baker RC: *Handbook of pediatric primary care*, Boston, 1996, Little, Brown.

Derchewitz RA: *Ambulatory pediatric care*, Philadelphia, 1993, JB Lippincott.

MMWR: Poliomyelitis prevention in the United States: recommendations and reports, *MMWR* 46(3):1, 1997.

CASE
8

OPENING SCENARIO

M'Tango Bali is a 45-year-old professor from a nearby university who is planning to spend a month in Central America in Belize working on a project and doing research. He makes an appointment to discuss a need for any immunizations for international travel. This episodic visit is his first visit to your office.

HISTORY OF PRESENT ILLNESS

"I plan to spend time in rural areas, living and working with people in the smaller villages. I will be living in people's homes and eating meals with them. I want to know if I need any immunizations and, in general, how to stay healthy. My field of study is education. I plan to spend much of my time working in schools, elementary through high school. This will be my first experience with field work. I have previously traveled out of the country but only to common tourist spots. I leave in 1 month."

MEDICAL HISTORY

Generally healthy. No hospitalizations or surgeries. Has had problems with cholesterol and has been on lovastatin (Mevacor) for the past 8 months. Last physcial examination: $1^1/_2$ years ago. Immunizations: Unsure of last tetanus, thinks it was 20 years ago when he went to college. No immunizations for hepatitis A or B.

FAMILY MEDICAL HISTORY

MGM: Died at 95 yr (osteoarthritis)
MGF: Died at 71 yr (lung cancer)
PGM: Died at 80 yr (natural causes)
PGF: Died at 77 yr (myocardial infarction [MI])
Mother: 70 yr (A&W)
Father: Died at 68 yr (MI)
One sister, one younger brother: 37, 41 yr (A&W)

SOCIAL HISTORY

Born in Tanzania and moved to the United States at age 5. Divorced for 2 years. Two children in high school who live with their mother. Nonsmoker. Moved here 5 months ago to take a position at the university. Works out at a gym 2 to 3 times a week, plus plays racquetball twice a week. Sleeps 7 hours per night.

MEDICATIONS

Lovastatin: 20 mg daily
Ibuprofen: 400 mg prn

ALLERGIES

None

REVIEW OF SYSTEMS

General: Denies appetite or weight changes; no unusual fatigue
HEENT: Denies headaches, blurry vision; wears glasses for reading; no complaints of hearing loss; mild seasonal hayfever; no history of asthma; no problems with frequent colds, sore throats, bronchitis
Cardiac: Denies chest pain; no history of palpitations, murmurs, hypertension; states cholesterol level of 271 $1^1/_2$ years ago; thinks low-density lipoproteins (LDLs) were a bit over 200 and high-density lipoproteins (HDLs) were within normal limits, cannot remember exact figures; worked on diet and exercise but the numbers did not change much; put on lovastatin 8 months ago; had normal liver function tests (LFTs) at 6 and 12 weeks but has not seen a provider since he moved here
Respiratory: No complaints of shortness of breath, dyspnea, cough
Gastrointestinal: Good appetite; trying a low-fat diet since diagnosed with high cholesterol $1^1/_2$ years ago but eats out often and finds it difficult to make good choices; no heartburn, ulcer, diarrhea, constipation; no history of exposure to hepatitis
Genitourinary: No problems with urination; no history of kidney problems; denies sexual problems
Musculoskeletal: Knee problem that bothers him periodically; the pain is dull, only somewhat bothersome on the inner part of his right knee; started about 10 years ago when he was running about 30 miles per week; no longer runs; only bothers him after vigorous, prolonged activity such as a full day of hiking; no locking; takes ibuprofen, 400 mg prn, and tries not to do 2 consecutive days of such activity; thinks he will do much walking

during this trip because transportation will be limited; possibly walking 5 to 10 miles per day when in the villages; also wants to hike into hills to explore Mayan ruins; worried that this may bother his knee

Neurological: No history of seizures, weakness, dizziness, syncope; no history of depression, psychiatric disorders

PHYSICAL EXAMINATION

Vital signs: Temperature: 98.2° F; *Pulse:* 72 beats/min; *Respirations:* 16 breaths/min; *BP:* 136/84 mm Hg
Height: 5' 11"; *Weight:* 200 lb
General: Healthy male who appears his stated age
Skin: No apparent lesions, rashes
Neck: No lymphadenopathy

Heart: Regular rate and rhythm; no murmurs, rubs, or gallops
Lungs: Clear to auscultation
Abdomen: Soft; no masses palpated; no hepatosplenomegaly
Extremities: Right knee: no bruising, swelling, erythema; no point tenderness, but client points to right medial aspect of the knee as area of aching and swelling after vigorous, prolonged physical activity; normal range of motion; no ballotment; negative bulge sign; negative McMurray and drawer tests (anterior and posterior); no cyanosis, clubbing, or edema
Neurological: Muscle strength testing: 5/5 of both lower extremities; deep tendon reflexes (biceps, triceps, patellar, ankle) 2+

ASSESSMENT   *Please indicate the problems or issues you have identified that will guide your care (preferably in list form):*

PLAN   *Please list your plans for addressing each of the problems or issues in your assessment:*

Community Clinic
Jeffrey A. Eaton, NP
Joyce D. Cappiello, NP

Name:_____ DOB_____
Address_____ Date_____

Rx

"label all unless indicated"
Refill:_____ times-- Do not refill ( )

Signed:_____
DO NOT TAKE THIS TO YOUR PHARMACIST

Community Clinic
Jeffrey A. Eaton, NP
Joyce D. Cappiello, NP

Name:_____ DOB_____
Address_____ Date_____

Rx

"label all unless indicated"
Refill:_____ times-- Do not refill ( )

Signed:_____
DO NOT TAKE THIS TO YOUR PHARMACIST

Community Clinic
Jeffrey A. Eaton, NP
Joyce D. Cappiello, NP

Name:_____ DOB_____
Address_____ Date_____

Rx

"label all unless indicated"
Refill:_____ times-- Do not refill ( )

Signed:_____
DO NOT TAKE THIS TO YOUR PHARMACIST

Community Clinic
Jeffrey A. Eaton, NP
Joyce D. Cappiello, NP

Name:_____ DOB_____
Address_____ Date_____

Rx

"label all unless indicated"
Refill:_____ times-- Do not refill ( )

Signed:_____
DO NOT TAKE THIS TO YOUR PHARMACIST

LEARNING ISSUES

In order to resolve this patient's problem, you will need to consider and address the following issues (you may generate additional issues as well):

- **How will you find the information this client is requesting?**
- **What resources will you use?**
- **How will you locate current information about disease prevalences?**
- **How extensive must your history and physical be?**
- **What immunizations, if any, will you recommend?**
- **What additional health information for traveling, if any, will you give him?**
- **Are there any other health concerns to attend to on this visit?**
- **What type of follow-up is indicated when on lipid-lowering agents?**

INITIAL IDEAS

Before you went into the room, you were probably thinking how you would find current, up-to-date travel information and whether this client's general health is adequate for travel. The latter will unfold as you do a history. The former will take some thought. Most textbooks contain travel information several years old. Infectious disease patterns may have changed since publication. The most up-to-date source, if you have a fax machine in the office, is the Centers for Disease Control and Prevention (CDC) Fax Information Service on International Travel at (404) 332-4565. First you will receive a faxed list of available reference documents on general travel information, disease risk and prevention by region of the world, disease outbreak bulletins, and additional topics, such as prescription drugs for malaria. Then you select from the menu which bulletins to order and these will be immediately faxed. All documents are current and updated as necessary. This information is also available on the Internet for those with this capability in your office at www.cdc.gov.

INTERPRETATION OF CUES, PATTERNS, AND INFORMATION

As you take this client's history, the "problem areas" that arise include his need to maintain health while traveling, knee pain after vigorous activity, his cardiovascular risk status, and his hay fever. Elevated total cholesterol and LDL levels and a family history of cardiovascular disease are definitely of concern. As you prioritize his needs for today, you know that the abnormal lipid levels have been addressed previously, so this will require less immediate attention. His need for immunization and/or prophylaxis is your main focus as well as examining his knee, which does not appear to be bothering him currently.

REVISED IDEAS

Focus on the knee pain:
- Right lateral collateral ligament strain
- Right lateral collateral ligament laxity
- Arthritis
- Anterior or posterior cruciate ligament tear

PHYSICAL EXAMINATION TECHNIQUES

Mr. Bali is not scheduled for a complete physical, but nevertheless, he is new to your practice and you will need some baseline data from his history and physical examination. You may then identify his health care needs and more properly advise him on immunizations for his upcoming travels. A basic auscultation of heart and lungs and palpation of the abdomen to rule out any major problems along with the knee examination is probably adequate for today. A follow-up visit can then be scheduled for a more complete examination to focus on his hypercholesterolemia and general health-maintenance needs.

DIAGNOSTIC OPTIONS

Regarding the knee problem, the physical examination was negative. With these findings and only occasional symptoms, diagnostic options such as an x-ray examination would render a low yield.

In terms of his elevated cholesterol level, discuss his plan for follow-up. Does he know specifically what laboratory testing was done at his last visit? Since he has been on lovastatin for 8 months, now seems an appropriate time for a fasting lipid profile. Liver enzymes need periodic monitoring while on lovastatin. He is certainly due for these studies since it is recommended that they be performed before initiating therapy and then every 4 to 6 weeks during the first 15 months.

THERAPEUTIC OPTIONS

Problem Number One

1. International travel: Generally, traveler's illnesses stem from two sources: mosquitoes and contaminated food or water. Consider how to reduce his risk in both areas.
2. A review of the current CDC recommendations (1996) for Central America:

a. *Malaria:* Malaria exists in many parts of Central America. In Belize the risk is prevalent in the rural areas, forest preserves, and offshore islands, including resort areas. There is no risk in the central coastal district. Given the itinerary of your client, malaria prophylaxis is indicated. The CDC states that most travelers to Central America who are at risk for malaria should take chloroquine. Chloroquine resistance has only been noted to the east of Panama. Although mefloquine (Larium) could be used, it is more typically used in areas of chloroquinine resistance.

b. *Yellow fever:* Yellow fever is rare in Central America, and immunization is not generally recommended. Prevention of mosquito bites is the best option.

c. *Dengue fever:* Dengue fever has been reported in all Central American countries, but no vaccine is available. Prevention of mosquito bites is the best option.

d. *Cholera:* A recent epidemic of cholera has swept through the entire Central American area. The risk of cholera to U.S. travelers is so low that it is questionable whether vaccination is of benefit. The vaccine confers only brief and incomplete immunity.

e. *Typhoid fever:* Travelers, such as this client, are especially at risk for typhoid fever when traveling to smaller cities, villages, or rural areas. Typhoid vaccine is recommended.

f. *Hepatitis A:* Travelers are at high risk for hepatitis A, especially if travel plans include extensive visits to rural areas, frequent close contact with local persons, or eating in settings of poor sanitation. Hepatitis A vaccine is recommended.

g. *Parasites:* No vaccine is available for parasites.

h. *Hepatitis B:* There is an intermediate risk of hepatitis B for all of Central America. The vaccine is recommended for health care workers whose activities might result in blood exposure, any traveler who may have intimate sexual contact with the local population, any traveler who stays for 6 months or longer in countries with a high rate of hepatitis B and will have contact with the local populations, or any traveler likely to seek medical, dental, or other treatment in local facilities during the stay. Further discussion with this client is necessary to assess his risk for hepatitis B. Generally, the hepatitis B vaccine is given with the first two injections 1 month apart and the third injection 6 months after the first. An accelerated dose of the Engerix brand of vaccine is approved at 0, 1, and 2 months; however, a fourth dose is recommended at 12 months to maintain long-term immunity (Jong and McMullen, 1995).

i. *Tetanus:* He is due for an update on his tetanus immunization.

j. *Polio:* Adults whose travel places them at increased risk of exposure to polio and have completed a previous series should receive one injectable adult or oral booster after the 18 years of age. The injectable form (IPOL or eIPV) is preferred for adults because of the slightly increased risk of acquiring the disease when given the oral form. The CDC does not list Belize as a high-risk area for polio.

k. *Measles-mumps-rubella (MMR):* Travelers born before January 1, 1957 are generally considered immune. Offer the vaccine, however, if there is reason to believe they are susceptible.

l. *Rabies:* In the United States, domestic cats and dogs account for only a minority of reported rabies cases, whereas wild animals convey most of the rabies risk. In Central America, however, bites from cats and dogs as well as wild animals represent a significant risk of rabies. A preexposure series of three injections on days 1, 7, and 21 (or 28) provides protective antibodies in more than 90% of recipients (Jong and McMullen, 1995). It is quite expensive and like many traveler's immunizations may not be covered under an insurance plan. A lower volume, intradermal (ID) rabies vaccine is less expensive but must be completed at least 3 weeks before starting malaria prophylaxis for full immunogenicity. If Mr. Bali chooses to forgo this vaccine, inform him that if he is bitten to have someone capture the animal for observation. The bite should be washed with soap and water, and he needs to contact the local public health department. Postexposure rabies prophylaxis consists of doses of human rabies immune globulin at days 0, 3, 7, 14, and 28. Many countries use vaccine made from animals, which is not currently recommended for use in the United States (Jong and McMullen, 1995). The best advice is, if bitten and human rabies immune globulin is not available, to go to a large medical center for appropriate treatment even if it means ending his trip earlier than planned and returning to the United States immediately.

m. *Motor-vehicle accidents:* Motor-vehicle accidents are the leading cause of death of travelers in developing countries. Nonfatal injuries occur in 1 of every 500 trips abroad. Encourage the traveler to rent a car with seatbelts or use the safest form of travel.

n. *Emergency first aid kit:* Take basic first aid supplies. All prescription medicine needs to be in the original, labeled container.

o. *Sexually transmitted diseases:* Travelers should be advised that human immunodeficiency virus (HIV) and other sexually transmitted disease are a worldwide problem. Carrying and using American-made latex condoms with nonoxynol-9 spermicide should be recommended.

p. *Serious injuries:* The U.S. embassy can be of assistance. The International SOS Assistance offers medical insurance covering medical evacuation, which can be purchased before travel (215) 245-4707.

3. Sample plan

a. Chloroquine: Take 500 mg weekly beginning 1 week before travel, weekly while traveling, and weekly for 4 weeks after return. Adverse effects: upset stomach, headache, dizziness, blurred vision, and itching. All symptoms are usually mild.

b. ViCPS (typhoid fever) vaccine (requires a booster every 2 years)

c. Hepatitis A vaccine

d. Hepatitis B vaccine if indicated (administer the first dose today and second dose in 1 month just before he leaves)

e. Tetanus immunization at this visit

NOTE: If your office does not stock or cannot order the vaccines, refer to a traveler's clinic if available.

4. Nonpharmacological interventions

a. Avoid mosquito bites: To prevent malaria, travelers must protect themselves from insect bites by wearing proper clothing and applying an insect repellent with DEET to exposed skin and clothing. Also, if possible, avoid high-risk situations, such as outdoor activities from dusk to dawn when mosquitoes bite and unscreened living accommodations. In spite of all protective measures, travelers may still develop malaria. Advise your client to see you if he has any flu-like illness for up to 1 year after returning home.

b. Traveler's diarrhea: Prevented best by drinking only bottled or boiled beverages (and ice cubes made from such); eating hot, cooked food; and eating fruits and vegetables peeled by the traveler himself. Cholera, typhoid fever, and hepatitis A are spread by contaminated food and water. If it occurs, moderate diarrhea of 2 to 3 unformed stools per day can be treated with loperamide (Imodium) or bismuth subsalicyclate (Pepto-Bismol). More severe diarrhea will need treatment with antibiotics such as Cipro, doxycycline, or trimethoprim sulfamethoxazole (TMP/SMX)(Bactrim or Septra). All diarrhea will require fluid replacement.

c. Do not walk with bare feet because several types of parasites can penetrate intact skin.

Problem Number Two

Knee pain: Knee pain is somewhat vague, and the diagnostic tests are negative. Recommend exercises to strengthen the quadriceps, which will decrease stress on the knee. A weight loss of 20 to 25 pounds would also reduce stress on the knee joint. Nonsteroidal antiinflammatory drugs (NSAIDS) will be helpful when the problem is acute.

Problem Number Three

Hypercholesterolemia may be an ongoing problem for him. If old records could be obtained, this would verify the lipid values. It appears that follow-up laboratory studies have not been performed in a timely fashion because of his relocation and need to find another provider. Liver-function studies and a repeat lipid profile are now needed. At this point, his medication regimen need not be changed. Urge him to continue with a low-fat diet and consider a referral to a nutritionist. Schedule a complete physical and health-maintenance appointment soon. Perhaps this can be scheduled when he returns for the second hepatitis B vaccination 1 month before departure.

References

Centers for Disease Control and Prevention: *Centers for Disease Control and Prevention International Travel Service*, Atlanta, 1996, Centers for Disease Control and Prevention.

Jong E, McMullen R: *The travel and tropical medicine manual*, Philadelphia, 1995, WB Saunders.

Recommended Reading

Buckley, Gertrude: Traveling healthy: a guide for counseling the international traveler, *Nurs Pract* 20(10):38, 1995.

CASE
9

11:45 AM
Martha Krauntz
Age 35 years

OPENING SCENARIO

Martha Krauntz is a 35-year-old female scheduled for an episodic visit for cold symptoms. She was seen in your office 5 years ago. Since then, she has been followed by her obstetrician/gynecologist.

HISTORY OF PRESENT ILLNESS

"I've had this cold for 3 to 4 days. My kids have it also. I'm going to be traveling on an airplane in 2 days and I'm worried about how I'll feel when flying. When I flew a few years ago, my ears really hurt and I didn't have a cold then. I've been taking some acetaminophen and pseudoephedrine (Sudafed) with some relief. I've been reading about Echinacea and vitamin C. Do you think either would help? How much should I take?" The patient complains of copious, clear to yellow nasal discharge, head stuffiness, sneezing, and mild cough. Occasional mild headache "all over." Denies frontal or maxillary pain, ear pain, or dental pain.

MEDICAL HISTORY

Generally healthy. Hospitalizations only for childbirth. No surgeries. No major medical problems.

SOCIAL HISTORY

Nonsmoker. Lives with husband and two children, ages 2 and 4. Works part-time as store clerk.

MEDICATIONS

Acetaminophen: 1000 mg q4h prn
Pseudoephedrine HCl: sustained release: 120 mg, 1 tab q12h for 2 days

ALLERGIES

None

REVIEW OF SYSTEMS

General: No chills, fever, body aches
HEENT: No history of environmental allergies, asthma; has 1 to 2 colds per year; has had sinus pain previously but has never been treated for a sinus infection; no ear infections since childhood; regular dental care
Cardiac: Denies chest pain, palpitations
Respiratory: Only occasional cough with this cold; no shortness of breath, no history of asthma
Gastrointestinal: No heartburn, nausea or vomiting, diarrhea, constipation

PHYSICAL EXAMINATION

Vital signs: Temperature: 98.6° F; *Pulse:* 72 beats/min; *Respirations:* 16 breaths/min; *BP:* 122/64 mm Hg
HEENT: No frontal or maxillary pain to palpitation and percussion; eyes watery; nasal mucosa swollen, red, no polyps; oral mucosa pink without lesions; pharynx slightly reddened, no purulent discharge noted; tonsils 2+; ears: no pain elicited; drums: good light reflex, landmarks visualized, no redness, retraction, or fluid noted; submandibular and submental nodes soft, slightly enlarged
Heart: Regular rate and rhythm; no murmurs, rubs, or gallops
Lungs: Clear to auscultation
Abdomen: Soft, no masses, no hepatosplenomegaly

ASSESSMENT   *Please indicate the problems or issues you have identified that will guide your care (preferably in list form):*

PLAN   *Please list your plans for addressing each of the problems or issues in your assessment:*

Community Clinic
Jeffrey A. Eaton, NP
Joyce D. Cappiello, NP

Name:_____ DOB_____
Address_____ Date_____

Rx

"label all unless indicated"
Refill:_____ times-- Do not refill ( )

Signed:_____
DO NOT TAKE THIS TO YOUR PHARMACIST

Community Clinic
Jeffrey A. Eaton, NP
Joyce D. Cappiello, NP

Name:_____ DOB_____
Address_____ Date_____

Rx

"label all unless indicated"
Refill:_____ times-- Do not refill ( )

Signed:_____
DO NOT TAKE THIS TO YOUR PHARMACIST

Community Clinic
Jeffrey A. Eaton, NP
Joyce D. Cappiello, NP

Name:_____ DOB_____
Address_____ Date_____

Rx

"label all unless indicated"
Refill:_____ times-- Do not refill ( )

Signed:_____
DO NOT TAKE THIS TO YOUR PHARMACIST

Community Clinic
Jeffrey A. Eaton, NP
Joyce D. Cappiello, NP

Name:_____ DOB_____
Address_____ Date_____

Rx

"label all unless indicated"
Refill:_____ times-- Do not refill ( )

Signed:_____
DO NOT TAKE THIS TO YOUR PHARMACIST

9 Discussion

LEARNING ISSUES

In order to resolve this patient's problem, you will need to consider and address the following issues (you may generate additional issues as well):

- **The value in incorporating questions regarding herbal use into your regular history-taking format**
- **Barriers to the use of herbal preparations by health care providers**
- **Current Food and Drug Administration (FDA) restrictions regarding the use of herbal medicine**
- **Important practice considerations if you were beginning to incorporate herbal products into your armamentarium**
- **Resources available to the practitioner in learning about herbal products**
- **Appropriate physical examination techniques**

INITIAL IDEAS

Answering Ms. Krauntz' questions about Echinacea in a research-based manner is difficult for most clinicians because standard medical and nursing journals infrequently report on such research.

INTERPRETATION OF CUES, PATTERNS, AND INFORMATION

A bacterial or viral pharyngitis seems unlikely since her major complaints are not throat related and physical examination shows only a mild erythema.

A sinusitis seems unlikely without findings of purulent discharge, persistant headache, or pain over the sinus area.

With influenza, one would expect more constitutional symptoms of aching, fever, nausea, or vomiting.

Bronchitis, too, seems unlikely based on the short duration of symptoms with only a mild cough. An allergic component seems less likely than a viral URI based on her lack of history of allergies and short duration of symptoms. The client's self-assessment of upper respiratory infection (URI) appears accurate.

Physical Examination Techniques

Appropriate techniques would focus on the upper and lower respiratory tracts: HEENT and lungs. While listening to the lungs, it is easy to listen to the heart. If you have not seen this person for a prior physical, it makes sense to have some baseline clinical data, especially before prescribing medications. The abdominal examination offers little useful clinical data since she has no gastrointestinal complaints and you have essentially ruled out influenza by history.

THERAPEUTIC OPTIONS

It seems that her main reasons for seeking care are how to be more comfortable on the airplane with this cold, whether alternative therapies may be helpful, and how to use alternative remedies.

1. The usual allopathic approach for a URI would be to treat the symptoms.

    a. Acetaminophen (extra strength) is helpful for the discomfort.

    b. Adrenergic topical decongestants (sprays) come in short-acting (3 to 4 hours) or longer-acting (8 to 10 hours), which occasionally cause stinging when first used. Topical decongestants can only be used for about 3 days or the likelihood of rebound phenomena increases. Atrovent nasal spray (an anticholinergic) 0.06% is indicated for the treatment of rhinorrhea associated with the common cold without the concern of rebound effect.

    c. Oral decongestants can cause an elevation of blood pressure, but that seems an unlikely response in this healthy woman with no previous history of high blood pressure. She could use whichever method she prefers.

    d. Antihistamines are helpful with allergic rhinitis but would be less effective than decongestants in the common cold. Combination cold preparations that may include antihistamines, decongestants, caffeine, pain relievers, and so on will be more expensive, have more side effects, and perhaps give less relief of symptoms. There is no evidence that expectorants are useful. If her cough becomes worse, a cough suppressant such as dextromethorphan may be taken at night. Antibiotics are not warranted in this uncomplicated viral infection.

2. What are the efficacy and safety of alternatives to this standard approach?

    a. *Vitamin C:* High doses of vitamin C have been a part of popular culture since the initial work of Linus Pauling. No consistent beneficial effect has been found in trials of large doses of vitamin C for the common cold. Smaller doses of daily vitamin C have an antioxidant effect that may be useful for long-term prevention of illness. Vitamin C (500 mg per day) seems reasonable to give an antioxidant effect and possibly help with the URI symptoms.

    b. *Zinc throat lozenges:* Zinc gluconate lozenges (13.3 mg) have been found to shorten the duration of the common cold. The lozenges curbed sore throats, nasal congestion and drainage, coughing, headache, and hoarseness, but they did not eliminate fever, muscle ache, scratchy throat, or sneezing. Side effects include an unpleasant taste experienced by the majority of users and nausea in about 20% of users. Lozenges are used every 2 hours while awake as long as symptoms last (Mossad, 1996).

    c. *Echinacea:* Echinacea is derived from coneflowers, a group of native American wildflowers. It's medicinal use was a part of Native American culture for hundreds of years. Echinacea became popular in Western culture when German chemists looking for new herbal remedies became interested in this plant, researched the active ingredients, and legitimized its medicinal uses. There have been hundreds of journal articles published on the chemistry, pharmacology, and clinical uses to date, but only a few are controlled, double-blind clinical trials. More studies have been done with the injectable form of Echinacea, but this form is not available in the United States. Other studies have focused on the topical application for a variety of skin conditions. Most of the research has been done on *E. purpurea* rather than *E. augustifolia* or *E. pallida*. This discussion will focus only on *E. purpurea*.

Echinacea's popularity is as an immune stimulator. The few tests on humans have shown Echinacea to exhibit clinically significant activation of macrophage and granulocyte activity with an increase of phagocytosis. Two placebo-controlled, double-blind studies with 100 influenza patients each showed a significant shortening of the duration of influenza and a reduction of the severity of the symptoms (Hobbs, 1994).

In another double-blind study with 650 students, Echinacea was used as a preventive measure and showed a reduction in the frequency of infection. A placebo-controlled, double-blind study with 108 human volunteers who had chronic URIs (more than 3 occurrences of such infections as otitis, rhinitis, tonsillitis, pharyngitis, laryngitis, bronchitis, pneumonia, or sinusitis in a half year) were given 4 ml of Echinacea in liquid form twice a day over an 8-week period. Compared with the placebo group, 36% more patients suffered no infections, the time between infections was lengthened, the duration of illness was shortened, and the severity of symptoms was lessened. The Echinacea preparation was well-tolerated, and patients with lowered T4/T8 ratios seemed to profit most from the treatment (Hobbs, 1994).

Echinacea appears to be a safe product. A number of toxicology studies have been done with animals showing no toxic effects. There are no reports of adverse reactions with humans with oral preparations. Contraindications include progressive systemic disease such as lupus, multiple sclerosis, diabetes mellitus, and tuberculosis because of the immune stimulant properties of Echinacea (Blumenthal, 1994).

Most of the worldwide research on herbal products is done in Germany and thus published in German in their scientific literature. Phytotherapy (herbal treatment) is part of the school of medicine in Germany, not an alternative medicine, although herbs are more frequently used as adjunct therapies rather than primary therapies. More than 70% of the general practitioners in Germany prescribe phytotherapy. The cost of most herbal products is covered under German national health insurance. This means there is a financial incentive for companies to spend millions of dollars to isolate the active ingredients in plants, develop a standardized extract (an extract guaranteed to contain a specific amount of a particular active ingredient), perform efficacy and safety studies, and bring it to market. Standardized extracts are useful because the concentration of active ingredients can vary greatly in different parts of a plant or even within the same part of the plant in different seasons, soils, or climates. The German *Commission E Monograph* contains probably the most accurate information available in the world on safety and efficacy of hundreds of herbs. English translations are available. However, the research articles that the *Monograph* uses to arrive at conclusions on doses and length of therapy are unavailable unless you are fluent in German. You must rely on other analysis of the research data.

The dosage information on Echinacea varies from study to study. Currently, the most popular Echinacea products are liquid extracts, freeze-dried extracts in capsules and tablets, simple herb powders in capsules and tablets, and fresh juice preparations. According to Wagner and Jurcic (Hobbs, 1994), immune reactions work by the law of all or nothing; that is, when immune modulators reach a critical dose, they lead to an immune response, which cannot be further increased by raising the dose and may even, in some cases, lead to immune suppression. They recommended 50 drops (about one dropperful), or 300 to 400 mg, of a dry extract 3 times daily (Hobbs, 1994).

This dose-dependent response was shown in one placebo-controlled, double-blind study by Braunig in 1992, which showed that 180 drops of an ethanolic extract significantly reduced the severity and duration of the symptoms of influenza, whereas 90 drops were no more effective than the placebo (Hobbs, 1994).

In another study by Jurcic in 1989, maximum immune stimulation was reached after 5 days, after which the immune stimulation began to subside even though the preparation was continued at the same dose (Hobbs,1994). However, the *Commission E Monograph* recommends that the preparation can be used for up to 8 weeks (Blumenthal, 1994). This is most likely based on the 4 ml bid, but it is not referenced. It appears that a safe dose, based on the information available, would be 300 to 400 mg (this seems a more standardized dose than counting 50 drops) of standardized dry extract in capsule form tid. The studies do not seem to clarify the optimal length of therapy. Use for 5 days seems to be safe and therapeutic, but the data is conflicting regarding its use beyond 5 days. A review of English summaries of the research suggests 5 days for acute problems and up to 8 weeks for chronic problems but does not clarify dosage for the longer regimen. This also conflicts with the in vitro research of optimal therapeutic effect within 5 days. Echinacea (300 mg po tid for 5 days) seems reasonable based on the available data.

3. Discussion of practice issues: Two extreme points of view on the use of herbal therapies focus on one side that says herbs are incapable of causing harm because they are natural and the other

side that believes herbs are ineffective and dangerous. The truth may be somewhere in the middle. Herbal medications may be gentler than other pharmaceuticals because they are less concentrated, but herbs do contain a variety of active ingredients that can have strong effects.

The FDA has only investigated and approved a small number of herbs for medicinal uses. The first FDA action with herbs was to approve about 250 herbs as food additives in 1958. These became generally recognized as safe because of their long history of use. No category for medicinal use of plants was established. More recently, the Dietary Supplement Health and Education Act of 1994 placed herbal medicines in the category of dietary supplements. A stipulation was added that no therapeutic claims could be made on the labels of any of these products. Literature about the dietary supplement must be displayed separately from the product. Thus it is important for health providers to ask their patients about their use of herbal products and then to know about or research accurate dosages. See Box 9-1 for a discussion about the legal considerations for recommmending herbal medicines.

The Commission on Dietary Supplement Labels is charged with making dietary supplement labels informative and accurate about health benefit claims while also promoting the safety and quality of the products. An office of dietary supplements within the National Institutes of Health has been established to promote the scientific study of dietary supplements to improve health care within the United States.

Costs are an important factor to consider since most alternative treatments are not currently reimbursable by health insurance.

Box 9-1 Discussion of Legal Considerations for the Practitioner Recommending Herbal Medicine

The following guidelines may help providers who are interested in safely incorporating herbal therapies into a medical practice:

1. Become educated in herbal medicine by attending workshops, courses, and conferences.
2. Do not dispense herbal preparations from your office.
3. Research and recommend only reliable manufacturers of herbal preparations with names and reputations. Ask for a company's medical and research department to obtain information on clinical trials and ask questions on how their products are obtained, dried, and manufactured. The L-tryptophan tragedy of a few years ago comes to mind. Several patients died of complications not from L-tryptophan itself but from using a product that was contaminated in the manufacturing process.
4. Standardized extracts should provide a standardized dose of active ingredients in each preparation, although the quality control is not as stringently regulated as the preparation of over-the-counter (OTC) and prescription medications. Labels on herbal products should state the active ingredients and the amount.
5. Keep at least one clinical trial on file in your office for each herbal remedy you choose to recommend to a patient.
6. Recommend only those herbal remedies of which you have knowledge.
7. Have the patient sign a consent form detailing herbal medicine recommendations for usual allopathic treatment.
8. Include direct questions about the use of alternative therapies, especially questions on the use of herbal products, when taking the history of all clients. Recent studies show that 34% of all Americans use herbal products (Eisenberg et al, 1993) but do not discuss this use with their clinician.
9. Have a referral list of knowledgeable herbalists.
10. As with any other medication, instruct clients to take only the recommended dosage and only for the length of time advised.
11. Caution against herbal use during pregnancy and breastfeeding. Adult doses will not apply to children.

Modified from Bascom A: *The right to more than one medical culture: incorporating herbal medicine into clinical practice for physicians and nurse practitioners,* Master's thesis requirement at the University of New Hampshire, 1997.

References

Bascom A: *The right to more than one medical culture: incorporating herbal medicine into clinical practice for physicians and nurse practitioners,* Master's thesis requirement at the University of New Hampshire, 1997.

Blumenthal M (editor), Klein S (translator): *Therapeutic monographs on medicinal plants for human use of special expert committee* (Federal Health Agency, Germany), Austin, Texas, 1994, American Botanical Council.

Eisenberg D et al: Unconventional medicine in the United States, *N Engl J Med* 328:246, 1993.

Hobbs C: Echinacea: a literature review: botany, history, chemistry, pharmacology, toxicology and clinical uses, *Herbalgram* 30:34, 1994.

Mossad S et al: Zinc gluconate lozenges for treating the common cold: a randomized, double-blind, placebo-controlled study, *Ann Intern Med* 125:81, 1996.

CASE
10

OPENING SCENARIO

The medical assistant tells you that a nursing home called to let you know that Ms. Lincoln's purified protein derivative (PPD) was negative. Ms. Lincoln is the patient of one of your associates who will be away for the next week and for whom you are covering. She was just admitted to the nursing home 3 days ago.

ASSESSMENT   *Please indicate the problems or issues you have identified that will guide your care (preferably in list form):*

PLAN   *Please list your plans for addressing each of the problems or issues in your assessment:*

Community Clinic
Jeffrey A. Eaton, NP
Joyce D. Cappiello, NP

Name:_____ DOB_____
Address_____ Date_____

Rx

"label all unless indicated"
Refill:_____ times-- Do not refill ( )

Signed:_____
DO NOT TAKE THIS TO YOUR PHARMACIST

C A S E
10 *Discussion*

LEARNING ISSUES

In order to resolve this patient's problem, you will need to consider and address the following issues (you may generate additional issues as well):

- **Tuberculosis (Tb) in the elderly**
- **Screening tests for Tb**
- **Changing treatments of patients other than your own**

INITIAL IDEAS

Ms. Lincoln is not your patient, but you are covering. You assume the PPD was done predominantly as a screening measure since many nursing homes and some states require a test as part of the admission process. You also know, however, that older people are more apt to be anergic and that this reaction may not actually represent the absence of infection.

INTERPRETATION OF CUES, PATTERNS, AND INFORMATION

There are several ways to handle this situation. Most will depend more on your philosophy regarding screening for Tb than they will on patient information. Probably the key piece of information that you need at this point is whether Ms. Lincoln had this as a screening test or if there is real concern that she may have Tb.

DIFFERENTIAL DIAGNOSIS

The differential diagnosis at this point is true-negative versus false-negative PPD.

DIAGNOSTIC OPTIONS

There are three options:

1. *Order a boosted PPD:* When an elderly person has been exposed to Tb many years previously, he or she may not react to PPD. Thus a second dose can be given. This is most effective between 1 week and 1 year after the first dose (Physicians' Desk Reference, 1997). Thus you could order a second dose of PPD to be planted intracutaneously 7 days after admission.

2. *Plant an anergy control:* Mumps and/or candida can be used. The assumption is that all people of this age have been exposed to these infections and that therefore they will all react. If a person does not react, then it is suspicious that they are anergic.

3. *Do nothing and leave the issue for Ms. Lincoln's primary provider:* This may be the best option. Chances are there is nothing that needs to be changed acutely for Ms. Lincoln and that the PPD can be boosted or an anergy panel done as easily and effectively when her primary provider returns.

This case raises the issue of how much should be done while "on coverage." This will vary based on the relationship of the providers and the acuity of the situation. You do not want to miss an opportunity for appropriate diagnosis and treatment and thus should not be hesitant to step in and offer appropriate treatment. On the other side of the discussion, however, is the context that a primary care provider has regarding the individual patient and the reasons behind treatment.

It may be important to establish Ms. Lincoln's status related to her PPD because if she does get exposed within the next year, she may appear to "turn positive" when in fact she is just demonstrating a boosted reaction.

If she does react, the issue then becomes whether she will need a course of isoniazid. Although some references do not recommend INH prophylaxis in an elderly person, that decision may be best made with the consultation of an infectious disease specialist.

References

Physicians' desk reference, Oradell, NJ, 1997, Medical Economics.

CASE
11

1:00 PM
Jake Marland
Age 8 1/2 months

OPENING SCENARIO

Jake Marland is an 8 1/2-month-old male on your schedule for an ear infection.

HISTORY OF PRESENT ILLNESS

(Obtained from mother)
"Jake was awake a lot last night, and I think he's been pulling at his right ear. Amoxicillin doesn't work for him. He had a cold about 4 days ago with a runny nose and a mild cough. I gave him acetaminophen for the cold and it seemed to get better. No one else at home is sick."

MEDICAL HISTORY

Normal spontaneous vaginal delivery. Apgar scores were 9 and 9. Had ear infections at 2 months (treated with amoxicillin), 3 months (treated with Bactrim), and 6 months (treated with Bactrim). Immunization record is shown in Table 11-1. Still had a mild effusion at 4-month well child check (WCC), but provider felt it was not worth treating. Developmental milestones are all within normal limits on previous visits. Currently he is able to sit well and has started to push himself backwards on the ground when he is on his stomach. Sleeps about 10 hours per night. Likes to fall asleep drinking a bottle but has been switched to water. Takes evening nap but often skips morning nap. Growth is indicated in Table 11-2.

FAMILY MEDICAL HISTORY

MGM: 51 yr (breast cancer diagnosed 4 years ago)
MGF: 54 yr (A&W)
PGM: 47 yr (A&W)
PGF: 46 yr (hypertension)
Mother: 26 yr (A&W)
Father: 25 yr (A&W)
One brother: 3 yr (A&W)

SOCIAL HISTORY

Lives with both parents and older brother (now 3 years old). Father works as a highway department employee.

Mother works part time at convenience store (four mornings per week). Jake attends the local daycare center when his mother is working. Jake was just approved for Medicaid. Father smokes 1/2 pack per day but is trying to quit and smokes primarily outside. Mother has never smoked.

Table **11-1** *Immunization Record for Jake Marland*

Vaccine	Date	Initials	Notes
DPT	2 mo	MDO	Tetramune
DPT	4 mo	MDO	Tetramune
DPT	6 mo	MDO	Tetramune
DPT			
Td			
Td			
OPV	2 mo	MDO	
OPV	4 mo	MDO	
OPV			
OPV			
MMR			
MMR			
HBV	2 mo	MDO	
HBV	4 mo	MDO	
HBV			
Hib	2 mo	MDO	Tetramune
Hib	4 mo	MDO	Tetramune
Hib	6 mo	MDO	Tetramune
Hib			

Table **11-2** *Growth of Jake Marland*

Measure	Age	Result	Percentile
Length	2 wk	20"	20%
	2 mo	22"	25%
	4 mo	24 1/4"	25%
	6 mo	26"	25%
Weight	2 wk	7 lb 12 oz	25%
	2 mo	9 lb	25%
	4 mo	12 lb 1 oz	25%
	6 mo	16 lb 1 oz	25%
Head circum-ference	2 wk	13 3/4 cm	40%
	2 mo	14 3/4 cm	40%
	4 mo	16 cm	35%
	6 mo	17 cm	30%

MEDICATIONS

None

ALLERGIES

None

REVIEW OF SYSTEMS

(Obtained from mother)

General: Good energy level

Skin: No itching or rashes

HEENT: No history of head injury; had about 3 colds (upper respiratory infections [URIs]) since birth; no allergy symptoms; five teeth present without gross defects

Neck: No lumps, goiters, or pain

Thorax: Mother denies evidence of shortness of breath

Cardiac: No shortness of breath with normal activity

Gastrointestinal: No vomiting, constipation, or diarrhea

Genitourinary: No odor to urine

Extremities: No sign of joint pain or swelling

Neurological: No seizures

Hematological: No excessive bruising; no history of transfusions

Nutrition: Eats from all four food groups; using commercial baby food and soft and ground table foods; utilizes Women, Infants, and Children (WIC) services; current formula is Enfamil with Iron, 28 ounces per day

PHYSICAL EXAMINATION

Vital signs: Temperature: 99.8° F (tympanic); *Pulse:* 98 beats/min; *Respirations:* 28 breaths/min

Weight: 15 lb, 5 oz (10th percentile)

General: Well nourished, well developed; in no acute distress; appears stated age

HEENT: Normocephalic without masses or lesions; pupils equal, round, and reactive to light; extraocular movements intact; moderate amount of clear discharge present in both eyes; no redness of conjunctiva; nares patent and noninjected; throat without redness or lesions; *right* tympanic membrane (TM) noninjected, cone of light crisp, mobility 4+/4+; *left* TM with bubbles apparent; mobility 2+/4+; very mild redness at the periphery only; cone of light diffuse

Neck: Supple without thyromegaly or adenopathy

Thorax: Clear to auscultation and percussion

Heart: Regular rate and rhythm; no murmurs, rubs, or gallops

Gastrointestinal: No hepatosplenomegaly; abdomen soft, nontender; bowel sounds normoactive

Extremities: Range of motion functionally intact; no cyanosis, clubbing, or edema

Neurological: Babinski reflex present

ASSESSMENT   *Please indicate the problems or issues you have identified that will guide your care (preferably in list form):*

PLAN   *Please list your plans for addressing each of the problems or issues in your assessment:*

Community Clinic
Jeffrey A. Eaton, NP
Joyce D. Cappiello, NP

Name:_____ DOB_____
Address_____ Date_____

Rx

"label all unless indicated"
Refill:_____ times-- Do not refill ( )

Signed:_____
DO NOT TAKE THIS TO YOUR PHARMACIST

Community Clinic
Jeffrey A. Eaton, NP
Joyce D. Cappiello, NP

Name:_____ DOB_____
Address_____ Date_____

Rx

"label all unless indicated"
Refill:_____ times-- Do not refill ( )

Signed:_____
DO NOT TAKE THIS TO YOUR PHARMACIST

C A S E
11 *Discussion*

LEARNING ISSUES

In order to resolve this patient's problem, you will need to consider and address the following issues (you may generate additional issues as well):

- **Signs and symptoms of acute otitis media (AOM)**
- **Diagnostic criteria of AOM including interpretation of otoscopic and pneumatic otoscopic findings**
- **Appropriate interval for recheck after AOM**
- **Choice of antibiotics for AOM**
- **Nonantibiotic treatment of AOM**
- **Prevention of AOM**
- **Treatment of recurrent AOM**
- **Diagnosis and treatment of otitis media with effusion (OME)**
- **Tympanic thermometer use in an 8 month old**
- **Teething**
- **Hearing loss and speech and language delay associated with persistent effusion**
- **Other complications of OM**

INITIAL IDEAS

- Recurrent AOM versus OME
- Symptoms related to teething, URI, or other viral etiology
- Teething as a cause of discomfort

INTERPRETATION OF CUES, PATTERNS, AND INFORMATION

Textbooks often describe the treatment for OM in a manner that makes decision making appear simple. However, dealing with Jake and his Mom shows it may not be that simple. There are several different reasonable approaches to Jake's care, and that must be kept in mind when evaluating the following information.

Jake's situation is unfortunately not uncommon. Jake's mother is concerned that he has an ear infection, and she has what she probably feels to be good experience in deciding whether Jake has an ear infection. This puts you in a challenging situation since you may now want to recommend something different for treatment. Several questions are probably occurring to you at this point. Did Jake ever really get rid of his effusion? Was the previous choice of antibiotics the best one? Does this child meet the criteria for prophylaxis? So what do I do now? Each one of these questions will be addressed separately.

1. *Did Jake ever really get rid of his effusion?* Effusion can persist for 3 months or longer after an episode of AOM. There was never a visit that Jake did not have an effusion. The possibility then exists that either this is the "same" effusion that Jake had at 2 months old or it had abated but recurred and this is the result of the second infection that occurred at 6 months of age.

2. *Was the previous choice of antibiotics the best one?* Amoxicillin is the drug of choice for almost all first ear infections. Based on a series of cultures the organisms that are most commonly found to cause AOM are *Streptococcus pneumoniae* (31%), *Haemophilus influenzae* (22%), and *Moraxella catarrhalis* (7%). About 33% of AOM cases had no bacterial isolate and group A streptococcus, enteric gram-negative bacteria, *Staphylococcus aureus,* and a few other miscellaneous organisms accounted for the remaining 7% (Johnson and Oski, 1997). The drug chosen should of course cover the most common organisms. Regional or local resistance patterns may also need to be considered.

A second issue that may be as important as the actual choice of antibiotics with the earlier infections was the way in which they were given. Did the parents ever even fill the prescription (especially since cost can be an issue, although amoxicillin and Bactrim are relatively inexpensive)? If they did, was the medication taken regularly and for long enough? If the medication was found unpalatable by the child, was a lot of it spit out and thus not effective? Did side effects cause the parents to stop the medication before it might have been fully effective? If this is a concern, then choice of another antibiotic treatment would have to address whatever the perceived problem was such as taste, cost, or inconvenience.

3. *Does this child meet the criteria for prophylaxis?* Prophylaxis is suggested when children have three ear infections within 6 months or four within 1 year. A reasonable case can be made either way for Jake's meeting the criteria. The benefit of erring on the side of supporting prophylaxis is that it may cut down on the recurrence of infections and possibly of complications. There are several different approaches to prophylaxis including amoxicillin or sulfisoxazole for medication therapy or myringotomy and tubes as surgical therapy. Trimethoprim sulfamethoxazole (TMP/SMX) combinations such as Bactrim are also used for this but do not have a Food and Drug Administration (FDA) indication for doing so. The relative efficacies of these prophylactic interventions are currently unclear. Other approaches such as beginning antibiotics at the first signs of a URI are also being recommended, but as of now there are no studies that show better or worse outcomes than traditional approaches to prophylaxis.

4. *So what do I do now?* The answer to this question will in large part be based on your assessment of the previous issues. Is Jake sick today? He does have a low-grade fever based on the tympanic thermometer reading, but there is controversy over the use of tympanic thermometers in children his age. It is also a possibility that his infection may have created an elevated reading because of the direct measurement of the TM and that the core temperature itself is not well reflected. Do you believe that all of his "infections" actually represented clinical infection versus persistent effusion? There are obviously several reasonable approaches to this case. One would be to obtain audiological evaluation of Jake and then base further actions on the presence or absence of hearing deficit.

What role should a tympanogram play in this case? You have a drum that is mobile but has decreased mobility. The tympanogram may give further evidence for the presence of effusion as well as allowing an objective measure on which to assess the presence or absence of change.

If you have questions about adherence to the treatment regimen or regional patterns of resistance, one more try with antibiotic therapy might be appropriate. The drug chosen would obviously have to have a different spectrum of activity and a profile that would maximize adherence such as once- or twice-a-day dosing, pleasing taste, reasonable cost and/or insurance coverage, and a lack of side effects.

One option that is only rarely used but does exist is a culture of the fluid in the ear. Since this requires a myringotomy, obviously the clinician would need to be comfortable with that skill.

Therapeutic options for Jake's OM will vary based on the diagnosis made. Some options are described later under Therapeutic Options.

The issue of teething has been raised. Jake does appear to have a problem with his ear, but the factors that kept him up last night are not certain. He has already cut through five teeth, but he has several more that may be in various stages of coming through the gums. The issue of whether teething can cause a fever is controversial. Baker (1997) says that a fever over 101° F should never be attributed to teething, but the empiric evidence of teething causing fever is difficult to obtain.

REVISED IDEAS

- AOM
- Persistent OME
- Possible teething

DIFFERENTIAL DIAGNOSIS

How do you decide between these diagnoses? If the treatment will be the same, then you may not need to decide. If this particular infection is felt to represent an AOM and the previous infections have been interpreted as two episodes with effusions that lasted 2 to 3 months, then a course of antibiotics would be appropriate. If the diagnosis is to be OME, then either observation or a course of antibiotics would be appropriate based on Agency for Health Care Policy and Research guidelines (AHCPR, 1994). If this is felt to be a persistent OME, then it has persisted long enough that further evaluation is appropriate.

Another form of AOM that is described is bullous myringitis in which a bleb forms between the anatomical layers of the TM. This finding may be associated with a mycoplasmal infection or any of the usual organisms that cause AOM. It is not present in this case, however, so you do not need to be concerned with it.

Although not direct causes of OM, certain other conditions that increase the probability of OM can be considered depending on other findings. Children with allergies, hypothyroidism, cystic fibrosis, cleft palate, obstructing adenoids, and nasopharyngeal masses may be at increased risk for AOM. You do not have any specific reasons to suspect these in Jake, but you should be vigilant for signs of any of them.

DIAGNOSTIC OPTIONS

1. *Tympanogram:* The tympanogram may provide additional information, but it may not change the approach to treatment. Some clinicians use the tympanogram to monitor for changes by doing interval readings.
2. *Trial of therapy:* This would be carried out if the clinician felt that previous treatment had been suboptimal based on organism resistance or treatment regimen adherence issues.
3. *Audiology:* Documentation of the presence of a hearing loss may provide impetus for further evaluation or surgical treatment.
4. *Ear/nose/throat (ENT) consult:* Effusions that persist longer than 12 weeks are unlikely to resolve spontaneously. Insertion of a polyethylene tube restores hearing and may prevent speech problems related to a persistent decrease in hearing from persistent OM.

THERAPEUTIC OPTIONS

Pharmacological

Is it worth one more try? If there is some question whether previous treatments were of insufficient frequency or duration, then a course of an antibiotic with a different spectrum and easier scheduling might be an option. This child has had amoxicillin and TMP/SMX (Bactrim). Unfortunately TMP/SMX is not always palatable, and the probability of taking the full amount for the complete course of the antibiotic may thus be decreased. Both amoxicillin and Bactrim may be inadequate for a beta-lactamase—producing organism. Roughly 80% to 90% of *M. catarrhalis* and 30% to 40% of *H. influenzae* are beta-lactamase producers (Sanford, 1996) and thus will be resistant to medications already attempted. Other options would be amoxicillin with a beta-lactamase inhibitor such as clavulanate (Augmentin) or a second- or third-generation cephalosporin. Cefaclor is a second-generation and cefixime is a third-generation cephalosporin. Cefixime (Suprax) provides once-a-day dosage and a pleasant taste but at a fairly high cost. It has wide coverage but with "holes," including *S. aureus* and *Enterobacter.*

Referral for audiology and/or ENT evaluation is another option, although most clinicians would try a beta-lactamase—inhibiting antibiotic first. Although relatively uncommon based on current information, speech and language delays and cholesteatomas are serious complications that may be avoided with appropriate intervention. The AHCPR (1994) recommendation is that children with effusion for greater than 3 months should have hearing testing. In small children, this may be difficult and may come down to clinical judgment.

Some clinicians recommend treating with a combination of antibiotic and oral steroids, although at this point there is controversy about this approach. Some have also theorized that a nonsteroidal anti-inflammatory drug (NSAID) like children's ibuprofen may decrease inflammation of the eustachian tube and thus improve drainage, although empiric evidence is lacking in this area as well.

Should antihistamines or decongestants be used in AOM? Most recommendations are to avoid antihistamines, but some clinicians recommend decongestants. They are possibly helpful and probably do not have negative effects on the resolution of the OM.

For Jake's teething issues, acetaminophen or ibuprofen are reasonable.

Educational

Bottle propping may be associated with AOM and thus should be discouraged. Passive smoke has also been associated with AOM, and parents should be encouraged to eliminate any exposure. The role of daycare is a little more complicated to address. Day care has been associated with a higher incidence of AOM, but some parents may already be dealing with guilt feelings regarding the placement in a daycare setting. Thus if the subject is addressed, it must be done with care and sensitivity.

Usually if prescribing antibiotics, an instruction is given to call if the child is not symptom free in 48 hours. This may or may not apply in this case, but if this was felt to be an acute infection, this instruction may be appropriate.

Other Nonpharmacological Options

As previously noted, it may be time to obtain consultation from audiology and/or otorhinolaryngology. Many clinicians feel that the potential problems with speech benefit from surgical intervention, although the empiric evidence in this area is not conclusive.

HEALTH PROMOTION/HEALTH MAINTENANCE

Jake is 8 months old. Will his mother bring him in for a 9-month WCC? If you have any concerns that she will not, a very brief discussion about feeding issues, safety (including syrup of ipecac), and the approach of stranger anxiety could be carried out. Jake should probably come back for a recheck of his ear in several weeks, but if you do refer him to ENT, the mother may feel that he already has been "checked by a doctor" so that a WCC is not necessary. Assessment for appropriate fluoride supplementation could also be carried out since it can be initiated at 6 months of age.

FOLLOW-UP

Follow-up will depend on the option chosen for treatment, although most clinicians would bring Jake back for his regular 9-month WCC so that appropriate developmental assessment and anticipatory guidance could be carried out. This would also allow a review of appropriate social issues.

References

Agency for Health Care Policy and Research: *Otitis media with effusion in young children,* AHCPR Pub No 94-0623, 1994.

Baker RC: *Handbook of pediatric primary care,* Boston, 1997, Little, Brown.

Johnson KB, Oski FA: Essential pediatrics, Philadelphia, 1997, JB Lippincott.

Sanford J, Gilbert DN, Sande MA: *The Sanford guide to antimicrobial therapy, Dallas,* 1996, Antimicrobial Therapy.

CASE
12

1:15 PM
Maurice Lamontagne
Age 64 years

OPENING SCENARIO

Maurice Lamontagne is a 64-year-old male who has not had any primary care for several years. When he tried to give blood last week, he was told that he was anemic. He called the office and asked for an appointment because of this. The office staff asked if you wanted him to have any laboratory tests. You ordered a complete blood count (CBC), which is now available (Table 12-1).

HISTORY OF PRESENT ILLNESS

"I've been a little more tired than usual, but I've been busy at work. I'm getting close to retirement, so I figured I was just slowing down a bit. Nothing else is unusual at all. I avoid doctors if I can. I feel pretty good, but I tire easily."

MEDICAL HISTORY

Inguinal hernia repair 20 years ago

FAMILY MEDICAL HISTORY

MGM: Deceased at 80 yr (pancreatic cancer)
MGF: Deceased at 77 yr (heart attack)

Table 12-1 Laboratory Work for Maurice Lamontagne

CBC	Result	Normal Range
WBC	8.2	4.5-10.8
RBC	3.85 L	4.20-5.40
Hgb	10.9 L	12.0-16.0
Hct	32.2 L	37.0-47.0
MCV	79.2 L	81.0-99.0
MCH	26.9 L	27.0-32.0
MCHC	33.4	32.0-36.0
RDW	16.4 H	11.0-16.0
Platelets	221	150-450
Segs	64	50-65
Lymphocytes	23 L	25-45
Monocytes	9	0-10
Eosinophils	4	0-4

PGM: Deceased at 60 yr ("women's problems")
PGF: Deceased at 74 yr (stroke)
Mother: 87 yr (A&W)
Father: Deceased 10 years ago at age 80 yr (heart attack)
Daughter: 39 yr (A&W)
One brother: 60 yr (alcoholism)
Four grandchildren: None with health problems

SOCIAL HISTORY

Married for 44 years. Works as a project foreman for landscaping portion of local nursery. Due for retirement soon. Smoking 1 pack per day. Alcohol: "A couple of beers in the evening."

MEDICATIONS

Multivitamin: i po qd

ALLERGIES

None

REVIEW OF SYSTEMS

General: Good energy level in the morning but tires easily; denies significant weight change, fevers, chills, or sweats
Skin: No itching or rashes
HEENT: No history of head injury; no corrective lenses; denies eye pain, excessive tearing, blurring, or change in vision; no tinnitus or vertigo; denies frequent colds, hay fever, or sinus problems
Neck: No lumps, goiters, or pain
Thorax: Denies shortness of breath, paroxysmal nocturnal dyspnea
Cardiac: No chest pain; no shortness of breath with normal activity
Gastrointestinal: No nausea, vomiting, constipation, or diarrhea; denies belching, bloating, and black or clay colored stools; no bright red blood per rectum; weight stable past 10 years
Genitourinary: No dysuria; no difficulty starting stream; urine seems a little darker lately
Extremities: Mild joint pain with significant activity
Neurological: No headaches, seizures
Endocrine: No polyuria, polyphagia, polydipsia; temperature tolerances good
Hematological: No excessive bruising; no history of transfusions

PHYSICAL EXAMINATION

Vital signs: Temperature: 98.4° F; *Pulse:* 98 beats/min; *Respirations:* 20 breaths/min; *BP:* 112/70 mm Hg
Height: 5' 10"; *Weight:* 172 lb
General: Well nourished, well developed; in no acute distress; appears younger than stated age
HEENT: Normocephalic without masses or lesions; pupils equal, round, and reactive to light; extraocular movements intact; skin and conjunctiva are slightly pale; fundi benign; nares patent and noninjected; throat without redness or lesions
Neck: Supple without thyromegaly or adenopathy
Thorax: Clear to auscultation and percussion

Heart: Regular rate and rhythm; no murmurs, rubs, or gallops
Gastrointestinal: No hepatosplenomegaly; abdomen soft, nontender; bowel sounds normoactive
Genitourinary: Normal male, circumcised, both testicles descended
Rectal: No masses; prostate smooth and not enlarged; stool is brown and guaiac negative
Extremities: Range of motion functionally intact; no cyanosis, clubbing, or edema
Neurological: Reflexes 2+ at Achilles, patellar, biceps, triceps, and brachioradialis; no Babinski signs present

ASSESSMENT   *Please indicate the problems or issues you have identified that will guide your care (preferably in list form):*

PLAN   *Please list your plans for addressing each of the problems or issues in your assessment:*

Community Clinic
Jeffrey A. Eaton, NP
Joyce D. Cappiello, NP

Name:_____ DOB_____
Address_____ Date_____

Rx

"label all unless indicated"
Refill:_____ times-- Do not refill ( )

Signed:_____
DO NOT TAKE THIS TO YOUR PHARMACIST

Community Clinic
Jeffrey A. Eaton, NP
Joyce D. Cappiello, NP

Name:_____ DOB_____
Address_____ Date_____

Rx

"label all unless indicated"
Refill:_____ times-- Do not refill ( )

Signed:_____
DO NOT TAKE THIS TO YOUR PHARMACIST

Community Clinic
Jeffrey A. Eaton, NP
Joyce D. Cappiello, NP

Name:_____ DOB_____
Address_____ Date_____

Rx

"label all unless indicated"
Refill:_____ times-- Do not refill ( )

Signed:_____
DO NOT TAKE THIS TO YOUR PHARMACIST

Community Clinic
Jeffrey A. Eaton, NP
Joyce D. Cappiello, NP

Name:_____ DOB_____
Address_____ Date_____

Rx

"label all unless indicated"
Refill:_____ times-- Do not refill ( )

Signed:_____
DO NOT TAKE THIS TO YOUR PHARMACIST

12 *Discussion*

LEARNING ISSUES

In order to resolve this patient's problem, you will need to consider and address the following issues (you may generate additional issues as well):

- **Anemia differential diagnosis**
- **Anemia workup**
- **Causes of anemia**
- **Alcoholism**
- **Interpretation of CBC**

INITIAL IDEAS

- Anemia secondary to dietary intake
- Anemia secondary to blood loss

INTERPRETATION OF CUES, PATTERNS, AND INFORMATION

There is evidence of an iron deficiency anemia (IDA) with a low mean corpuscular volume (MCV), although thalassemia or sideroblastic anemia cannot be ruled out with current evidence.

Mr. Lamontagne is a 64-year-old man. He indicates that he drinks a couple of beers in the evening, but you of course do not have any objective corroboration of that and might suspect that he may be drinking more. If he is drinking heavily, his dietary intake may not be adequate. Alcoholics, however, often have a greater problem with vitamin B_{12} and folate intake and absorption, and they thus present with a macrocytic anemia. He has a brother who is an alcoholic, so that puts him at a somewhat greater risk for alcoholism.

You also know that the incidence of certain cancers, including colon cancer, increases with age. This is a diagnosis that could cause blood loss and one that you will not want to miss. If he is drinking heavily, he could also have a gastrointestinal bleed.

His urine has seemed a little darker lately, which could mean an increase in blood or bilirubin in the urine. Bilirubin might indicate a liver dysfunction.

REVISED IDEAS

- Alcoholism
- Peptic ulcer disease
- Gastrointestinal cancer
- Liver dysfunction

DIFFERENTIAL DIAGNOSIS

1. IDA: As mentioned previously, low dietary intake of iron is possible but would be of less concern than a blood loss anemia. This requires that a second differential diagnosis process be instituted

simultaneously with the first. Both the differential for anemia and the differential for blood loss need to be addressed. The most common cause in Mr. Lamontagne's age group would be gastrointestinal bleeding. Other possibilities such as urinary loss could also be explored, although unless gross hematuria is present, blood loss is usually not enough to cause anemia.

2. Sideroblastic anemia: If the ferritin and serum iron levels are high, then this could be a possibility.

3. Thalassemia: In thalassemia the RDW is often normal, so this lowers the probability. This would also be a very late diagnosis for thalassemia. If no other answer is found for the IDA, then hemoglobin electrophoresis or consultation could be considered.

4. Anemia of chronic disease (ACD): If the etiology is not found in a blood loss or a dietary intake problem, then consideration of ACD might be a next logical consideration. Renal disease screening (blood urea nitrogen [BUN] and creatinine to start), total iron binding capacity (TIBC), and investigation of other chronic systemic conditions should be done. The diagnosis will be dependent on finding another chronic disease that has caused his anemia.

DIAGNOSTIC OPTIONS

The CAGE questionnaire could be used to try to increase data around alcohol use.

A decreased serum ferritin level will rule out sideroblastic anemia and basically rule in IDA because it is highly sensitive and specific for IDA (Goroll, May, and Mulley, 1995). Once you have established that it is an IDA, a reticulocyte count may be helpful in this case. If it is high, it is very consistent with a blood loss anemia. If there are not enough iron stores (as in a nutritional deficiency), new red blood cells (RBCs) will not be formed. If it is low, then a nutritional lack (or blood loss that has been going on long enough to deplete iron stores) could be considered. It is probably necessary in this age group to look for a colon cancer no matter what. Thus a gastroenterology consult for colonoscopy might be obtained. Some clinicians might opt for fecal occult blood testing (FOBT), but the risks and benefits should be considered before doing so.

A urinalysis should be ordered because of his dark urine and a chemistry profile (reimbursement has become more problematic for "panels," so specific tests could also be ordered) and LFTs are also reasonable tests both to look for an ACD as well as possible liver changes that could have caused the urine changes.

If he had abdominal pain or other signs of pancreatic cancer, an ultrasound could be considered.

THERAPEUTIC OPTIONS

Pharmacological

Oral iron could be considered, but sources of bleeding should be ruled out first. Since you know his anemia is fairly mild and he is not symptomatic, waiting for the laboratory workup to return is reasonable.

Educational

Mr. Lamontagne should be counseled about his dietary intake, although waiting for the laboratory workup to be completed is appropriate. Decreasing alcohol intake because of his family history may be appropriate, although there is no real evidence that two drinks per day does any harm and in fact may have some protective benefit for heart disease.

Other Nonpharmacological Options

As noted above, a colonoscopy may be indicated. The issue of using FOBT as an alternative is a complicated one. Two issues that contribute to this are the variation in adherence to collection procedures by patients and the issue of the sensitivity of the test. The sensitivity (the probability of calling a positive a positive) for FOBT has usually been based on its detection of cancers. This has been reported to range from 26% to 92% (US Preventive Services Task Force, 1996). This may not be adequate sensitivity to provide the clinician with comfort that a problem would be detected. FOBT may be a useful adjunct to colonoscopy since it may detect bleeding that is above the reach of the colonoscope.

HEALTH PROMOTION/HEALTH MAINTENANCE

It is probably best to hold off until the laboratory workup is completed, but you could then consider an update of his tetanus-diphtheria (Td) immunization, a pneumococcal vaccine, a cholesterol screening, and recommendations of injury prevention, dental care, and physical activity.

FOLLOW-UP

If a gastointestinal consult is obtained, have the patient call you after he sees the gastroenterologist, and then follow-up can be discussed.

References

Goroll AH, May LA, Mulley AG: *Primary care medicine,* Philadelphia, 1995, JB Lippincott.

US Preventive Services Task Force: *Guide to clinical preventive services,* Baltimore, 1996, Williams & Wilkins.

OPENING SCENARIO

Jerome Wilson is a 47-year-old male on your schedule for a follow-up visit. He had an annual examination 6 months ago (see note) with elevated lipid levels. He was started on the American Heart Association (AHA) Step II diet with an exercise plan. The results of his lipid profile drawn 3 days ago are shown in Table 13-1.

Note of Jerome Wilson's Visit 6 Months Ago

REASON FOR VISIT

Jerome Wilson is a 47-year-old male scheduled for a complete physical examination. It is has been 3 years since his last physical with you.

HISTORY OF PRESENT ILLNESS

"I am planning to increase my exercise level by joining a local fitness club. I thought it would be a good idea to schedule a physical before doing this. I feel fine and have not had any change in my health."

MEDICAL HISTORY

No hospitalizations or surgery. Seen twice in the past for bursitis of the left shoulder, which required steroid injections. No hypertension, coronary artery disease (CAD), or diabetes mellitus (DM).

FAMILY MEDICAL HISTORY

Mother: 71 yr (hypercholesterolemia, surgery at age 65 for vascular occlusion in the leg)
Father: 71 yr (Alzheimer's disease for 3 years)
Sister: 47 yr (current diagnosis of breast cancer)
Grandparents: All died many years ago; he does not know causes of death

SOCIAL HISTORY

Lives with wife and 3 children, ages 3, 8, and 12. Works as a certified public accountant in a large accounting firm. Nonsmoker for 15 years. Four drinks of alcohol per week. Three cups of coffee per day. Golfs two to three times a week in good weather.

MEDICATIONS

None

ALLERGIES

None

REVIEW OF SYSTEMS

General: States energy level is good; sleeps well; feels healthy but stressed keeping up with family and work responsibilities
Skin: Dry, itchy areas on scalp
HEENT: Denies problems with hearing; recently began to use reading glasses; sees dentist regularly
Thorax: Denies any chest pain, shortness of breath, cough, or dyspnea on exertion
Gastrointestinal: No heartburn, nausea, abdominal pain; occasional constipation with occasional painful hemorrhoid; no rectal bleeding
Genitourinary: No dysuria, frequency, hesitancy, nocturia
Extremities: No current joint pain, but occasionally (every few months) notes transient joint pain in knees, wrists, and fingers; uses aspirin or acetaminophen (Tylenol) when needed
Neurological: No headaches; denies depression, memory changes

PHYSICAL EXAMINATION

Vital signs: Temperature: 98.0° F; *Pulse:* 72 beats/min; *Respirations:* 16 breaths/min; *BP:* 136/74 mm Hg
Height: 5' 8"; *Weight:* 160 lb; *BMI:* 24
General: Healthy-appearing male who appears his stated age
Skin: Dry, scaly patches (approximately 6 areas ranging 1/2 to 1 cm in size on scalp); no other lesions
HEENT: Pupils equal and reactive to light, extraocular movements intact, fundi benign; nares patent and non-injected; throat without redness or lesions
Neck: Supple without thyromegaly or adenopathy
Heart: Regular rate and rhythm; no murmurs, rubs, or gallops
Lungs: Clear to auscultation
Gastrointestinal: Abdomen soft, nontender, without

hepatosplenomegaly; bowel sounds normoactive; rectal without masses; stools negative for occult blood
Genitourinary: No lesions or discharge noted; no testicular masses; no hernias noted; prostate firm, no nodules or enlargement
Extremities: Range of motion functionally intact; no redness, pain, or swelling noted; no edema, cyanosis, clubbing
Neurological: Reflexes 2+ at Achilles, patellar, biceps, triceps, brachioradialis; no Babinski signs

Chemistry Profile for Jerome Wilson

Test Name	Result	Normal Range
Calcium	9.0	8.4-10.2 mg/dl
Phosphorus	4.4	2.7-4.5 mg/dl
Glucose	90	70-105 mg/dl
BUN	21	6-26 mg/dl
Creatinine	1.4	0.7-1.6 mg/dl
BUN/creatinine ratio	15	6-35
Uric acid	5.5	3.4-7.0 mg/dl
Cholesterol	281	150-200mg/dl
Triglycerides	205	50-175 mg/dl
Total protein	7.7	6.9-8.2 g/dl
Albumin	4.4	3.4-5.3 g/dl
Globulin	3.3	2.0-4.0 g/dl
A/G ratio	1.3	1.0-2.2
ALP	89	39-117 U/L
LDH	192	118-273 U/L
AST (SGOT)	18	0-37 U/L
ALT (SGPT)	23	0-40 U/L
Total bilirubin	0.5	0-1.0 mg/dl

Urinalysis for Jerome Wilson

Appearance	Clear
Color	Yellow
SG	1.010
pH	5.5
Protein	Negative
Glucose	Negative
Ketones	Negative
Blood	Negative
Nitrite	Negative
Bilirubin	Negative
Leukocytes	Negative

ASSESSMENT
- Hyperlipidemia
- Seborrheic dermatitis
- Recurrent joint pain
- Constipation with recurring hemorrhoid
- S/P bursitis left shoulder
- Family history of hypercholesterolemia

PLAN
- AHA Step II diet; dietitian referral
- Exercise: Muscle strengthening program at gym with slow, gentle progression to avoid joint pain; swimming recommended for aerobic activity; learn to check pulse and target zone
- Stress reduction
- Ketoconazole-containing shampoo
- Increase fiber and water in diet
- Return in 6 months for fasting lipid profile and review of lifestyle changes

Table 13-1 Lipid Profile for Jerome Wilson

Test	Result	Normal Range
Cholesterol	257	150-200 mg/dl
Triglycerides	174	50-175 mg/dl
High-density lipoproteins	38	35-55 mg/dl
High-density lipoproteins/ cholesterol	15	15.4-24.7 mg/ml
Low-density lipoproteins	204	0-190 mg/ml

INTERVAL HISTORY
Works out at a health club 3 days a week, swims 3 days a week, and does a muscle strengthening program with machines twice a week. Remains a nonsmoker and has two to three drinks of alcohol per week. Continues to work in a high-pressure job.

REVIEW OF SYSTEMS
General: States he met with the dietitian for two visits; he spoke with her right after the visit of 6 months ago and then 1 month later; he feels he has changed his diet significantly but has difficulty making wise choices when eating out
Skin: Scalp problem improved with ketoconazole shampoo; no longer needs to use shampoo

Heart: Denies chest pain

Lungs: Denies shortness of breath, cough, dyspnea on exertion

Gastrointestinal: Continues to have occasional constipation with occasional flare up of his hemorrhoid

Extremities: No recent joint pain; thinks his program of muscle strengthening at the gym may be helping this

PHYSICAL EXAMINATION

Vital signs: Temperature: 97.6° F; *Pulse:* 70 beats/min; *Respirations:* 16 breaths/min; *BP:* 130/70 mm Hg

Skin: No patches on scalp

Heart: Regular rate and rhythm; no murmurs, rubs, or gallops

Lungs: Clear to auscultation

ASSESSMENT   *Please indicate the problems or issues you have identified that will guide your care (preferably in list form):*

PLAN   *Please list your plans for addressing each of the problems or issues in your assessment:*

Community Clinic
Jeffrey A. Eaton, NP
Joyce D. Cappiello, NP

Name:_____ DOB_____
Address_____ Date_____

Rx

"label all unless indicated"
Refill:_____ times-- Do not refill ( )

Signed:_____
DO NOT TAKE THIS TO YOUR PHARMACIST

Community Clinic
Jeffrey A. Eaton, NP
Joyce D. Cappiello, NP

Name:_____ DOB_____
Address_____ Date_____

Rx

"label all unless indicated"
Refill:_____ times-- Do not refill ( )

Signed:_____
DO NOT TAKE THIS TO YOUR PHARMACIST

LEARNING ISSUES

In order to resolve this patient's problem, you will need to consider and address the following issues (you may generate additional issues as well):

- **Reasons for and against baseline electrocardiogram (ECG) and/or exercise tolerance testing before starting an exercise program**
- **How does a clinician effectively promote behavioral and lifestyle changes?**
- **Time frame for repeating a lipid profile**
- **Current research on when to initiate or not to initiate lipid-lowering agents**
- **Choice of which type of lipid-lowering agents and why**
- **Monitoring and follow-up of lipid-lowering agents**

INITIAL IDEAS

- Elevated lipids (risk factor for cardiovascular disease)
- Cardiovascular disease

INTERPRETATION OF CUES, PATTERNS, AND INFORMATION

Mr. Wilson's risk factors for cardiovascular disease, however, are less serious than many males his age since he is a nonsmoker, has an appropriate weight for his height, and has a negative history for hypertension and DM. It seems he has made a deliberate effort to work on lowering dietary fat and cholesterol. His exercise level has increased significantly over the past 6 months from his previous sedentary lifestyle. His life remains stressful as are the lives of many people his age. Managing the demands of the workplace and a busy family can leave little relaxation time. He seems committed to improving his health.

DIAGNOSTIC OPTIONS

Are there other laboratory tests that you want to order either to screen for disease or for baseline measurements? If you decide to start him on a lipid-lowering agent, will you need baseline liver function studies?

At his first visit, the decision was consciously made to not order a baseline ECG or exercise stress testing before his beginning an exercise plan. This was based on current recommendations as outlined in the *Guide to Clinical Preventive Services* (US Preventive Services Task Force, 1996). There is insufficient evidence to recommend for or against screening middle-age and older men and women for asymptomatic CAD with resting ECG, ambulatory ECG, or exercise ECG. Recommendations against routine screening may be made on other grounds for persons who are not at high risk of developing symptomatic CAD. These grounds include the limited sensitivity and low predictive value of an abnormal resting ECG in asymptomatic persons and the high costs of screening and follow-up. The exercise ECG is more accurate than the resting ECG. Although asymptomatic persons with a positive exercise ECG are more likely to experience an event than those with negative tests, longitudinal studies following such patients from 4 to 13 years have shown that only 1% to 11% will suffer an acute myocardial infarction (MI) or sudden death. As with resting ECG, the majority of events will occur in those with a negative exercise test result (US Preventive Services Task Force, 1996). The American College of Sports Medicine concludes that virtually all sedentary individuals can begin a moderate (not vigorous) exercise program safely (Kenney, Humphrey, and Bryant, 1995).

THERAPEUTIC OPTIONS

Pharmacological

When do you make the decision to begin lipid-lowering agents? Will lipid-lowering agents not only lower lipids but prevent cardiovascular disease? To what degree are they cost effective? The AHA *Comprehensive Risk Reduction in Patients With Coronary and Other Vascular Disease* guidelines suggest considering drug therapy when low-density lipoproteins (LDLs) are between 100 and 130 and to definitely start if LDLs are over 130 (American Heart Association, 1995).

The National Cholesterol Education Program (NCEP) varies somewhat from the AHA guidelines (National Institute of Health, 1993) in regard to LDLs:

No CAD and <2 risk factors	>190 after >6 mo dietary therapy	Goal: 160
No CAD and >2 risk factors	>160 after >6 mo dietary therapy	Goal: 130
No CAD or other atherosclerotic disease	>130 after 6-12 wk of maximal dietary therapy	Goal: <100

Mr. Wilson would be a candidate for lipid-lowering drug therapy with any of the above criteria. Three recent studies have studied the benefit of lipid-lowering agents in reducing both morbidity and mortality from CAD.

The Scandinavian Simvastin Survival Study (4S) was the first prospective randomized-controlled clinical study that showed the benefit of aggressive lipid management. It was a 5-year study that enrolled subjects who had either angina or a previous MI and serum total cholesterol levels between 212 and 309 mg/dl. Compared with the placebo group, treatment with simvastin was associated with a 30% reduction in overall mortality (Pedersen et al, 1994).

The Cholesterol and Recurrent Events (CARE) study looked at individuals post-MI who had only mild cholesterol elevations. These individuals also benefited from lipid-lowering agents. The rate of MI decreased by 24%, and stroke decreased by 31% compared with placebo, but no difference in overall survival rates between the treated and placebo groups was noted (Sachs et al, 1996).

The third study that shed light on this issue of primary prevention, and which is most applicable to Mr. Wilson, is the West of Scotland Coronary Prevention Study (WOSCOPS). This study involved 6500 men with no history of MI and with LDL levels between 174 and 232 mg/dl who were randomized to placebo or pravastatin and then followed for an average of 5 years. It was estimated that 70% to 90% of the study subjects had at least two risk factors for CAD. No women were studied. Compared with placebo, the rate of fatal or nonfatal MI was reduced by 31% and total mortality by 22% in the pravastatin treated group. The WOSCOPS trial investigators also concluded that dietary modification was an essential component of treatment (Shepherd et al, 1995).

With these studies, there is growing evidence that lipid-lowering agents make a difference in men with a history of cardiovascular disease. They also have proved to be a preventive therapy for those *at risk* for cardiovascular disease. The cost effectiveness is more difficult to assess.

Cost effectiveness is a function of benefit gained compared with the cost expended. Medications to lower LDL cholesterol become relatively less cost effective as the underlying level of risk declines, since the cost of intervention remains the same but less benefit is obtained. The optimal cost-effective threshold for LDL-lowering therapy is not currently known; such drug therapy is not likely to be cost effective with two or less risk factors as is the case with men with isolated elevated LDL level (Schwartz, 1996).

This may have been part of the reason why the American College of Physicians (ACP) recommended against cholesterol screening in low-risk individuals. Such screening will not be cost effective if it leads to the initiation of pharmacological therapy in low-risk individuals. Just when the management of lipid disorders began to seem clear, the ACP issued guidelines that advocate cholesterol screening only among limited-age and limited-risk groups. These guidelines vary radically from the NCEP guidelines and also from the ACPs own previous guidelines.

The ACP rejected the appropriateness of screening for high-density lipoproteins (HDLs) and triglycerides because they have little effect on cholesterol management. They also no longer recommend screening men under the age of 35 or women under the age of 45. The ACP concluded from their data that the short-term risk of developing coronary heart disease is low in these groups (even when the cholesterol is elevated) and that screening is not cost effective unless they have at least two risk factors for coronary heart disease such as DM, hypertension, history of smoking, a history of occlusive peripheral arterial disease, or an inherited lipid disorder.

Even in groups in which the ACP did recommend cholesterol screening (men ages 35 to 65 and women ages 45 to 65), screening is categorized as appropriate but not mandatory. Between the ages of 65 and 75, the lack of clinical data on the benefit of cholesterol reduction and the potential dangers of pharmacotherapy refute routine screening in this group. Screening past age 75 was not recommended.

What is the response to this? The ACP is criticized for assuming the following:
1. Widespread screening will lead to the overuse of cholesterol-lowering medications rather than using screening as a tool to guide dietary intervention. Screening may well be cost effective if it leads to increased emphasis on lifestyle modification.
2. The ACP looked solely at mortality as an end point rather than including improvements in morbidity.
3. Some recent studies of older adults point toward the benefits of cholesterol-lowering therapy.
4. The belief that cholesterol-lowering therapy can be delayed because reductions in cholesterol levels can be achieved more quickly with medications than previously thought puts the client at needless risk for a cardiovascular event (DeDonato, 1996).

The new ACP guidelines may not bring about changes in current prescribing practices of most clinicians, but they certainly shape the debate on the effectiveness of cholesterol monitoring and intervention. The ACP appears to be trying to provide a voice in the debate between those who would advocate widespread screening based on little clinical data and those who would demand comprehensive clinical trial data before implementing screening and treatment programs for any age group.

Decision Making   As is often the case, clinicians must make decisions based on imperfect information.

Mr. Wilson had a lipid profile repeated at 6 months with continued elevation of cholesterol and LDL levels. His triglycerides have dropped to 174 and his HDL level is 38. An appropriate assessment at this point is that lifestyle modifications are not adequate alone but should be continued with the addition of medications.

There are a number of drugs from which to choose. Bile sequestrants are effective in lowering LDL levels but can raise triglycerides and have the gastrointestinal side effect of constipation. This patient already has problems with constipation and hemorrhoids, so this may not be the best choice.

Niacin is a relatively inexpensive over-the-counter (OTC) drug that lowers cholesterol and triglycerides. It is started in low doses of 100 to 300 mg tid to maximum doses of 6 g/day. Small doses of aspirin may reduce the side effect of flushing.

Lopid (gemfibrozil 600 mg bid) was initially marketed for type IV and V hyperlipidemias, but the Helsinki Trial, a 5-year trial of asymptomatic men aged 40 to 55 with cholesterol >200 mg, supported its use as initial therapy in type II hyperlipidemia. If used in individuals with elevated cholesterol and triglycerides, the drug may cause either an increase or decrease in LDL levels. This research has shown that this drug is effective in decreasing morbidity and mortality in CAD. It has low toxicity and is less expensive compared with some of the statins. It has the disadvantage of bid dosing and also requires periodic liver function tests (LFTs).

The statins reduce LDL levels more than any other class of medications, but they are not as potent as niacin for triglyceride or HDL levels. The fibric acids are primarily effective for those patients with high triglyceride levels, whereas the bile acid sequestrant's effectiveness is primarily limited to LDL reduction. The statins, although expensive, are highly potent for LDL reduction and have minimal side effects.

The statins (HMG-CoA reductase inhibitors) are widely used today and have the advantage of once-a-day dosing. They are expensive, although some of the newer statins cost surprisingly less than the older preparations. Baseline and regular LFTs and CPK are recommended. The statins lower total cholesterol, decrease triglycerides slightly, and increase HDL levels in some individuals. All of the most recent studies have used statins as the therapeutic agent. Our knowledge of the long-term effects of lipid-lowering agents is derived primarily from the use of statins.

If medications are prescribed, a recheck of lipids and a follow-up visit at 3 months would be appropriate. Medications can then be adjusted upward if necessary.

Low-dose aspirin is an optional and additional treatment. Its use has been studied with post-MI patients showing good results. Current research suggests that aspirin is helpful not only for its blood thinning effects but also for its antiinflammatory properties. Cost effectiveness is not a major consideration here since aspirin is very low cost. This fact often encourages a clinician to try this therapy, even though the long-term data on the value of prevention in lower-risk individuals is not as well established.

Mr. Wilson can continue to address the issues of stress and the benefits of dietary modification and exercise. Mr. Wilson needs positive feedback for the effect he has made in changing his activity level and diet.

References

American Heart Association: *Consensus panel: preventing heart attack and death in patients with coronary disease,* Dallas, 1995, AHA.

DeDonato R, editor: The cholesterol controversy: how far should screening go? *Clin Rev* 6, 10, 91, 1996.

Kenney WL, Humphrey RH, Bryant CX: *American College of Sports Medicine's guidelines for exercise testing and prescription,* ed 5, Baltimore, 1995, Williams & Wilkins.

National Institute of Health; National Heart, Lung, and Blood Institute: *Second report of the expert panel on detection, evaluation, and treatment of high blood cholesterol in adults,* NIH Pub No 93-3095, Bethesda, Md, 1993, NIH.

Pederson TR et al: Randomized trial of cholesterol lowering in 4444 patients with coronary heart disease: the Scandinavian Simvastin Survival Study (4S). *Lancet* 344:1383, 1994.

Sachs FM et al: The effect of pravastatin on coronary events after myocardial infarction in patients with average cholesterol levels, *N Engl J Med* 335:1001, 1996.

Schwartz J: The cost-effectiveness of cholesterol-lowering therapy: a guide for the perplexed, *J Clin Outcome Manage* 3, 6, 48, 1996.

Shepherd J et al: Prevention of coronary heart disease with pravastatin in men with hypercholesterolemia, *N Engl J Med* 333:1301, 1995.

US Preventive Services Task Force: *Guide to clinical preventive services,* ed 2, Washington, DC, 1996, US Preventive Services.

CASE
14

OPENING SCENARIO

Dolores Sanchez is a 16-year-old female scheduled for a complete physical, including a gynecological examination. This is her first visit to your practice. She desires contraception.

HISTORY OF PRESENT ILLNESS

"I would like a prescription for the pill. My boyfriend and I have used condoms for a while, but I want something more effective. Some of my friends use the shot but have gained weight. I don't want to gain weight. Will the pill make me gain weight?" Ms. Sanchez states that she has been sexually active on an infrequent basis over the past year. Now has a steady partner and has been having intercourse approximately twice a week for the past 2 months. Last month there were some times he didn't use a condom and she became very worried about pregnancy. Her last menstrual period (LMP) (10 days ago) was regular and normal in amount and length of flow, so she does not think she is pregnant. Her partner has used condoms consistently since her LMP.

MEDICAL HISTORY

Describes herself as healthy but would really like to lose 15 pounds. Has had all the usual childhood immunizations: Measles-mumps-rubella (MMR), poliovirus vaccine, diphtheria-pertussis-tetanus (DPT). Had chicken pox at 3 years of age. Has not had hepatitis B immunization. Last tetanus-diphtheria (Td) was at 5 years of age. No hospitalizations, surgeries, or major medical problems.

FAMILY MEDICAL HISTORY

MGM: 65 yr (breast cancer)
MGF: 67 yr (lung problems, nicotine addiction)
PGM: 70 yr (high cholesterol)
PGF: Deceased at 65 yr (myocardial infarction [MI])
Mother: 40 yr (asthmatic, nicotine addiction)
Father: 42 yr (hypertension, hypercholesterolemia)
Three brothers: 14, 18, 20 yr (A&W)

SOCIAL HISTORY

Smokes 1 pack per day. Started smoking at age 13. High school sophomore; likes school and maintains B grades. Lives at home with both parents. Works part-time in a convenience store. Denies drug use. Occasional beer with friends. CAGE questions: negative responses. Not in high school sports, has physical education twice a week, no other regular exercise. Uses seat belts. Denies history of domestic violence.

MEDICATIONS

Occasional ibuprofen: 400 mg for menstrual cramping.

ALLERGIES

None

REVIEW OF SYSTEMS

General: Alert, healthy appearing young female
HEENT: Ear infections as a child but not since age 10; denies hayfever, frequent colds, nasal discharge, sinus pain; no dental problems but does not have regular preventive dental care
Cardiac: No history of heart murmur or heart problems
Respiratory: Denies any difficulty with breathing, asthma, or bronchitis
Gastrointestinal: Denies heartburn, abdominal pain, constipation, diarrhea, rectal bleeding; no history of liver or gallbladder disease
Genitourinary: Menarche: age 12; regular 28- to 30-day cycles; menses last 5 days with cramping the first day; takes 400 mg of ibuprofen with relief; denies intermenstrual or postcoital spotting or dyspareunia; no complaints of vaginal discharge, itching, or burning; denies urinary pain or frequency
Neurological: Headache on first day of menses, which is relieved by ibuprofen; no history of seizures.
Endocrine: States she is fatigued on the 3 days a week that she works after school because she must stay up late to finish homework; is not fatigued if she has 8 hours of sleep each night; no history of diabetes
Extremities: No complaints; no history of injuries, muscle pain, or joint pain

CASE 14   93

PHYSICAL EXAMINATION

Vital signs: Temperature: 98° F; *Pulse:* 70 beats/min; *Respirations:* 16 breaths/min; *BP:* 120/64 mm Hg
Height: 5' 6"; *Weight:* 140 lb; *BMI:* 23
General: Healthy, alert-appearing teenager
Skin: No lesions or rashes; mild facial acne
HEENT: Pupils equal and reactive to light; eardrums: no redness, good light reflex, landmarks visualized; pharynx: no redness; no visible caries
Neck: Thyroid: no enlargement noted

Heart: Regular rate and rhythm; no murmurs, rubs, or gallops
Lungs: Clear to auscultation
Breasts: No skin changes, retraction, or masses noted
Abdomen: Soft, no masses; no hepatosplenomegaly
Pelvic: Labia: no lesions, erythema, discharge; vagina: scant amount of clear mucus; cervix closed, no redness or lesions; uterus: anteverted, anteflexed, small, smooth, nontender; adnexa: nonpalpable, nontender; rectal: no visible lesions or hemorrhoids seen

ASSESSMENT   *Please indicate the problems or issues you have identified that will guide your care (preferably in list form):*

PLAN   *Please list your plans for addressing each of the problems or issues in your assessment:*

Community Clinic
Jeffrey A. Eaton, NP
Joyce D. Cappiello, NP

Name:_____ DOB_____
Address_____ Date_____

Rx

"label all unless indicated"
Refill:_____ times-- Do not refill ( )

Signed:_____
DO NOT TAKE THIS TO YOUR PHARMACIST

Community Clinic
Jeffrey A. Eaton, NP
Joyce D. Cappiello, NP

Name:_____ DOB_____
Address_____ Date_____

Rx

"label all unless indicated"
Refill:_____ times-- Do not refill ( )

Signed:_____
DO NOT TAKE THIS TO YOUR PHARMACIST

Community Clinic
Jeffrey A. Eaton, NP
Joyce D. Cappiello, NP

Name:_____ DOB_____
Address_____ Date_____

Rx

"label all unless indicated"
Refill:_____ times-- Do not refill ( )

Signed:_____
DO NOT TAKE THIS TO YOUR PHARMACIST

Community Clinic
Jeffrey A. Eaton, NP
Joyce D. Cappiello, NP

Name:_____ DOB_____
Address_____ Date_____

Rx

"label all unless indicated"
Refill:_____ times-- Do not refill ( )

Signed:_____
DO NOT TAKE THIS TO YOUR PHARMACIST

LEARNING ISSUES

In order to resolve this patient's problem, you will need to consider and address the following issues (you may generate additional issues as well):

- **What are the laws in your state regarding the provision of contraceptive services to minors?**
- **How do a provider and client work together to decide on an appropriate contraceptive method?**
- **How do you screen a client (by history, physical examination, and diagnostics if needed) to ensure that oral contraceptives (OCs) are a safe method for her?**
- **What components of the physical examination are appropriate for this visit?**
- **How do you choose an appropriate initial contraceptive?**
- **Is her history of smoking an issue with the use of OCs?**
- **How do you address her concern regarding her weight?**
- **What type of follow-up is indicated?**
- **What health-maintenance issues need to be addressed?**

INITIAL IDEAS

As you review the chart before entering the examination room, you might expect to see a healthy but nervous female. Most young women at this age feel somewhat conflicted about their emerging sexuality. She may come from a strong religious background that does not approve of intercourse before marriage, yet modern culture certainly does not promote such constraints. Remember, this is her first pelvic examination and most likely her first physical examination without her parents present.

In the majority of states, parental consent is not required for contraception, sexually transmitted disease (STD) treatment, and pregnancy care or termination. You need to know the laws in your state regarding the provision of contraception without parental consent. Nevertheless, encourage minors, if appropriate, to discuss this decision with parents.

If you as a provider are not comfortable providing contraception to a minor, then perhaps you can refer her to a clinician who will do so.

INTERPRETATION OF CUES, PATTERNS, AND INFORMATION

As you begin the interview, your general sense that this visit will focus on contraception and wellness issues is confirmed. You learn that Ms. Sanchez has been concerned about her weight for the past few years, feeling that she would like to weigh 15 pounds less. This is a strong factor in her contraception decision and may be a factor in her continued use of a method. You will want to explore this issue further.

Discuss the need for regular, daily pill-taking if she should choose OCs. If she assures you that she can remember to take a pill on a daily basis because she is very motivated to avoid pregnancy, perhaps OCs may be an appropriate method for her. If not, then a long-acting hormonal method may be more effective for her.

Assess any risk for immediate health concerns such as the possibility of current pregnancy or STD. Less immediate but equally important is to assess risk of potentially unhealthy lifestyle behaviors such as smoking, alcohol and drug use, depression, domestic violence, seat belt use, and immunization update.

Positive reinforcement of her decision to prevent an unplanned pregnancy may help reduce her nervousness and increase the likelihood that she will return to you for follow-up of any concerns. Urge her to call you with any concerns regarding her contraceptive method before discontinuing it.

Her history and physical examination were negative for any contraindications to OC use. Serious health risks from OC use are lower for young women under 20 than any other age group, even if they are smokers. The combination of OC use and smoking does not significantly increase the risk of side effects (i.e., cardiovascular events) until after age 35 (Hatcher et al, 1994).

Her maternal grandmother had a diagnosis of breast cancer. Is this a concern with prescribing OCs to Ms. Sanchez? Because of the long latency between exposure to a carcinogen and clinical manifestations of cancer, the final word is not in on OCs and cancer. Numerous epidemiological studies have been performed on the risk of breast cancer in pill users, but it remains to be seen whether an increased risk can be repeatedly shown for any subgroup of women (Hatcher et al, 1994). Ms. Sanchez's inherited risk would be higher if the relative involved were a first degree relative, such as a mother or sister. From current knowledge of the relationship between OC use and breast cancer, it seems that OCs are a safe option.

DIAGNOSTIC OPTIONS

Are there any tests you want to order for Ms. Sanchez? STD screening is appropriate to consider. The genprobe test is a widely available screening test for both chlamydia and gonorrhea with a sensitivity of 75% to 85% and a specificity of 97% and 98%. The newer polymerase chain reaction (PCR) tests have a sensitivity of 95% and specificity of 98% but are more expensive (Ravel, 1995). Both chlamydia and gonorrhea can be asymptomatic and lead to pelvic inflammatory disease (PID) and its sequelae, so it is worthwhile to have a high index of suspicion.

It seems that any risk of pregnancy is low given her history of a normal LMP and protected coitus since then. Some providers will automatically order a pregnancy test if there has been a history of unprotected coitus even if the LMP was normal. The most sensitive pregnancy tests need 7 to 10 days of pregnancy to be accurate. If you decide to order a test, it will give accurate information on conception during her last menstrual cycle but may be too early to be accurate for this cycle. You will need to decide whether this is worth doing at this point or just wait until her next menses.

A Pap smear is usually done at the annual gynecological examination. It is not essential that it be performed at this visit and could be deferred until the time of the follow-up visit. If deferring the Pap and pelvic examination lessens the anxiety for the client and is the factor that will encourage her to come in for the visit, then it is worthwhile to postpone it for a few months.

In 1993, the Food and Drug Administration (FDA) approved changes in OC labeling in both clinician prescribing information and the patient package insert to allow deferral of the pelvic examination if deemed appropriate by the clinician. This change was in response to the following situations where the pelvic examination might need to be deferred:

1. There are some teenagers who wish to use OCs but have avoided going to a clinician out of fear of a pelvic examination.

2. Some women are seen for medical care during their menstrual period, and often the advice of the clinician is to avoid a full physical examination, including a pelvic examination, because of the

interference of menstrual blood with cervical cytological sampling. Often a woman has to reschedule her visit for a full physical examination and is not able to use OCs during that time.

3. There are some women who wish to begin OC use but who experience long delays in the scheduling of an appointment for a full physical examination. If those women were able to have a shorter visit where a medical history was taken, informed consent was given, and pill use was initiated, then they are protected from an unplanned pregnancy while they wait for the appointment for the physical examination (Grimes, 1993). Since Ms. Sanchez made this appointment for a full gynecological examination, she is most likely expecting a Pap and pelvic examination today.

The rectal examination offers little to the workup and is a very uncomfortable physical examination technique. If the uterus cannot be palpated because of a retroverted position, then a rectal examination may help the provider assess the uterus. With Ms. Sanchez, her uterus is anteverted and easily palpated, so additional testing is not necessary for assessment. The digital rectal examination is of limited value as a screening test for colorectal cancer. Ms. Sanchez is certainly not in the age group in which there is concern about colon cancer.

THERAPEUTIC OPTIONS

Pharmacological Options for Contraception

How will you decide which of the many pills on the market to prescribe? Start with the reasonable assumption that you want to prescribe the lowest effective dose to reduce the incidence of side effects and still prevent pregnancy. All low-dose combined OCs on the market provide equivalent contraceptive efficacy (Hatcher et al, 1994). There are so many pills on the market that it is reasonable to limit your choices to a few selections and to then familiarize yourself with these pills. Low-dose pills, the most commonly prescribed pills, usually contain 35 μg or less of ethinyl estradiol, although the progestational component varies in both dose and type of steroid. Generally, a low-estrogen pill with a low-progestin and low-androgenic effect is a good initial choice. Low and moderate potency pills are listed in Table 14-1.

Table **14-1** *Potency of Low-Dose Combination Oral Contraceptives*

LOW ANDROGENIC/PROGESTATIONAL		
Ovcon	35 μg ethinyl estradiol	0.4 mg norethindrone
Brevicon	35 μg ethinyl estradiol	0.5 mg norethindrone
Ortho-Cept	30 μg ethinyl estradiol	0.15 mg desogestrel
Modicon	35 μg ethinyl estradiol	0.5 mg norethindrone
Desogen	30 μg ethinyl estradiol	0.15 mg desogestrel
Ortho-Cyclen	35 μg ethinyl estradiol	0.25 mg norgestimate
Ortho Tri-Cyclen	35 μg ethinyl estradiol	0.18, 0.215, 0.25 mg norgestimate
MODERATE ANDROGENIC/PROGESTATIONAL		
Allesse	20 μg ethinyl estradiol	0.10 mg levonorgestrel
Loestrin 1/20	20 μg ethinyl estradiol	1.0 mg norethindrone acetate
Demulen	35 μg ethinyl estradiol	1.0 mg ethynodial diacetate
Ortho-Novum 7/7/7	35 μg ethinyl estradiol	0.5, 0.75, 1.0 mg norethindrone
Ortho-Novum	35 μg ethinyl estradiol	1.0 norethindrone
Norinyl 1/35	35 μg ethinyl estradiol	1.0 norethindrone
Tri-Norinyl	35 μg ethinyl estradiol	0.5, 1.0, 0.5 mg norethindrone
Tri-Levlen	30 μg ethinyl estradiol	0.05, 0.075, 0.125 mg levonorgestrel
Triphasil	30 μg ethinyl estradiol	0.05, 0.075, 0.125 mg levonorgestrel

Modified from Mishell D, editor: Guidelines for OC selection, *Dialogues Contraception* 4:7, 1996a.

It is difficult and confusing to understand the relative potency of progestins in various pills. For example, 0.15 μg of levonorgestrel is actually more potent than 0.4 μg of norethindrone. Norethindrone (Ortho products), norethindrone acetate (Loestrin formulations), and ethynodial diacetate (Demulen formulations) are similar in potency, whereas levonorgestrel is 10 times (or more depending on the effect studied) more potent (Hatcher et al, 1994).

Pills also have androgenic effects that impact their side-effect profile. How do you learn this information about OCs? The androgenic effect of pills is not noted in the label or product information insert. Charts are available in various sources that list and compare their bioavailablity and side-effect profile.

Go back to the premise of trying to choose a low-estrogen, low-progestin, low-androgenic pill. What other issues are involved? OCs are generally monophasic, meaning the same dose is in each pill each day of the month, or triphasic, meaning there are three varying doses of hormones in the pill pack. Triphasic pills are newer than monophasic preparations, are very popular, and are widely prescribed. For a short time, one biphasic pill was marketed, but it has been replaced by triphasics. Triphasics are good pills, but there are no proven advantages for triphasic compared with monophasic formulations (Mishell, 1996a).

The 20 μg estrogen pills have a similar efficacy rate to the 30 to 35 μg pills in preventing pregnancy. The lower dose of estrogen may be associated with a somewhat higher incidence of breakthrough bleeding (Mishell, 1996b).

Since Ms. Sanchez is healthy, she really could use any low-dose pill, but will any factors affect this choice? The concern about weight gain (an androgen-related side effect) is a common reason why adolescents discontinue OCs. In clinical studies of OCs with the newer low progestins, norgestimate, and desogestrel, the maximum mean weight gain after 1 year of use was $1/2$ pound. Few studies compare the low-androgen pills with medium- or high-androgen pills. A U.S. multicenter trial of a norgestimate and a desogestrel monophasic pill showed a discontinuation rate of 1% due to perceived weight gain (Mishell, 1996a). There appear to be more data on the newer, lower-androgen pills, but possibly she would do well on any low androgen pill.

Of the newer low-androgen preparations, recent studies have shown that desogestrel and gestodene (not available in the United States) increases the risk of nonfatal venous thrombosis from 10 to 15/100,000 to 20 to 30/100,000. The risk for healthy, nonpregnant women is 4/100,000, and the risk for pregnant women is 60/100,000. Although the increased risk is very low, you must decide how much risk is acceptable. Norgestimate was not studied.

Ms. Sanchez mentioned cramps. Is it possible to prescribe a pill to lessen menstrual cramping? In the majority of cases, any low-dose OC provides effective treatment for dysmenorrhea (Mishell, 1996a).

Will OCs have any effect on her premenstrual headache? Headaches are common in women taking the pill as well as women not taking the pill. There are very few controlled studies on common headaches (nonmigraines) in OC users, particularly with respect to formulation. There is no clear reason to prescribe one OC formulation over another for her premenstrual headache.

What about her family history of high cholesterol (value not known)? Older OCs with high doses of progestin with high-androgenic activity were associated with a decrease in high-density lipoproteins (HDLs) and an increase in low-density lipoproteins (LDLs), yet their use did not appear to increase cardiovascular risk. The newer progestins, as well as the older 0.5 mg norethindrone OCs, have the opposite effect, but any decrease of atherosclerosis is yet to be demonstrated (Hatcher et al, 1994)..

What about her cigarette smoking? The risk of MI increases in smokers over the age of 35 who are on any formulation of OCs. This risk would not apply to Ms. Sanchez, but she should be counseled to stop smoking for many other health-related reasons.

What about the mild acne noted on examination but not mentioned by Ms. Sanchez? All combined OCs lower serum testosterone levels through a number of mechanisms that should improve acne (Hatcher et al, 1994). Recently, Ortho Tri-Cylen was approved by the FDA for the treatment of acne. This was an unusual event for a contraceptive method to be approved for the treatment of a noncontraceptive health concern.

Based on the review of the above concerns, a low-dose pill with norgestimate or norethindrone seems reasonable for an initial choice. Studies have been more extensive with the newer formulations than the latter, which have been on the market for many years. It may not mean the pills have fewer side effects but that comparative studies are lacking.

It is helpful to discuss the advantages of pill use as well as the side effects. In addition to their effectiveness, safety, and beneficial effects on acne and menstrual cramping, OCs offer protection from PID, ectopic pregnancy, and ovarian and endometrial cancers (Hatcher et al, 1994).

Prescribing decisions are also influenced by the price of pills or by what is available on your formulary. Health maintenance organizations (HMO) and family planning clinics have prescribing formularies that often limit pills to several types. You, as the provider, must then choose pills from this list. Low-dose combination pills are generally comparably priced at the pharmacy, although at least one manufacturer is offering substantial discounts on OCs if you subscribe to its wholesale buying club available at selected pharmacies.

Pharmacological Options for Headaches

If OCs do not provide premenstrual headache relief, then continue with ibuprofen at the first sign of premenstrual symptoms. Prescription nonsteroidal antiinflammatory drugs (NSAIDs) may offer relief if the over-the-counter (OTC) products do not. Counsel her to call in the unlikely situation that the headaches worsen after starting the OCs.

Severe pill-induced headaches may be an early warning sign of a stroke and need careful evaluation but would be very rare in a healthy young woman such as Ms. Sanchez. Symptoms such as blurred vision, loss of vision, nausea, vomiting, or weakness in an extremity deserve attention.

Educational

1. *Smoking cessation plan:* The following has been adapted from the Agency for Health Care Policy and Research guidelines (1996). Their expert panel reviewed evidence from clinical studies to create a guide on smoking cessation. Recent data show that the role of the health care provider is critical in preventing clients from initiating tobacco use or quitting if they already smoke. Clients who are told by their provider to quit smoking are nearly twice as likely to prepare to quit as those who had never been so advised.

a. **ASK:** First ask the question, Do you smoke? In a 1993 survey of 12,000 individuals between the ages of 10 and 22, only 25% stated that a doctor, dentist, or nurse had said anything to them about quitting smoking (Gilpin, 1993). At least Ms. Sanchez had the question asked of her.

b. **ADVISE:** What is the next step? Be clear: "I think it is important for you to quit smoking now, and I will help you any way I can." Speak clearly: "As your clinician, I need you to know that quitting smoking is the most important thing you can do to protect your current and future health." Personalize your advice.

c. **ASSIST:** The next step is to work with Ms. Sanchez in developing a smoking cessation plan. Start with simple interventions:

(1) Set a quit date, ideally within 2 weeks.

(2) Inform family and friends of the plan to quit and ask for support.

(3) Remove cigarettes from your home, car, etc., and avoid smoking in these areas.

(4) If she has previously tried to quit, review these attempts: What helped? What led to relapse?

(5) Anticipate where the challenges will be, particularly during the critical first few weeks. For example, if she usually smokes with friends after school, how will she handle this?

(6) Drinking alcohol is strongly associated with relapses, and should be discouraged in all teenagers.

(7) Having other smokers in the household hinders successful quitting. Explore this issue with her.

   d. Intensive measures: Most hospitals and/or communities offer specific smoking cessation programs, but most are likely geared to adults, not teens. Pharmacological approaches such as nicotine gum and the patch are now available over the counter.

2. *Alcohol use:* What does she mean by an occasional drink? In most states, she is old enough to have a driver's license. Does she ever drink and drive? Does she ride with friends who have been drinking?

3. *STD protection:* Have you given her clear advice regarding the continued need for condom use for protection against STDs even though she will now be on the pill?

4. *Sleep:* Counsel her to get more sleep.

5. *Immunization status:* The teen years are an excellent time to begin the hepatitis B series. If she followed the usual schedule of childhood immunizations, her last tetanus shot was probably at age 5. This would make her due again at age 15. Has she had this update? When was her last MMR?

6. *Dental care:* Does she floss and brush each day? Can she be convinced of the value of regular cleaning and preventive care? Is cost an issue?

7. *Dietary habits:* A quick 24-hour recall can be helpful in assessing her diet, especially since she is concerned about her weight.

8. *Exercise habits:* Since she is concerned about weight, would she exercise regularly? How can she establish such a pattern?

9. *Accident prevention:* Does she give positive feedback concerning regular use of seatbelts? Does she wear a bicycle helmet if biking?

FOLLOW-UP

1. When would you like to see her back? A 3-month recheck is common practice. Breakthough bleeding is common in the first few months of use. Nausea and breast tenderness are other complaints seen initially. These symptoms usually resolve by the third month of use, and if not, a pill change can be discussed at that time.

2. Review pill taking and how to make up for missed pills. Remind Ms. Sanchez that the most risky time to miss pills is just before or after the 7-day pill-free interval. Extending this pill-free interval a few days may be enough to allow ovulation to occur (Hatcher, 1995). Advise her to be sure to purchase her next pill pack in advance so she will not be late in starting each new pill pack.

3. What will you focus on at the follow-up visit? The following mnemonic may be helpful for assessing the rare, serious side effects of OC use:
- **A:** Abdominal pain
- **C:** Chest pain
- **H:** Headaches
- **E:** Eye problems
- **S:** Severe leg pain

4. Has the pill affected her weight? Review her dietary and exercise plan along with her progress with smoking cessation.

5. Check her vital signs.

6. Monitoring her blood pressure is a primary focus of this visit even though the likelihood of developing hypertension at her age is low.

7. If side effects develop, refer to a resource that has charts of types and doses of hormones. The pocket edition by Dickey (1994) is indexed by patient complaint. This guide is particularly helpful when a patient returns with a pill complaint. Then the potency charts can be used to choose an alternative OC based on research or cumulative clinical expertise to reduce the likelihood of the side effect.

References

Agency for Health Care Policy and Research: *Smoking cessation clinical practice guideline.* Silver Springs, Md, 1996, Agency for Health Care Policy and Research Clearing House.

Dickey R: *Managing oral contraceptive patients,* ed 8, Durant, Okla, 1994, Essential Medical Information Systems.

Gilpin EA et al: Physician advice to quit smoking: results from the 1990 California Tobacco Survey, *J Gen Intern Med* 8:549, 1993.

Grimes D, editor: Delay of pelvic exam when prescribing OCs, *The Contraception Report IV* 5:4, 1993.

Hatcher R, editor: When do missed pills count the most? providers, patients may be surprised, *Contraceptive Technology Update* 16(6):69, 1995.

Hatcher R et al: *Contraceptive technology,* ed 16, New York, 1994, Irvington.

Mishell D, editor: Guidelines for OC selection, *Dialogues in Contraception* 4:7, 1996a.

Mishell D, editor: Estrogen doses of oral contraceptives: what are the choices? *Dialogues in Contraception* 4:8, 1996b.

Ravel R: *Clinical laboratory medicine,* ed 6, St Louis, 1995, Mosby.

CASE
15

OPENING SCENARIO

Maria O'Malley is a 13-year-old female who has been seen previously in your practice. She comes today accompanied by her mother for evaluation of right ankle pain, which has bothered her for the past 2 weeks.

HISTORY OF PRESENT ILLNESS

"My right ankle has been bothering me for 2 weeks. I don't remember any specific event that caused the ankle to begin hurting. It only hurts when I'm playing soccer, running and jumping, and kicking the ball. It also hurts when I am ice skating with my precision skating team. It hurts while I am playing sports, but the pain goes away as soon as I finish practice. It doesn't hurt when I'm at home; just when I am playing sports, so I tend to forget about it when I get home. When I remembered to tell my mom, she tried to get me to take naproxen and put ice on it, but I didn't do that very often." She denies any swelling and describes the pain as dull and nonradiating, a 4 to 5 on scale of 1 to 10 when the ankle is bothering her. She denies previous injury.

MEDICAL HISTORY

A review of her past visits shows that she has been followed for routine care only. She is up-to-date on all immunizations. Most recent physical examination was 6 months ago. Menarche 1 year ago. Has denied any need for contraception. No surgeries or hospitalizations. Last menstrual period (LMP) was 1 week ago.

FAMILY MEDICAL HISTORY

Mother: 45 yr (A&W)
Father: 50 yr (hypertension and arthritis)
Two brothers: 9, 17 yr (A&W)

SOCIAL HISTORY

Eighth grade student who lives with both parents and two brothers. Honor role student. Nonsmoker. States no alcohol or drug use.

MEDICATIONS

Occasional naproxen

ALLERGIES

None

PHYSICAL EXAMINATON

Vital signs: Temperature: 98.2° F; *Pulse:* 88 beats/min; *Respirations:* 20 breaths/min; *BP:* 102/50 mm Hg
Height: 5' 6"; *Weight:* 125 lb
General: Young adolescent female who appears healthy in no acute distress
Musculoskeletal: Right ankle: no swelling, redness, ecchymosis; pain localized over the right distal tibial-fibula joint with some radiation proximally and distally into the midfoot with activity; tenderness palpated over the anterior tibiofibular ligament; this is made worse with internal and external rotation of the foot; nontender over the anterior talofibular, calcaneofibular, and posterior talofibular ligaments; Achilles tendon is nontender; no proximal fibula tenderness; tender to resisted peroneal stress; ankle range of motion is limited only in dorsiflexion; sensory and motor examinations intact distally; Left ankle: no swelling, redness; full range of motion; no tenderness noted.

ASSESSMENT   *Please indicate the problems or issues you have identified that will guide your care (preferably in list form):*

PLAN   *Please list your plans for addressing each of the problems or issues in your assessment:*

Community Clinic	Community Clinic
Jeffrey A. Eaton, NP	Jeffrey A. Eaton, NP
Joyce D. Cappiello, NP	Joyce D. Cappiello, NP

Name:_____ DOB_____

Address_____ Date_____

Rx

Name:_____ DOB_____

Address_____ Date_____

Rx

"label all unless indicated"
Refill:_____ times-- Do not refill ( )

Signed:_____
DO NOT TAKE THIS TO YOUR PHARMACIST

"label all unless indicated"
Refill:_____ times-- Do not refill ( )

Signed:_____
DO NOT TAKE THIS TO YOUR PHARMACIST

LEARNING ISSUES

In order to resolve this patient's problem, you will need to consider and address the following issues (you may generate additional issues as well):

- **Key questions in a focused history of an ankle injury**
- **Important physical examination techniques for an ankle injury**
- **Difference between an inversion and eversion ankle sprain**
- **Ligaments in the ankle that are most commonly injured**
- **Ligament stability tests**
- **Decision making regarding ordering an x-ray examination with an ankle injury**
- **Sensitivity and specificity of the Ottawa Ankle Rules?**

INITIAL IDEAS

This seems to be an insidious injury of the ankle either caused by, or aggravated by, athletic activity. The differential diagnosis will focus on orthopedic causes of injury such as fracture, tendinitis, sprain. In a less straightforward presentation, you might include a broader differential of compartment syndrome, tumor, rheumatic disease, or connnective tissue disease.

INTERPRETATION OF CUES, PATTERNS, AND INFORMATION

How will you decide among the various differential diagnoses? What are the elements of the physical examination? How do you decide whether to order an x-ray examination?

The diagnosis will be made using your history-taking skills, knowledge of anatomy, function of the joint, and possibly radiography. The history will focus on the following:

1. What was the mechanism of injury? Where was the pain initially? Over 80% of all ankle sprains are inversion injuries where the ankle suddenly turns into plantar flexion and inversion, which will cause a person to feel a sharp pain on the anterolateral aspect of the ankle. With this injury, the anterior talofibular ligament is the first ligament to be affected. If the sprain is more severe, the calcaneofibular ligament is also affected (Fig. 15-1).

2. Did you hear a pop, snap, or crack? This would increase the likelihood of severe injury.

3. Were you able to walk immediately after the injury? This would decrease the likelihood of severe injury.

4. Have you injured your ankle before?

The physical examination will utilize your usual examination techniques of observation and palpation. Notice any areas of bruising and swelling. While Ms. O'Malley is sitting on the examination table with legs hanging over the end in a relaxed position, observe any noticeable difference in the

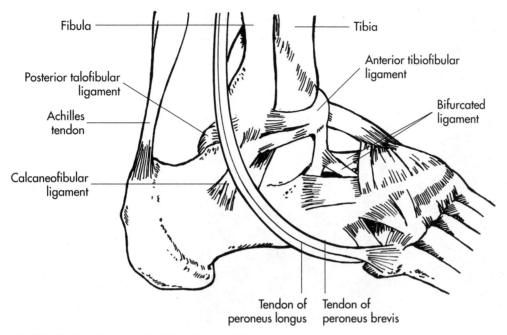

Fibula

Tibia

Posterior talofibular
ligament

Anterior tibiofibular
ligament

Achilles
tendon

Bifurcated
ligament

Calcaneofibular
ligament

Tendon of
peroneus longus

Tendon of
peroneus brevis

Fig. **15-1** The lateral ligaments (viewed from the lateral side).

amount of inversion on the affected side compared with the uninjured ankle. Can she move her ankle through normal range of motion?

Palpation

1. Start your examination away from the area of injury, leaving the most painful part for last. This helps the patient overcome the tendency to flinch when touched near an injury. Squeeze the mid-shaft of the fibula since pain felt here may indicate a fracture, interosseus membrane damage, or tibia-fibula ligament damage.
2. Palpate the following ligaments:
   a. Deltoid
   b. Anterior tibiofibular
   c. Anterior talofibular
   d. Calcaneofibular
   e. Posterior talofibular ligament and peroneal tendon
   f. Achilles tendon
3. Key bony areas for palpation are as follows:
   a. Posterior edge of both malleoli (palpating the posterior edge avoids confusion with ligamentous tenderness)
   b. At least 6 cm of the distal fibula so you will not miss a spiral fracture
   c. Navicular bone
   d. Base of the fifth metatarsal
4. Special maneuvers: Often the client with a severe injury cannot tolerate the following tests with a severe injury. With a less severe injury, these techniques for assessing ankle laxity might add diagnostic information:
   a. Eversion stress: Stress the deltoid ligament by moving the calcaneus and talus into eversion.
   b. Anterior drawer test (Fig. 15-2): Hold the ankle in slight plantar flexion. One hand holds the lower tibia and exerts a slight posterior force while the other grasps the posterior aspect of the

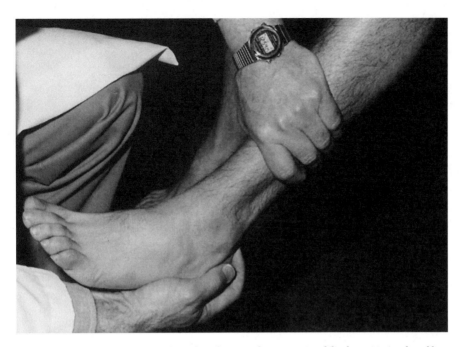

Fig. **15-2** An anterior drawer test can be performed to assess ligamentous instability by positioning the ankle at approximately 20 degrees of flexion, holding the tibia back with one hand, and pulling forward on the ankle mortise with the opposite hand. Excess excursion, which is often associated with a clunk, may suggest instability. (From Hawkins RJ: Musculoskeletal examination, St Louis, 1995, Mosby.)

calcaneus and tries to bring the calcaneus and talus forward on the tibia. If there is significant forward movement, then the anterior talofibular ligament has ruptured. Also test for instability in a posterior direction by moving the tibia forward on a fixed heel.

c. Inversion test: The heel is brought into inversion while the heel is stabilized. If a severe lateral ligament injury exists, a spongy, indefinite end point will be felt. This test is often too painful to perform.

5. Compare the affected side with the unaffected side because some people have ankle laxity without injury (Hoppenfeld, 1976).

With an early adolescent, you must think about fractures that could extend into the growth plate. Ms. O'Malley reached menarche 1 year ago, but the epiphyses may take 2 years to close. Salter I fractures of the growth plate, however, are more common with direct trauma.

DIAGNOSTIC OPTIONS

Is an x-ray examination necessary for every ankle injury? Traditionally, x-ray examinations have been ordered for virtually all ankle injuries, and approximately 85% of these films are negative for fractures. Ankle films are low-cost, high-volume procedures and can contribute to high health care costs as much as high-cost, low-volume procedures. It is estimated that $500 million is spent annually on ankle x-ray examinations in North America.

If many ankle films are unnecessary, then how do you decide on an appropriate candidate? The Ottawa Ankle Rules (Box 15-1) published in 1994 developed, studied, and proved the validity of certain physical examination findings in determining the necessity for x-ray examination. They have 100% sensitivity, meaning no fractures were missed, but they had 50% specificity for the ankle and 77% for the foot. Their use still resulted in negative x-ray examinations, but cost and waiting time have been reduced in the study.

Box 15-1 Ottawa Ankle Rules

1. An ankle series is only required if there is pain in the malleolar zone and any of these findings:
   a. Bone tenderness at the posterior edge or tip of the lateral malleolus
   b. Bone tenderness at the posterior edge or tip of the medial malleolus
   c. Inability to bear weight both immediately and later (weight bearing was defined as a patient taking 4 steps without assistance [two steps on each extremity] no matter how much they limped)
2. X-ray examinations of the foot are required only if there is any pain in the midfoot zone and any of these findings are present:
   a. Bone tenderness at the base of the fifth metatarsal
   b. Bone tenderness at the navicular bone
   c. Inability to bear weight immediately and later when examined

From Stiell I et al: Implementation of the Ottawa Ankle Rules, *JAMA* 271(11):827, 1994.

These criteria have proved to be very useful in assessing the need for films. Will it be helpful with this client? Ms. O'Malley has pain in the malleolar zone and has bone tenderness at the tip of the lateral malleolus, which meets the criteria for x-ray examination. The Ottawa Ankle Rules study excluded individuals younger than age 18 and those whose ankle injury occurred more than 10 days previously, so this criteria will not necessarily be applicable.

Although not pertinent to this case, the Ottawa Ankle Rules may not be reliable where patient assessment is difficult, such as with intoxication, head injury, multiple painful injuries, or diminished sensation resulting from neurological deficits.

X-ray Report

See the anterolateral x-ray film in Figure 15-3. The radiograph reveals an incomplete stress fracture of the lateral malleolus of the distal fibula at the level of the ankle mortise. It is important to realize that a stress fracture may not be visible on ordinary x-ray film for at least 2 weeks after symptoms begin.

Plan

Ms. O'Malley now needs immobilization of the ankle for 2 to 3 weeks and a follow-up visit. Many primary care offices refer all clients with fractures to an orthopedic office since they do not have the various braces and casting available. This will depend on the protocols of individual offices.

Educational

Communicate all of this clearly to Ms. O'Malley and her mother. At the age of 13, she may be reluctant to wear some type of brace or cast and limit her activity unless she clearly understands the situation.

Most schools and coaches require a written note from the provider to excuse a student from physical education activities or sports. Later, when she returns to physical activity, she will need another note specifically outlining any graded return to full activity.

Stress fractures of the lower third of the fibula tend to be more prevalent in the beginning jogger or in the athlete who switches from another sport to jogging. Also, 10% of females develop stress fractures as compared with only 1% of males. It is thought this might be due to the often lower level of previous athletic activity and lack of adequate conditioning of females. It is possible that the injury of Ms. O'Malley began as a tendinitis. Chronic fatigue and inflammation of the muscles, ligaments, and tendons may have contributed to the stress fracture. In this case, Ms. O'Malley was not involved in sports over the summer and then went into an intense soccer program in the fall. This is something to keep in mind if you have the opportunity to see young athletes for preseason sports physicals. It is an excellent time to discuss conditioning.

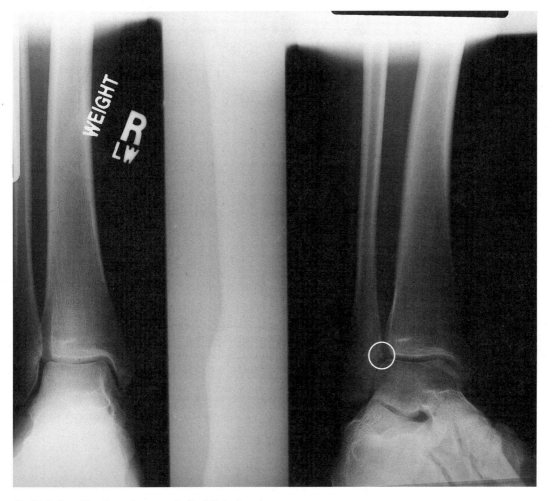

Fig. **15-3** X-ray film of stress fracture to the distal fibula *(arrow)*.

References

Hawkins R: *Musculoskeletal examination,* St. Louis, 1995, Mosby.

Hoppenfeld S: *Physical examination of the spine and extremities, Norwalk,* 1976, Appleton & Lange.

Stiell I et al: Implementation of the Ottawa Ankle Rules, *JAMA* 271(11):827, 1994.

CASE
16

OPENING SCENARIO

Liang Wang is a 13 1/2-year-old female scheduled for a follow-up acne visit. Her facial blemishes have not gotten better, and she is requesting a dermatology referral.

HISTORY OF PRESENT ILLNESS

"I was here about a month ago for a camp physical (see note). I was started on erythromycin 2% topical twice a day after cleansing with benzoyl peroxide 5%. I didn't feel that I was having any results after 3 weeks, so I tried some Cleocin T that had been prescribed for one of my friends. Cleocin was only slightly more effective than erythromycin. I do not want another topical; another friend of mine had a pill and that worked much better. I have been avoiding chocolate because my mother told my I should, and that seems to have helped a little." Her blemishes don't change related to menses. She has a few areas of acne on her back, but it is mostly on her face and chin.

MEDICAL HISTORY

No hospitalizations or accidents. Immunizations up-to-date for diphtheria-pertussis-tetanus (DPT), *Haemophilus influenzae* type b (Hib), poliovaccine, and measles-mumps-rubella (MMR).

FAMILY MEDICAL HISTORY

MGM: Diabetes mellitus (DM), onset at about 60 years old
Mother: 33 yr (A&W)
Father: 34 yr (A&W)

SOCIAL HISTORY

High school student. Plays soccer. Academically strong. Attends dances. Denies current sexual activity. Denies any alcohol use. Is a nonsmoker.

MEDICATIONS

Erythromycin and Cleocin as described under History of Present Illness.

ALLERGIES

None

REVIEW OF SYSTEMS

General: Denies fatigue or night sweats
HEENT: Denies diplopia, blurring, hearing impairment, sore throats
Cardiac: Denies chest pain, peripheral swelling
Respiratory: Denies shortness of breath, dyspnea on exertion
Gastrointestinal: Denies anorexia, nausea, vomiting, constipation, diarrhea, black or clay colored stools
Genitourinary: Notes that her periods are somewhat irregular with alternating every 28 days and the next about every 42 days; menarche at age 11; denies dysuria, hematuria
Muscoluskeletal: Denies joint or back pain
Hematological: Denies excessive bruising

PHYSICAL EXAMINATION

Skin of face has a moderate distribution of comedones, a few of which are cystic. Back comedones are also present.

Camp Physical Examination for Liang Wang from 1 Month Ago

Vital signs: Temperature: 97.4° F; *Pulse:* 66 beats/min; *Respirations:* 16 breaths/min; *BP:* 90/38 mm Hg
Height: 5' 1"; *Weight:* 97 lb
HEENT: Head is normocephalic, atraumatic; pupils equal, round, and reactive to light; extraocular movements intact; tympanic membranes are observable without excessive cerumen; nares are patent without redness or exudate; throat is noninjected; tongue is midline; palate rises symmetrically; teeth are in adequate repair; multiple facial comedones, a few of which are cystic.
Neck: Supple without thyromegaly, adenopathy, or carotid bruits
Heart: Regular rate and rhythm; no murmurs, rubs, or gallops
Lungs: Clear to auscultation and percussion
Breasts: Examination is deferred related to age and indications
Back and chest: A few comedones
Abdomen: Soft, nontender; no hepatosplenomegaly

Extremities: No cyanosis, clubbing, or edema;
Neurological: Reflexes are 2+ at the biceps, triceps, brachioradialis, patellar and Achilles; no Babinski signs present; strength and sensation are symmetrical

ASSESSMENT   *Please indicate the problems or issues you have identified that will guide your care (preferably in list form):*

PLAN   *Please list your plans for addressing each of the problems or issues in your assessment:*

Community Clinic
Jeffrey A. Eaton, NP
Joyce D. Cappiello, NP

Name:_____ DOB_____
Address_____ Date_____

Rx

"label all unless indicated"
Refill:_____ times-- Do not refill ( )

Signed:_____
DO NOT TAKE THIS TO YOUR PHARMACIST

Community Clinic
Jeffrey A. Eaton, NP
Joyce D. Cappiello, NP

Name:_____ DOB_____
Address_____ Date_____

Rx

"label all unless indicated"
Refill:_____ times-- Do not refill ( )

Signed:_____
DO NOT TAKE THIS TO YOUR PHARMACIST

Community Clinic
Jeffrey A. Eaton, NP
Joyce D. Cappiello, NP

Name:_____ DOB_____
Address_____ Date_____

Rx

"label all unless indicated"
Refill:_____ times-- Do not refill ( )

Signed:_____
DO NOT TAKE THIS TO YOUR PHARMACIST

Community Clinic
Jeffrey A. Eaton, NP
Joyce D. Cappiello, NP

Name:_____ DOB_____
Address_____ Date_____

Rx

"label all unless indicated"
Refill:_____ times-- Do not refill ( )

Signed:_____
DO NOT TAKE THIS TO YOUR PHARMACIST

LEARNING ISSUES

In order to resolve this patient's problem, you will need to consider and address the following issues (you may generate additional issues as well):

- Acne classification and treatment
- Adolescent developmental issues
- Chinese culture and medicine
- Appropriate use of consultants
- Menarche and menstrual patterns in a young adolescent
- Adolescent immunizations and health promotion

INITIAL IDEAS

- Acne vulgaris: Idiopathic
- Acne vulgaris: Related to hormonal problem
- Overall perception of health issues
- Irregular periods: Normal variant? Abnormal hormone levels?

INTERPRETATION OF CUES, PATTERNS, AND INFORMATION

Are there cultural issues that you need to consider? Is Ms. Wang more (or less) concerned about body image than other patients in your practice because of her cultural background. Ms. Wang is of Chinese heritage, and you must decide the significance of that fact by exploring its meaning with her. She may perceive herself as being "completely American," or she may have a strong belief in herbal or other Chinese medicinal therapies. You should be sensitive to her heritage without having unfounded assumptions.

DIFFERENTIAL DIAGNOSIS

Since Ms. Wang essentially has three potentially separate problems, a differential diagnosis for each is discussed.

1. *Acne vulgaris: Idiopathic or related to hormonal problem:* Restated, this differential could be, "Are there serious problems that first present with acne symptoms?" Although they are not common, the answer is yes (Kelso and Hall, 1994). They generally also include other signs of androgen excess such as facial hair and masculinization. A clinician should be alert for signs of problems such as Cushing's syndrome, adrenal and ovarian tumors, or polycystic ovary disease. Acne may also be caused by certain drugs. Ms. Wang denies other medications other than the erythromycin or Cleocin, but steroid use or oral contraceptives (OCs) would be possible causes. Acne can also be rated as mild, moderate, or severe (Fig. 16-1).

2. *Overall perception of health:* Do you need to be concerned about Liang's weight since she is on the lower end of her IBW range? There is a reasonable chance that this is genetic, and exploring

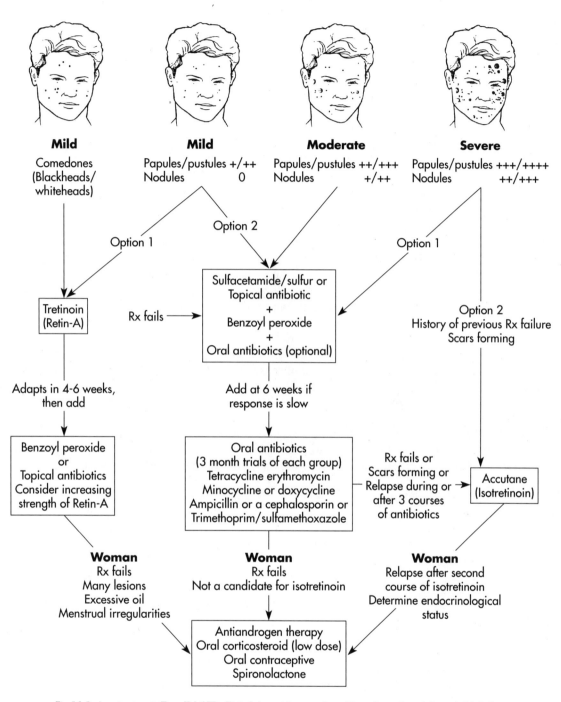

Fig. **16-1** Acne treatment. (From Habif TP: *Clinical dermatology: a color guide to diagnosis and therapy,* ed 3, St Louis, 1996, Mosby.)

her parents and siblings weights is a good place to start. Although a remote possibility, Ms. Wang could have an eating disorder, and you should be vigilant with all adolescents.

Has she had weight loss, or has she always been thin? Does she consider herself thin? Physical findings such as bradycardia; hypotension; hypothermia; dry, cracked, red skin; loss of female body contours; and thinning of scalp hair can all be signs of anorexia nervosa. Bulimia might be suspected if dental changes, parotid enlargement, and hair loss were present. People with bulimia often are a "normal" weight. Given her thorough history and physical examination, these are probably not a major concern with Ms. Wang, but in any young female who is below IBW, vigilance for other signs that would indicate an eating disorder is appropriate. Early intervention with family, psychological, or cognitive therapy may be helpful. Medication such as antidepressants are also used in treatment of eating disorders.

3. *Irregular periods: Normal variant?* Abnormal hormone levels? This actually may just be a normal variant. Periods are often irregular for about 2 years after menarche. Ms. Wang's periods have actually developed something of a regular pattern, so they may not even fit the definition of irregular periods. They are probably most important to consider in Ms. Wang for two reasons:

a. How do they relate to her acne? Is there some hormonal change that could be causing both problems? Is her acne related to her periods as far as when it flares?

b. You need to decide whether Ms. Wang's irregular periods are a concern to her, indicating that she might be pregnant. She did not bring it up until questioned, so it may not be a serious concern of hers. Malnutrition could cause a change in periods, although it does not appear that Ms. Wang's periods were ever any more normal than they are now.

c. Further information relating to the presence of cramps or heavy flow may allow appropriate interventions.

d. Sexuality issues may come up appropriately in this discussion.

DIAGNOSTIC OPTIONS

1. *Acne vulgaris: Idiopathic or related to hormonal problem:* After physical examination and history minimize the probability of potential hormonal pathologies, a trial of a new therapy is probably the approach that most clinicians would use.

2. *Overall perception of health:* Monitor patterns of weight gain or loss.

3. *Irregular periods: Normal variant? Abnormal hormone levels?* Exploration of the need for contraceptive counseling or intervention would be the first step, and then only if the problem was persistent or worsened would there be any need for consultation.

THERAPEUTIC OPTIONS

Acne vulgaris

Pharmacological The usual place to start in acne care is with Benzoyl peroxide 5%. Starting with a higher percentage may actually cause worsening of symptoms initially since it will irritate the skin and create redness. One option would be to increase the strength of Benzoyl peroxide to 10%.

The next step after a simple cleansing approach is to add a topical antibiotic. Cleocin T or erythromycin are both reasonable approaches, but in general they should tried for 6 weeks or so before progressing to the next step. Retin-A (Tretinoin) at 0.025% is a reasonable next step, and then oral antibiotics. Ms. Wang has asked to try oral antibiotics or for a dermatology referral. Many clinicians in this case would prescribe a course of oral tetracycline (TCN). Some references recommend TCN only for adolescents 14 or older. Others indicate that TCN is safe after the age of 8 (Nurse Practitioner Prescribing Reference, 1997), so it is probably reasonable in Ms. Wang, but some clinicians would be cautious and choose another approach. TCN will clear her acne more quickly, and avoids the need for a dermatology consult at this point.

In patients with moderate or more severe acne, earlier use of oral antibiotics may be appropriate.

Recently, a birth control pill, Ortho Tri-Cyclen, has received FDA approval for a new indication in the primary treatment of acne. This is an amazing event because this is the first time that OCs have received a noncontraceptive indication. Providers have known for years that OCs often help clear acne, so the improvement of acne was often a positive side effect of using the pill for contraception. Now providers can feel comfortable providing OCs solely for acne. It is possible that any low androgenic OC on the market will provide improvement of acne, but Ortho Tri-Cyclen is the only pill that has been brought before the FDA and received this indication. The *Physicians' Drug Reference* lists this consideration for use in young women age 15 and older. By listing a higher age, the company avoids the question of how young is too young to prescribe the pill. There is some theoretical concern regarding the initiation of OC use shortly after menarche and increasing the rate of epiphyseal closure. Since menarche occurred about 2 1/2 years ago for Ms. Wang, there is little medical concern about beginning OC use at this time.

The use of an OC would also regulate her menses if this is an issue with Ms. Wang. Although her somewhat irregular menses are common in teenagers, this pattern is not generally an indicator of an underlying gynecological problem. Certainly you would want to discuss OC therapy with Ms. Wang and her parents to decide if it would be appropriate for her.

Educational She will want to seek out noncomedogenic cosmetics. Cosmetics that are noncomedogenic will usually be well marked.

Dietary modification for acne is somewhat controversial. There is no current evidence that foods cause acne, however there are still many people, both clinicians and nonclinicians, who believe that they are related. A reasonable middle ground is to tell Ms. Wang that if she notices that there are any foods that seem to make her break out that she should avoid them but that otherwise there are no dietary modifications needed.

You also may want to take the opportunity to caution Ms. Wang in the future from taking other peoples medications. A practical explanation of the risks will probably be more useful than a dogmatic prohibition.

Other nonpharmacological options Herbal therapies from a Chinese medicine practitioner may be something that Ms. Wang or her family may want to try. Integrating these into an overall approach will require some knowledge of those herbs and their effects. Working with the Chinese medicine practitioner may be possible, but language and scientific theory issues may present challenges.

Overall Perception of Health and Irregular Periods

At this point the diagnostic and therapeutic options would be the same: to watch and wait. Use of OCs to regulate menses could be considered in the future, but they are probably not necessary for several more years unless there was a concern about pregnancy.

HEALTH PROMOTION/HEALTH MAINTENANCE

Immunizations to consider at this visit include the following:

1. Hepatitis B: This is especially important in teenagers since they may be on the verge of sexual activity (if they have not already begun). Unfortunately this is an expensive vaccine. Some states cover the cost for teens, but others do not.

2. Varicella zoster virus (VZV) vaccine: VZV vaccine could be considered if she did not have a documented case of chicken pox or previous vaccination. She will require the two-dose schedule since she is receiving it as a teen. Again, this is a fairly expensive vaccine, so not all clinicians will want to take advantage of the opportunity. If there is doubt about her immunity status, a VZV antibody titer could be checked.

3. Tuberculosis (TB) testing: TB testing would be considered based on the prevalence of TB in the community.

4. Tetanus-diphtheria (Td): She will be just about 10 years from her last dose since in all probability she received it before school at about age 4 or 5. She could hold off for another year or so, but getting it now might prevent the need to go an emergency room after an at-risk wound. She will be coming in for follow-up, so it could also be done at a later date.

5. MMR: You need to make sure that she has received her second dose of MMR.

If Ms. Wang had been (or was planning on traveling soon) to another country, then an exploration of further immunization needs would be necessary.

Depression/Anxiety/Suicide Screening

Since these are common problems among adolescents, some level of screening is appropriate. The HEADSS mnemonic can be helpful to guide an adolescent well visit:

- **H:** Home
- **E:** Education
- **A:** Alcohol
- **D:** Drugs
- **S:** Sexuality
- **S:** Suicide

If these areas are covered, problems will often surface. Denials do not, of course, guarantee that problems are not present, and the clinician should be vigilant for problems in these areas in all adolescents. -

Safety

Adolescents should be encouraged to use seatbelts. They also should think about safety around drinking alcohol. This includes not only alcohol avoidance but also not riding with someone who has been drinking and planning ahead to avoid being placed in that situation.

FOLLOW-UP

If oral antibiotics are chosen, a follow-up in 4 to 6 weeks will allow them time to be effective.

References

Murphy JL, editor: *Nurse Practitioner Prescribing Reference*, New York, 1997, Prescribing Reference.

Kelso T, Hall RP: *Review of acne and its treatment*, Durham, NC, 1994, Glaxo.

2:45 PM
Tess Ireland
Age 45 years

OPENING SCENARIO

Tess Ireland is a 45-year-old female on your schedule with a complaint of heartburn. She has been followed in your practice for several years. Her last physical examination was 9 months ago. Her most recent visit was 2 ½ weeks ago.

HISTORY OF PRESENT ILLNESS

"I've had severe heartburn for 10 to 12 days. I saw you 2 1/2 weeks ago (see note) when I had a left elbow problem and you prescribed some medication for 10 days. During the last few days of treatment I began to develop severe heartburn, pain in my lower chest, and a feeling of stomach acid coming up my throat. I assumed this was due to the medication. I stopped drinking coffee (reluctantly) and tea and began to take Maalox. This helped, but the symptoms have not yet resolved even though I have finished the medication."

Note From 2 1/2 Weeks Ago

REASON FOR VISIT

This 45-year-old woman known to your practice presents with a 10-day history of medial left elbow pain with some radiation down into the ring and little fingers. She has tried Naproxen 200 mg (2 tabs tid) for the past week without significant improvement. She aggravated the elbow pain this past weekend by skiing and driving a long distance in her car. She had a similar bout 6 months ago, which was resolved with ice and over-the-counter (OTC) nonsteroidal antiinflammatory drugs (NSAIDs).

PHYSICAL EXAMINATION

There is no erythema, ecchymosis, atrophy, or deformity in the left upper extremity. She has a positive Tinel's sign over the ulnar nerve of the left elbow. No weakness noted. Left elbow, forearm: no erythema, ecchymosis, atrophy, or deformity. No pain with range of motion or palpatation. Right arm: no significant findings.

ASSESSMENT

• Ulnar neuritis

PLAN

• Avoid local pressure.
• Try Ketoprofen 200 mg po qd for 10 days.
• Return for follow-up if symptoms persist.

MEDICAL HISTORY

Healthy individual. Physical examination and gynecological examination done 9 months ago in your office. No surgeries or major illnessess.

FAMILY MEDICAL HISTORY

Mother: 77 yr (Parkinson's disease)
Father: Deceased at 54 yr (myocardial infarction [MI])
Three paternal uncles with heart disease
Sister: 52 yr (A&W)
Three brothers: (one brother had MI at age 34 but is now age 50 and doing well)

MEDICATIONS

Daily multivitamin

ALLERGIES

None

REVIEW OF SYSTEMS

General: States energy level good; sleeps well, usually 7 hours per night; tries to eat low-fat diet and exercise regularly; recreational bicyclist; bikes approximately 75 miles each week in nice weather; it was thought that this had started the neuritis
HEENT: No problems with cold, flu, or asthma but is complaining of a cough for 5 days; she thinks this is unusual since she does not have any upper respiratory infection (URI) symptoms; the cough is more of a "clearing of my throat" and is worse at night; is not bothered by a sore throat; nonsmoker; no known environmental toxin exposure; denies eye, ear, throat, or dental pain
Thorax: Denies any chest pain, shortness of breath, lightheadedness, dyspnea on exertion; is coughing frequently during day and at night; finds the cough is less if she uses extra pillows

Gastrointestinal: No nausea, vomiting, abdominal pain, diarrhea, constipation, or blood in stools

Genitourinary: Regular menses; last menstrual period (LMP) 3 weeks ago; uses diaphragm regularly

Extremities: Neuritis of left elbow "about 75% improved"; continues to ice area approximately once a day and is riding bicycle less; noticing other things that bother her elbow (carrying heavy objects in left arm and driving car); tries not to rest elbow on armrest of car door; if she has to use pressure with her left hand on the steering wheel it bothers her elbow

Neurological: No paresthesia in left hand

PHYSICAL EXAMINATON

Vital signs: Temperature: 98.0° F; *Pulse:* 68 beats/min; *Respirations:* 16 breaths/min; *BP:* 130/68 mm Hg

Height: 5' 6"; *Weight:* 140 lb

General: Healthy-appearing female

HEENT: No frontal or maxillary tenderness; nasal mucosa: red, clear exudate; tympanic membranes: crisp cone of light, landmarks visible; pharynx: no redness or lesions noted

Neck: Supple without thyromegaly, lymphadenopathy

Heart: Regular rate and rhythm; no murmurs, rubs, or gallops

Lungs: Clear to auscultation

Abdomen: Soft, no masses; no pain elicited with palpation including the epigastric area; no hepatosplenomegaly

Extremities: No erythema, atrophy, deformity noted in left upper extremity; Tinel's sign remains slightly positive over ulnar nerve in left elbow; no lower extremity edema

Neurological: Sensory function intact to light touch in left upper and lower extremity and equal to right arm

ASSESSMENT   *Please indicate the problems or issues you have identified that will guide your care (preferably in list form):*

PLAN   *Please list your plans for addressing each of the problems or issues in your assessment:*

Community Clinic	Community Clinic
Jeffrey A. Eaton, NP	Jeffrey A. Eaton, NP
Joyce D. Cappiello, NP	Joyce D. Cappiello, NP
Name:_____ DOB_____	Name:_____ DOB_____
Address_____ Date_____	Address_____ Date_____
Rx	Rx
"label all unless indicated"	"label all unless indicated"
Refill:_____ times-- Do not refill ( )	Refill:_____ times-- Do not refill ( )
Signed:_____	Signed:_____
DO NOT TAKE THIS TO YOUR PHARMACIST	**DO NOT TAKE THIS TO YOUR PHARMACIST**

CASE
17 *Discussion*

LEARNING ISSUES

In order to resolve this patient's problem, you will need to consider and address the following issues (you may generate additional issues as well):

- **Pertinent history**
- **Pertinent diagnostic tests needed, if any**
- **Cytochrome P-450 enzyme**
- **Available therapeutic options**
- **Nonpharmacological options**
- **Unresolved problems from prior visits**

INITIAL IDEAS

Heartburn, or reflux, is most likely at the top of your differential diagnosis. Ms. Ireland is not associating cough with the heartburn, but you know this may be the case. Also consider other etiologies of her cough, such as the possibility of a cardiac origin of her complaints. The chief complaint of this visit is heartburn, but continuing neuritis is also on her problem list.

INTERPRETATION OF CUES, PATTERNS, AND INFORMATION

The pertinent history includes the recent use of an NSAID, the typical reflux symptoms of substernal pain (which is worse after lying down), some relief of symptoms with antacids, and a cough. A history of occasional heartburn also increases the likelihood of reflux.

DIAGNOSTIC OPTIONS

What type of workup is indicated to establish a diagnosis? What type of tests, if any, are needed? When thinking of a gastroesophageal reflux problem, the typical diagnostic tests to consider and their relative value include a barium swallow and endoscopy.

The barium swallow identifies anatomical lesions, but it has limited ability to detect mucosal abnormalities. The advantages are that it is widely available and relatively inexpensive. The diagnostic accuracy of radiography is 25% when esophagitis is mild, 82% when it is moderate, and 99% when it is severe (DeVault and Castell, 1995). Since Ms. Ireland has had symptoms for only 1 to 2 weeks, you can assume that any esophageal changes are mild. Therefore this test would have a low accuracy rate for her.

Endoscopy with biopsy is the gold standard for identifying mucosal injuries and anatomical lesions. The down side is that total endoscopy costs may be as much as three times those of the barium swallow. You must make a decision whether the expensive gold-standard test is needed with Ms. Ireland at this point.

pH ambulatory monitoring is frequently performed by gastroenterologists as a standard test in the workup of reflux, but this test is not commonly available in a primary care office. Specialists see the worst cases of any given disease, so their workup may be different from the workup of a primary care provider. With Ms. Ireland's short duration of symptoms, you might hold off on a gastroenterology referral.

Thinking through the various diagnostic options available, consider the cost/benefit aspect of testing versus empiric therapy. Empiric therapy has the advantages of low cost and convenience weighed against the possible risks of misdiagnosis or delayed diagnosis. What can be missed? Although an early cancer is always a concern, it seems unlikely given her acute onset of symptoms, the relatively short duration, and the clear history of symptoms starting with NSAID use. If you are suspicious of an ulcer, then a complete blood count (CBC) and a check of stools for occult blood are options. A check of stools for occult blood is probably a good idea anyway. If a careful history discloses symptoms consistent with uncomplicated gastroesophageal reflux disease (GERD) as with this woman, then no further testing is needed before beginning empiric therapy (DeVault and Castell, 1995).

Could any of these symptoms be of cardiac origin? Again, her presenting complaints seem clearly related to NSAID use, but with her family history of cardiac disease, you need to carefully consider this in the differential diagnosis. An office electrocardiogram (ECG) as a basic diagnostic test might lower any suspicion of cardiac disease, but the sensitivity is limited. If she is actually having substernal pain while in the office, the ECG could be quite helpful in ruling out any cardiac involvement.

There may be other etiologies of her cough. An allergic response could cause a postnasal drip, which leads to cough at night. It is generally accepted that GERD and asthma are connected, but the exact nature of the relationship is yet to be determined. Asthma may promote GERD, and GERD may provoke asthma (Sullivan and Samuelson, 1996). GERD-induced asthma may result from either aspiration of gastric contents into the lung with consequent bronchospasm or activation of a vagal reflex arc from the esophagus to the lung causing vasoconstriction (Kahrilas, 1996). Many more asthmatics have GERD than have GERD-induced asthma. A few key history questions and auscultation of her lungs should help to rule out asthma.

Laryngitis, cough, frequent throat clearing, or sore throat without identifiable allergic or infectious causes can be complications of longstanding GERD. With chronic symptoms such as these, it is important to examine the pharynx and larynx.

REVISED IDEAS

- GERD (NSAID induced)

THERAPEUTIC OPTIONS

GERD

Treatment goals for Ms. Ireland will focus on relieving symptoms and healing the irritation of the esophageal mucosa to prevent long-term stricture formation and Barrett's esophagitis. Medication use seems appropriate since she is uncomfortable enough to come see you and has tried some lifestyle changes such as reducing caffeine use.

The H_2 receptor antagonists are the most commonly used and prescribed drugs for this condition because they are effective in relieving symptoms and healing the mucosa and are relatively inexpensive with few side effects.

Antacids are also effective in improving reflux in mild disease. Since Ms. Ireland was experiencing difficulty taking antacids on a regular basis, the ease of carrying a small bottle of pills with her versus a larger bottle of liquid medicine may help compliance. Also, diarrhea is a common complaint with magnesium-containing antacids. This will remain a good option for prn use. Another type of antacid is Gaviscon, which is a chewable aluminum and magnesium compound that forms a viscous foam that floats on the surface of gastric secretions. Theoretically, this foam forms a mechanical barrier, which decreases the amount of material that can be refluxed into the esophagus, although published efficacy rates are conflicting (Koda-Kimble and Young, 1995).

The acid pump inhibitor drugs, such as omeprazole and lansoprazole, are more effective than the H_2 blockers but have more drug interactions because of the inhibition of the cytochrome P-450 enzyme system. In spite of this, they are generally well tolerated but costly. In this case, with short-term symptoms rather than a long-standing condition, these drugs would not generally be chosen as a first-line medication. They could be considered down the road if there is no response to therapy.

Cisapride (Propulsid) is in the prokinetic category of drugs and has just been approved as a first-line medication. More typically it is used as a second-line drug after trying the H_2 blockers. Diarrhea is a common side effect that may necessitate reducing the dose or stopping the medication. Again, this drug inhibits the cytochrome P-450 enzyme system, so there is potential for many drug interactions. The use of other prokinetic agents, such as bethanechol and metoclopramide hydrochloride, are limited because of adverse reactions.

The treatment options have been narrowed to the H_2 blockers. This gives you four choices: cimetidine (Tagamet), ranitidine (Zantac), famotidine (Pepcid), or nizatidine (Axid). Any of these drugs will work and can be considered for Ms. Ireland. Cimetidine is the least expensive but has more drug interactions because of its effect on the cytochrome P-450 system, whereas famotidine and nizatidine have no appreciable effect on this system. Since Ms. Ireland is not on any other daily medications, this is not a major concern. She will be using this medicine for 6 to 8 weeks, so the theoretical possibility exists that other drugs might be prescribed for her during this time. Cimetidine and ranitidine (to a lesser extent) interact with alcohol. Famotidine does not appear to do so. In the history, it is noted that Ms. Ireland drinks 1 to 2 glasses of wine approximately three times a week. In addition to this, cimetidine is very short acting, necessitating more frequent dosing. Since there are several drugs from which to choose, it seems appropriate to choose the most cost-effective drug with a minimum of side effects.

If there is no improvement after a 6-week trial of a H_2 blocker, then either switch to an acid pump inhibitor (many clinicians would do this), increase the dose (DeVault and Castell, 1995) or refer to a gastroenterologist.

Nonpharmocological Interventions Stop prescription NSAIDs and avoid any OTC NSAIDs. The following are the usual recommendations for lifestyle changes although not necessarily research based:

1. Elevate the head of the bed by 6 inches with blocks to use gravity for improvement of acid clearance at night.
2. Avoid the recumbent position for 3 hours after eating.
3. Reduce or eliminate coffee intake, including decaffeinated coffee and tea.
4. Dietary factors such as fatty food, citrus products, chocolate, peppermint, onions, and garlic have been proven in research studies to increase reflux. They may be aggravating her NSAID-caused heartburn.
5. Fortunately she is a nonsmoker. Give positive reenforcement for this.

Elbow Neuritis

She gives you a fairly clear history of what is aggravating the elbow, but perhaps there are additional aggravating activities she has not yet considered. Can she continue to adjust her lifestyle? She states about 75% improvement of symptoms, so it seems reasonable for her to continue with symptomatic therapy.

The NSAIDs have been discontinued due to the development of GERD. A trial of acetaminophen and ice may control the discomfort.

Have Ms. Ireland return to the office if symptoms are not resolved in several weeks.

HEALTH PROMOTION/HEALTH MAINTENANCE

Ms. Ireland is a regular patient in the office with a physical examination 9 months ago. If you attended to the health-maintenance issues at that visit, she should be current with most screening tests and immunizations.

References

DeVault K, Castell D: Guidelines for the diagnosis and treatment of gastroesophageal reflux disease. *Arch Intern Med* 155:2163, 1995.

Kahrilas P: Gastroesophageal reflux disease, *JAMA* 276,12, 993, 1996.

Koda-Kimble M, Young L: *Applied therapeutics:* the clinical use of drugs, ed 6, Vancouver, 1995, Applied Therapeutic.

Sullivan C, Samuelson W: Gastroesophageal reflux: a common exacerabating factor in adult asthma, *Nurs Pract* 12, 11, 82, 1996.

OPENING SCENARIO

Michael Smith is a 24-year-old male scheduled for a complete physical examination. This is his first visit in your office.

HISTORY OF PRESENT ILLNESS

"I have intermittent episodes of diarrhea, abdominal discomfort, bloating, and on occasion constipation. Often I eat and then 5 minutes later have gas and bloating. I hate mornings. I try to sleep late but I can't. I feel sick every morning. I'm bloated, nauseous, have watery stools, and have to look for a bathroom when away from home. This is difficult because currently I'm in a class that requires an outdoor experience. I'm expected to spend time doing research in the mountains, which means day hikes without a nearby bathroom. It's a nightmare. I would do overnight camping trips in this program if this were not such a problem.

"I don't know what size clothes to buy because I need a larger size for the days I have a lot of bloating, but if I have a few good days, then I wear a size smaller." The patient feels as if he is not evacuating his bowels completely. He has three to five semiformed stools per day. Stools are often urgent. Rarely has mucus in his stools. No blood in stools. Symptoms are almost daily. The only thing that helps is lying down. Does not wake at night to have a bowel movement.

Was seen elsewhere for this problem 1 year ago. At that time he was diagnosed with giardia. His stool cultures were negative, but the diagnosis was made presumptively based on his history of extensive world travel. He was treated with a trial of metronidazole and did not improve.

Symptoms have been present since at least his freshman year in high school. He did not realize his bowel patterns were atypical until he lived in a dorm as an undergraduate in college. Then he learned what was normal by observing his peers. He denies laxative use.

MEDICAL HISTORY

No hospitalizations or surgery. Up-to-date on all childhood immunizations including tetanus 5 years ago. No hepatitis A or B immunizations. His only past health concerns have been abdominal pain, bloating, and diarrhea. No history of colon problems, colon cancer, or gallbladder disease.

FAMILY MEDICAL HISTORY

MGM: 70 yr (A&W)
MGF: 71 yr (hypertension)
PGM: 66 yr (breast cancer)
PGF: 67 yr (arthritis)
Mother: 45 yr (A&W)
Father: 47 yr (A&W)
One sister: 19 yr (A&W)

SOCIAL HISTORY

Good relationship with girlfriend. Sees parents frequently. They are understanding of this problem. Is currently a graduate student with a hectic lifestyle. Previously worked on a cruise ship, which took him all over the world. Drank a lot of alcohol as a college student, which gave him loose stools. Rarely has a drink now. Denies intravenous (IV) drug use or other drug use. Nonsmoker. Exercises regularly, which helps reduce symptoms somewhat.

MEDICATIONS

None. Infrequent antibiotic use: thinks he had penicillin for a strep throat in high school and amoxicillin for a sinusitis 3 years ago.

ALLERGIES

None

REVIEW OF SYSTEMS

General: Good appetite with no weight loss; no fatigue; no fever, chills; no blood transfusions; sleeps 7 hours per night
Skin: No lesions or rashes
HEENT: Denies any vision problems; no allergies; sees dentist twice a year; no ear or hearing problems
Cardiac: No chest pain, dyspnea of exertion, palpitations
Respiratory: No shortness of breath, dyspnea, cough, or asthma
Gastrointestinal: Frequent nausea, no vomiting; frequent heartburn

Genitourinary: Sex life affected slightly because sometimes he feels sick and just wants to "be still"; no dysuria or frequency; heterosexual; denies homosexual or bisexual contact

Extremities: No joint pain or swelling, arthritis, myalgias

Endocrine: No skin or hair changes; temperature tolerances good

Neurological: No weakness, seizures; occasional "stress" headache relieved by acetaminophen; denies depression but states sometimes that this health problem "gets him down"

Nutritional: Eats one meal a day in the evening; when life is more settled, he eats regularly and makes better food choices; red meat firms up stool; last night had a huge steak and potato with blue cheese dip, which caused diarrhea; for lunch had some corn chips, which caused cramps; for breakfast, had cereal and milk, which again caused bloating; milk alone does not seem to bother him

PHYSICAL EXAMINATION

Vital signs: Temperature: 98.0° F; *Pulse:* 70 beats/min; *Respirations:* 16 breaths/min; *BP:* 120/80 mm Hg

Height: 5' 11"; *Weight:* 175 lb; *BMI:* 24

General: Well nourished, well developed

Skin: No rashes, lesions, scars

HEENT: No redness or lesions of eyes; extraocular movements intact; Ear: no discharge; tympanic membrane intact, crisp cone of light; Nose: no exudate, polyps; Mouth: no lesions, good dentition

Neck: No lymphadenopathy or thyromegaly

Heart: Regular rate and rhythm; no murmurs, rubs, or gallops

Lungs: Clear to auscultation

Abdomen: Soft, no masses, no hepatosplenomegaly; slight, diffuse tenderness in lower abdomen; Rectal: empty, no masses, normal anal tone, no anal fissures or hemorrhoids

Genitourinary: Without palpable inguinal nodes; circumcised penis; without lesions, edema, erythema, masses of genitalia; testes palpated without masses, tenderness; negative direct inguinal hernia

Extremities: No edema; pedal pulses palpable bilaterally

Neurological: Cranial nerves 2 through 12 intact

ASSESSMENT   *Please indicate the problems or issues you have identified that will guide your care (preferably in list form):*

PLAN   *Please list your plans for addressing each of the problems or issues in your assessment:*

Community Clinic
Jeffrey A. Eaton, NP
Joyce D. Cappiello, NP

Name:_____ DOB_____
Address_____ Date_____

Rx

"label all unless indicated"
Refill:_____ times-- Do not refill ( )

Signed:_____
DO NOT TAKE THIS TO YOUR PHARMACIST

Community Clinic
Jeffrey A. Eaton, NP
Joyce D. Cappiello, NP

Name:_____ DOB_____
Address_____ Date_____

Rx

"label all unless indicated"
Refill:_____ times-- Do not refill ( )

Signed:_____
DO NOT TAKE THIS TO YOUR PHARMACIST

Community Clinic
Jeffrey A. Eaton, NP
Joyce D. Cappiello, NP

Name:_____ DOB_____
Address_____ Date_____

Rx

"label all unless indicated"
Refill:_____ times-- Do not refill ( )

Signed:_____
DO NOT TAKE THIS TO YOUR PHARMACIST

Community Clinic
Jeffrey A. Eaton, NP
Joyce D. Cappiello, NP

Name:_____ DOB_____
Address_____ Date_____

Rx

"label all unless indicated"
Refill:_____ times-- Do not refill ( )

Signed:_____
DO NOT TAKE THIS TO YOUR PHARMACIST

CASE
18 Discussion

INITIAL IDEAS

Before you enter the room, you are thinking of the various bowel problems that can occur from acute to chronic:

- Infectious organisms
- Parasitic bowel disease
- IBS
- Cancer

INTERPRETATION OF CUES, PATTERN, AND INFORMATION

It is immediately apparent from his history that this is not an acute diarrhea (meaning a diarrhea of sudden onset with symptoms for less than 1 week) but a chronic diarrhea.

His young age and absence of blood in the stool makes cancer less likely. Frequent travel to other countries stands out in your mind as a reason for bacterial or parasitic bowel disease. His interest in outdoor activities may put him in areas of giardia outbreak; however, his symptoms began while in high school, which seems to be before the traveling began and a common age for the onset of IBS.

Although you have not ruled out the possibility of infectious organisms, you are also thinking of inflammatory or irritable bowel problems or possibly lactose intolerance.

He is not currently, nor has been in the recent past, on medications, so an antibiotic or other medication side effect seems less likely.

Since he denies laxative abuse (and this occurs mostly in women), it can be put lower on the differential list.

The physical examination may reveal complications of the diseases on the differential list, such as weight loss with a malabsorption, erythema nodosum, arthritis in inflammatory bowel disease (IBD), and rectal abscess and fissures in Crohn's disease.

Tenderness may be present in the lower abdomen. The rectal examination is usually unremarkable except for tenderness. Areas of focus with the physical examination include the skin, gastrointestinal, and musculoskeletal areas.

REVISED IDEAS

- Inflammatory bowel disease (IBD)(Crohn's or ulcerative colitis)
- IBS
- Lactose intolerance
- Sorbitol intolerance
- Celiac sprue
- Infectious diarrhea
- Malabsorption

DIAGNOSTIC OPTIONS

What tests, if any, will help narrow the focus?

1. A test of *stool for occult blood,* if positive, suggests a mucosal disruption as seen in ulcerative colitis and Crohn's disease.

2. A *complete blood count* (CBC) will help rule out a microcytic anemia. A small of amount of blood loss can occur without causing changes in the CBC. If negative, it does not necessarily rule out bleeding, but it makes it less likely. The white blood cell (WBC) count or erythrocyte sedimentation rate (ESR) may be elevated in diverticulitis but not in IBS. If the differential showed an elevated eosinophil count, a parasitic infection is possible.

3. *Fecal leukocytes* are absent in infectious processes that do not invade the mucosa such as in viral illness, diarrhea from drugs or toxins, noninvasive *E. coli,* and cholera. Salmonella, shigella, amoeba, and helicobacter are invasive organisms and usually lead to production of leukocytes as does IBD. If the stool is negative for blood and fecal leukocytes, this is a very encouraging sign.

4. A *blood sugar test* would rule out the remote possibility of a diabetes mellitus-related diabetic gastroenteropathy in this healthy-appearing young man. This seems unlikely, but the test is inexpensive.

5. *Stool cultures* and a test of *stool for ova and parasites* can diagnose parasites and giardia. Up to three stool specimens are ordered because giardia may not be passed consistently in the stool. Thus multiple specimens from varying days are usually necessary. There is a remote possibility that he is harboring a parasite that still has not been identified since he has had extensive world travel. *Entamoeba histolytica* testing may need to be special ordered since it is often not part of a routine parasite screen. A *Clostridium difficile* titer would also pick up *C. difficile,* more commonly seen after recent antibiotic use.

6. A *sigmoidoscopy* can be used to look for IBD, but may not be every clinician's first-line test in a young person. In a young person with no other health problems, a negative family history of colon cancer, and no worrisome symptoms like bleeding or weight loss, you could treat empirically and postpone the flexible sigmoidoscopy. If he were closer to 50 years of age, had a family history of colon cancer, a new onset of symptoms, bleeding, or weight loss to suggest a malabsorption condition or cancer, then a flexible sigmoidoscopy and perhaps a barium enema would be indicated.

7. Lactose intolerance can be diagnosed by a *hydrogen breath test,* which is found in gastroenterologists' offices but not in many primary care offices. A simple test called the "89 cent milk test" can be used. Mr. Smith can drink a quart of milk and then record his symptoms. This volume of milk is usually enough to induce symptoms in even mildly susceptible individuals. Alternatively, a trial of a diet free of milk and milk products for 3 weeks is often an adequate test for lactose intolerance. With this trial the patient must be vigilant in reading food labels since lactose is often an unexpected ingredient in many foods. If all the symptoms disappear on a lactose-free diet, then the diagnosis is lactose intolerance. If partial improvement occurs, this suggests a lactose intolerance in addition to another bowel disorder.

8. Sorbitol sensitivity is diagnosed by a *food diary* and eliminating and adding food to the diet.

How do you diagnose IBD? The diagnosis can be made exclusively on clinical grounds. The criteria in Box 18-1 have a high sensitivity and specificity. Mr. Smith's symptoms definitely meet these criteria.

There are other clues based on the patient history: (1) diarrhea is usually worse after breakfast and (2) a feeling of incomplete evacuation and symptoms do not bother him at night. The latter is characteristic of IBS, whereas sufferers of IBD are often awakened at night with symptoms.

REVISED IDEAS

These revised ideas are based on history and physical examination findings:

- IBS (based on history)
- Parasites and giardia (cannot rule out until laboratory results are available)
- Lactose intolerance

Since Mr. Smith thinks he can tolerate milk, lactose intolerance is lower on the list. Parasites and giardia also seem lower on the list since he was previously treated for giardia without improvement. The one diagnosis that remains high on the list is IBS.

Most individuals with IBS come to see health providers after their symptoms have been present for years. The major complaints are pain and altered bowel habits. The pattern of symptoms varies from person to person, but the pattern is fairly consistent for each individual.

THERAPEUTIC OPTIONS

Keep in mind while planning care that IBS is a condition of a hyperactive colon of unknown etiology that is aggravated by a person's environment. Dietary factors, which Mr. Smith stated for him were certain types of foods and irregular eating habits, are important. He has learned that regular meals reduce symptoms but has not figured out how to eat regularly given his schedule.

As with many IBS sufferers, certain foods increase his symptoms. Caffeine, carbonated beverages, and spicy foods are frequent offenders. Gas, in the form of belching or flatus, is a frequent complaint. About $1/4$ to $1/2$ of people with IBS also complain of heartburn, which suggests that IBS is not just a problem of the colon but also of the upper gastrointestinal system.

Bran, specifically, has been shown to increase the size of the stool and the frequency of the passage of the stool. This helps the person who has constipation problems. Some find that there is an increase in flatulence with adding high fiber, and they are usually already complaining of bloating. If patients can tolerate it, the adverse effects of bran will clear in a few weeks.

Box 18-1 Criteria for Diagnosis of IBS

Continuous or recurrent symptoms over several months of the following:

1. Abdominal pain or discomfort relieved with defecation or associated with a change in the frequency or consistency of the stool and/or
2. An irregular or varying pattern of defecation at least 25% of the time, consisting of two or more of the following:
   - Altered stool frequency
   - Altered stool consistency
   - Straining
   - Urgency
   - Feeling of incomplete evacuation
   - Passage of mucus with stool
   - Bloating or feeling of distention

From Manning A et al: Towards a positive diagnosis of irritable bowel, *Br Med J* 2:653, 1978.

Hydrophilic colloids such as Metamucil or LA Formula are especially useful in those clients with alternating diarrhea and constipation. Because of their hydrophilic qualities, they tend to bind water and decrease the fluidity of the diarrheal stools. One to two tablespoons of the powder are given with meals two to three times a day and gradually decreased to once a day as symptoms improve. Thin individuals should take it after meals because it can suppress the appetite, and obese individuals should take it before meals. Other individuals prefer Citrucil, finding it better tolerated and helpful for both diarrhea and constipation. Peppermint is a natural relaxant of the gut. Peppermint tea or altoid mints can be helpful.

Assess fluid intake. Is the patient with diarrhea drinking the recommended 6 to 8 glasses of water per day?

Individuals with significant diarrhea may obtain relief with an antidiarrheal agent such as loperamide HCl (Imodium).

The efficacy of most medications to prevent or treat gas and/or distention have been low. Over-the-counter (OTC) simethicone or charcoal capsules are helpful for some individuals. The clinical experience with antispasmodic drugs has also been disappointing. Persons likely to experience some benefit from these drugs are those whose symptoms are brought on by meals and have tenesmus. Dicyclomine hydrochloride (Bentyl), 20 to 40 mg qid, or hyoscyamine sulfate (Levsin), tid or qid, 30 minutes before meals is often used. Since Mr. Smith's symptoms are worse after meals, this might offer some relief.

Reenforce that mucus in the stools is caused by the increased motility and is not a sign of infection. It can sometimes be a sign for malabsorption conditions such as celiac sprue.

This patient complained of occasional heartburn, which might be relieved if the IBS improves. The treatments suggested for IBS such as hyoscyamine sulfate and peppermint relax the lower esophageal sphincter and may make reflux worse. Inform Mr. Smith about this and see how he does. More likely, Mr. Smith might need a trial of an H_2 blocker. If symptoms persist or continue to recur or more severe complaints develop, then he may need a prokinetic agent, an acid pump inhibitor, or endoscopy.

Educational

Although IBS is a physical disorder, it is often triggered or made worse by stress and emotional factors.

Many people have areas of the body where stress is held. For some it is the neck or shoulders, for others it is the gut. In one study, 70% of the general population reported that they suffered from changes in bowel function in reaction to stressful situations. Over half of this group also experienced stomach pain under stress (Drossman et al, 1982). IBS patients seem to suffer more and may actually have lower stress-tolerance levels. For those who recognize the gut as their stress point, they need to think through any connections between what is happening in their lives and exacerbations of IBS. Identifying the connection is the first step; the second is identifying stress-management techniques that will work and then practicing these techniques. Sometimes it means making lifestyle changes to eliminate the stress; other times it means trying to adjust reaction to stress. Identifying priorities and continuing to think about these priorities is important. Learning relaxation techniques, meditation, assertiveness training, and time-management techniques are a few possibilities. Physical exercise can help with constipation and is also a way for many individuals to decrease stress.

Food alone does not cause IBS, but like stress, it can trigger symptoms. A food diary for a short time may help to identify any foods that trigger symptoms. There is no list of forbidden foods since each person will vary in what they can or cannot tolerate. Include beverages, especially alcohol, in the food diary as well as any medications, time of day, location, mood, and symptoms. A pattern may emerge of triggers or of what contributes to the times that the patient is feeling good. Keep in mind when having a flare-up that it may not be the food as much as what was happening in the surroundings while eating that food. For example, it may not be the glass of orange juice and piece of toast eaten for breakfast as much as that it was "eaten on the run" while trying to finish a paper and get to class on time. Encourage Mr. Smith to try to schedule a regular time to move his bowels.

Reenforce with patients that this is not a serious disease like cancer, nor will it turn into cancer or ulcerative colitis. It is not a life-threatening disease, nor is it "all in his head." There is no "quick fix" for IBS, but it can be managed to decrease the recurrences. You, as the health provider, can teach Mr. Smith how to identify triggers, modify his diet according to his needs, prescribe medications if needed, and share coping strategies and stress-reduction techniques.

FOLLOW-UP

A follow-up visit in 3 to 4 weeks seems appropriate.

References

Manning A et al: Towards a positive diagnosis of irritable bowel, *Br Med J* 2:653, 1978.

Drossman D et al: Bowel patterns among subjects not seeking health care, *Gastroenterology* 83:529, 1982.

Recommended Reading

Shimberg EF: *Relief from IBS,* New York, 1988, Ballantine. (This is an excellent paperback to recommend to patients. It is an easy-to-read, comprehensive look at IBS.)

C A S E
19

OPENING SCENARIO

Timothy Gifford is a 4-year-old male on your schedule for possible head lice. His family is present. Timmy and his brothers have dirt on their lower arms and faces.

HISTORY OF PRESENT ILLNESS

(Obtained from mother)

"Timmy has head lice. He got rid of them when I used some medication I had left over from one of my older kids who had lice, but the people next door didn't get their kids treated, so Timmy got them again. I need something for him and for all the rest of us too. If you could give us the stuff that doesn't require picking off the nits I'd appreciate it." Timmy and his mother deny any other irritated, open, or itching areas on his body.

MEDICAL HISTORY

None

MEDICATIONS

None

ALLERGIES

None

PHYSICAL EXAMINATION

Vital signs: Temperature: 97.2° F; *Pulse:* 88 beats/min; *Respirations:* 22 breaths/min

Weight: 51 lbs

HEENT: Small, white "balls" clinging to his hair shafts scattered all over his head; they are approximately 1/16" from the scalp; no lice are seen; his head is slightly red, and there are three to four open areas of scratching lesions without purulent drainage; no nits seen in eyelashes; no cervical adenopathy; conjunctiva are without redness or discharge.

Cardiac: Regular rate and rhythm

Respiratory: Clear to auscultation

Extremities: No lesions seen on arms and trunk

ASSESSMENT   *Please indicate the problems or issues you have identified that will guide your care (preferably in list form):*

PLAN   *Please list your plans for addressing each of the problems or issues in your assessment:*

Community Clinic
Jeffrey A. Eaton, NP
Joyce D. Cappiello, NP

Name:_____ DOB_____
Address_____ Date_____

Rx

"label all unless indicated"
Refill:_____ times-- Do not refill ( )

Signed:_____
DO NOT TAKE THIS TO YOUR PHARMACIST

Community Clinic
Jeffrey A. Eaton, NP
Joyce D. Cappiello, NP

Name:_____ DOB_____
Address_____ Date_____

Rx

"label all unless indicated"
Refill:_____ times-- Do not refill ( )

Signed:_____
DO NOT TAKE THIS TO YOUR PHARMACIST

LEARNING ISSUES

In order to resolve this patient's problem, you will need to consider and address the following issues (you may generate additional issues as well):

- **Evaluation of scalp problems in children**
- **Treatment options in patients with head lice**
- **Reimbursement issues in prescribing practices**
- **Educational needs of the family with head lice**
- **Health promotion and immunization in an episodic visit in a 4 year old**

INITIAL IDEAS

- Head lice
- Dandruff or eczema
- Scabies
- Allergic reaction to previous treatment (less probable)

INTERPRETATION OF CUES, PATTERNS, AND INFORMATION

On obtaining a history of the reason for the visit, you found that family members were also possibly affected and that a neighbor was felt to be the source of the infection. The fact that the child had already been treated once with "success" makes you wonder whether this is a reinfection or possibly a reaction to the previous treatment (pyrethins such as RID can cause an allergic-type reaction). Timmy's apparent scratching of his head causes you concern that there may be a superimposed bacterial infection even though you have found no evidence at this point. On physical examination, you look at the hair and see findings that are most consistent with head lice. There are nits (egg cases) present. You can confirm that these are nits with a Wood's lamp since they will fluoresce. You are not sure, however, whether these are housing potential lice or are merely empty remnants from the earlier treatment. You will look at the location on the hair shaft, and if they are still quite close to the scalp, you will be more suspicious that this represents recent infestation since they are attached to the hair shaft and will grow out along with the hair.

It is not clear whether the family has sought prescription treatment. Is it because of the failure of the previous treatment or a need for prescription treatment to obtain reimbursement coverage? A delicate exploration of this issue is probably appropriate.

REVISED IDEAS

- Head lice
- Bacterial infection related to scratching
- Financial issues
- Reaction to the previous treatment

DIFFERENTIAL DIAGNOSIS

1. *Head lice:* This is well supported with current information. The presence of nits may be pathognomonic.
2. *Scabies:* This does not usually go above the scalp line except in infants. He has no complaints of lesions elsewhere, so scabies is effectively ruled out.
3. *Dandruff or eczema:* The presence of nits makes these improbable.
4. *Kerion:* This is an inflamed, boggy lesion of the scalp caused by a strong immunological reaction to a fungal infection. This is improbable based on the current evidence.

DIAGNOSTIC OPTIONS

Probably the most appropriate diagnostic option is a trial of therapy. If he does not respond, he can return and you can reconsider you diagnosis and treatment at that time.

THERAPEUTIC OPTIONS

Pharmacological

Avoid RID since it may be a factor in the irritation. If permethrin (Nix) was used before, it may still be appropriate to reuse it with more family members treated and other measures before going to lindane (Kwell). Nix is the most appropriate choice, especially if the mother is pregnant (or there is any chance that she is). Repeating in 7 days is recommended by some clinicians and in this case may be appropriate. Kwell could be used if you really suspect treatment failure with Nix, there is no chance of pregnancy, or if the other drugs are not going to be reimbursed and thus the prescriptions would not be filled (Kwell is less expensive). It is not really appropriate to prescribe one drug rather than another because of reimbursement if you truly believe the nonreimbursible drug is best, but you also need to be pragmatic about whether the prescription will be filled.

You will need to think about several other issues. Should you give a prescription that will allow all family members to be treated? How do you feel about giving prescriptions for people who are not officially your patients? Do the formulary or regulations in this state allow you to do so? Is this a different case than others since it is an over-the-counter (OTC) drug that might be chosen? If they had called and asked for a prescription over the phone, would you have given it to them?

A little diphenhydramine (Benadryl) at bedtime may help Timmy itch less and sleep better.

If skin infection is present, a penicillinase-resistant synthetic penicillin such as dicloxacillin is recommended by Sanford, Gilbert, and Sande (1996) and Uphold and Graham (1994). Timmy is 51 lbs (about 23 kg), so 1.5 teaspoons (93.75 mg since the solution is 62.5 mg/5 ml) of dicloxacillin qid would deliver 375 mg/day. The recommendations for dicloxacillin are 12.5 to 25 mg/kg/day, and this would deliver 16.3 mg/kg/day. Erythromycin would be an alternative.

Educational

A handout may be an excellent approach, especially since the room is a bit confusing with all the people there. You need to be aware of literacy issues, however, and may want to have "low-literacy" materials available. Information written at a sixth grade level is a good aim. Even people that are good readers can benefit from a simple, straightforward approach on a topic with which they have little if any familiarity.

Most educational handouts on lice include the following:.
1. Lice are about the size of a sesame seed and are rarely seen because they avoid light.
2. Lice lay many eggs, which are called nits, and these nits attach to the base of a hair. The eggs hatch after 1 to 2 weeks, but the white egg cases remain attached to the hair shaft.
3. Itching is the major symptom that is caused by the bite of a head louse.
4. Lice do not jump or fly. They are only contracted by person-to-person contact or contact with personal items, such as combs, bed clothing, or clothes.

5. Head lice prefer a clean scalp, so they are not a sign of uncleanliness. Some say the healthiest lice are found on the healthiest people.

6. Treatment must include humans, surroundings, and personal items.

7. If using Nix, it is not necessary to remove the nits since they will have been killed. To do so for cosmetic reasons can be achieved by using a comb dipped in a solution of vinegar and water.

8. Machine wash all washable items in hot water and dry in a hot dryer.

9. Things that cannot be washed (such as stuffed toys) may be dried in a hot dryer for 20 minutes or sealed in a plastic bag for 10 days.

10. Boil plastic items for 10 minutes or wash in Nix.

11. Hair cuts are an option, but to eliminate all nits, a buzz cut is necessary and is a personal decision of the child and/or family.

12. Vacuum rugs.

13. Do not use insecticide sprays.

14. Kids should be kept out of school or daycare until the initial treatment is completed.

15. Parents should report the occurrence to the school or daycare setting so other children can be checked.

16. Head lice are not reportable to state or local officials in most states.

Other Nonpharmacological Options

The mother has specifically asked that she not have to remove the eggs, but you may want to give her a fine-toothed comb and encourage her to do so anyway. If Timmy comes back, it will be easier to tell if nits are new or not. If you do not remove the nits, you may also be able to tell whether they are new by their distance up the shaft of the hair. The other factor here is that some schools or daycares have a no nits policy. Timmy is too young to be in school, but the topic should be explored.

Another consideration is how the issue of the neighbor, who is felt to be reinfesting the children, will be treated. Most clinicians would suggest that Timmy's family encourage them to get treatment or avoid them to avoid reinfestation.

HEALTH PROMOTION/HEALTH MAINTENANCE

If you do not have the information in the chart, you may want to ask at least a quick question about ongoing care and immunizations. If finances are a problem for this, you may be able to refer the mother to appropriate sources. If immunizations were well behind, there is no reason that you could not update them today. No matter what, you can let the mother know that Timmy will need some immunizations before school, and this will make a follow-up visit more probable.

Whether you decide to deal with it today, you need to come up with some sort of a plan to assure ongoing care.

Any anticipatory guidance done today would probably focus on safety issues such as seat belts, poisoning, and accident avoidance or protection (such as bicycle helmets). You could ask about issues like sleep, nutrition, or discipline in a very general way, and if they are a problem, encourage a follow-up visit.

FOLLOW-UP

Timmy should be seen for a 4-year well child check. Immunizations can be updated for preschool, and newer vaccines such as varicella zoster vaccine can be discussed.

References

Sanford JP, Gilbert DN, Sande MA: *The Sanford guide to antimicrobial therapy,* Dallas, 1996, Antimicrobial Therapy.

Uphold CR, Graham MV: *Clinical guidelines in family practice,* Gainesville, Fla, 1994, Barramarrae.

CASE
20

OPENING SCENARIO

Rita Davison is a 54-year-old female known to your practice for many years. She is on your schedule today for problems with blood sugar levels.

HISTORY OF PRESENT ILLNESS

"My blood sugar levels have been higher. My usual blood sugar levels are in the 100 to 150 range, and I have had several over 200 in the past week or so." You review her home glucose monitoring chart (Table 20-1).

MEDICAL HISTORY

You review her old chart and find that she has a 10-year history of Type II diabetes mellitus (DM) controlled by a 1500-calorie American Dietetic Association (ADA) diet and Micronase 2.5 mg po qd in the am. She tells you that she has been taking ibuprofen 400 mg every 4 hours or so for the past 3 or 4 days because she was playing more tennis and her back was starting to ache. Other than that, her history has been unremarkable.

MEDICATIONS

Micronase: 2.5 mg po qd in AM
Ibuprofen: 400 mg po q4h prn (over-the-counter [OTC] 200 mg tabs, two every 4 hours) taken for the past 2 weeks

PHYSICAL EXAMINATION

Vital signs: Temperature: 98.6° F; *Pulse:* 84 beats/min; *Respirations:* 24 breaths/min; *BP:* 144/86 mm Hg
Height: 5' 5"; *Weight:* 152 lb

Table **20-1** *Home Glucose Monitoring Chart for Rita Davison*

Day	Time	Result
8 days ago	7 am	210
8 days ago	4 pm	267
7 days ago	7 am	199
6 days ago	7 am	202
6 days ago	12 noon	274
6 days ago	8 pm	188
5 days ago	4 pm	211
5 days ago	8 pm	289
4 days ago	7 am	220
4 days ago	4 pm	145
3 days ago	12 noon	178
2 days ago	7 am	183
2 days ago	4 pm	244
1 day ago	7 am	197
1 day ago	4 pm	203
1 day ago	8 pm	184
This morning	7 am	190

ASSESSMENT   *Before you begin the physical examination, what are your current ideas for what may be causing her elevated blood sugar level?*

PLAN   *What is your plan for further data collection?*

Community Clinic
Jeffrey A. Eaton, NP
Joyce D. Cappiello, NP

Name:_____ DOB_____
Address_____ Date_____

Rx

"label all unless indicated"
Refill:_____ times-- Do not refill ( )

Signed:_____
DO NOT TAKE THIS TO YOUR PHARMACIST

Community Clinic
Jeffrey A. Eaton, NP
Joyce D. Cappiello, NP

Name:_____ DOB_____
Address_____ Date_____

Rx

"label all unless indicated"
Refill:_____ times-- Do not refill ( )

Signed:_____
DO NOT TAKE THIS TO YOUR PHARMACIST

Community Clinic
Jeffrey A. Eaton, NP
Joyce D. Cappiello, NP

Name:_____ DOB_____
Address_____ Date_____

Rx

"label all unless indicated"
Refill:_____ times-- Do not refill ( )

Signed:_____
DO NOT TAKE THIS TO YOUR PHARMACIST

Community Clinic
Jeffrey A. Eaton, NP
Joyce D. Cappiello, NP

Name:_____ DOB_____
Address_____ Date_____

Rx

"label all unless indicated"
Refill:_____ times-- Do not refill ( )

Signed:_____
DO NOT TAKE THIS TO YOUR PHARMACIST

CASE
20 Discussion

LEARNING ISSUES

In order to resolve this patient's problem, you will need to consider and address the following issues (you may generate additional issues as well):

- **DM monitoring**
- **Causes of hyperglycemia**

INITIAL IDEAS

Elevated blood sugar level
- Could she have an occult infection (especially an asymptomatic urinary tract infection [UTI])?
- Is she adhering to her diet?
- Has her activity level changed?
- Is she taking her medication?
- Could something be interfering with her medication?

INTERPRETATION OF CUES, PATTERNS, AND INFORMATION

There is very limited information available. However, the information that is available will guide you in the decision-making process regarding what additional data needs to be collected. Current key information includes the following:
- Changes in blood sugar levels
- Possible changes in activity pattern: Possibly an increase in playing tennis (or a decrease related to pain)
- Increase in ibuprofen intake

DIFFERENTIAL DIAGNOSIS

Your hypotheses reflect the most probable reasons that blood sugar level increase. Your top two hypotheses are probably the following:

1. Infections commonly raise blood sugar levels, and she could have occult infection (especially an asymptomatic UTI).
2. You question whether she is adhering to her diet.
   Also consider the following possibilities:
3. Is there some reason that she has stopped taking her Micronase? Is she having side effects from it? Is she developing a tolerance to the Micronase so that she needs a higher dosage?
4. Has she gained weight, and/or has her exercise pattern changed?
5. Does she have severe emotional or physical stress?
6. Is her meter in calibration?
7. Has she started another medication that interferes with Micronase?
8. Is her DM progressing so that she needs an increase in dosage?
   The following are relatively low on your differential:

9. Thyroid dysfunction: This would have to be hyperthyroidism, which is not a high probability but definitely occurs.

10. Somogyi phenomenon: This is a lower probability since blood sugar levels are not having dramatic changes, and this is usually associated with Type I DM.

You find no evidence that Motrin can cause hyperglycemia, although you do see that it can cause hypoglycemia rarely.

DIAGNOSTIC OPTIONS

Clearly your examination should be focused on those things that will help you determine why her blood sugar levels have elevated:

1. Ask her about symptoms of UTI or other infection and consider doing a urine dip.
2. Ask her if she has been adhering to her diet and consider a 24-hour (or longer) diet diary if this is still an issue.
3. Ask her about her Micronase and how she has been taking it.
4. Ask her about her weight and exercise patterns.
5. Ask her about her emotional and physical stressors.
6. Ask her what she does to assure that her meter is in calibration and check her blood sugar levels in the office or order a fasting blood sugar (FBS) to try to get a control.
7. Ask her if she has started any other prescription or nonprescription drugs.
8. Check for complications of DM, but realize that these occur from long-term changes and that the correlation to this brief change in blood sugar levels is going to be very low.
9. You will want to be sure that her ophthalmology, vascular, neuropathy, and extremity status is checked regularly.

Since the other things are relatively low on you differential, you will probably take no action on them currently, but consider them further if your current investigation does not reveal a probable cause for the changes in her blood sugar levels, or take them into consideration in your long-term plans.

Other Issues

How much control will you attempt in this patient? Uphold and Graham (1994) suggest acceptable levels as the following:

Fasting plasma glucose	Less than 140
Postprandial blood glucose	Less than 200
Glycosylated hemoglobin	Around 7

Based on these values, further investigation of Ms. Davison's blood sugar levels is appropriate.

How will you monitor her long-term control? Will you use glycosylated hemoglobin? Is fructosamine a useful test? Some clinicians suggest that fructosamine may be an alternative to the glycosylated hemoglobin. It gives a 2-week reflection of blood sugar levels and is usually less expensive than a glycosylated hemoglobin (Ham and Sloane, 1997).

HEALTH PROMOTION/HEALTH MAINTENANCE

What other health-maintenance issues should be addressed in the case of Ms. Davison (probably at a follow-up appointment)? She is 54 years old, so appropriate monitoring of cholesterol and high-density lipoproteins (HDLs), mammograms, Pap smears, immunizations, blood pressure screening (especially since she was mildly elevated today), fecal occult blood testing (FOBT), and a discussion of hormone therapy would be appropriate. She should also be encouraged to use seat belts and smoke detectors (US Preventive Services Task Force, 1996).

What will you do to help her achieve her ideal body weight range (which is about 112 to 138 lb)? She is 152 lb, so she should lose about 14 lb. A dietary referral may be helpful, and exercise is appropriate, although she may need help to choose the best approach to exercise. Exercise should be for 20 to 45 minutes at least 3 days per week (Uphold and Graham, 1994).

FOLLOW-UP

How often will you bring her back for rechecks? In general, she should be on at least an annual recall. In this particular case, some contact, either through an office visit or by phone, should take place in about 3 weeks to ensure that her blood sugars are coming under better control. As with all patients, she should be instructed to call if she has worsening symptoms or any other concerns.

References

Ham RJ, Sloane PD: *Primary care geriatrics,* St Louis, 1997, Mosby.

US Preventice Services Task Force: *Guide to clinical preventive services,* Baltimore, 1996, Williams & Wilkins.

Uphold CR, Graham MV: *Clinical guidelines in family practice,* Gainesville, Fla, 1994, Barramarrae.

OPENING SCENARIO

Jay Leeds is a 13-year-old male who presents with a 2-day history of progressive pain in his right hemiscrotum.

HISTORY OF PRESENT ILLNESS

He denies fever, dysuria, urinary frequency, or scrotal trauma. He is not sexually active. No gross hematuria. He rates the pain as a 6 on a scale of 1 to 10. He has mild nausea but no vomiting. He took acetaminophen for the pain with minimal relief. Pain is made somewhat worse by activity but is constant.

MEDICAL HISTORY

Jay has had no major illnesses.

SOCIAL HISTORY

He lives with both parents and his 8-year-old sister.

MEDICATIONS

None

ALLERGIES

None

REVIEW OF SYSTEMS

No other complaints.

ASSESSMENT   *How will the previous information guide your physical examination?*

PLAN   *Depending on that information, how will your assessment and plan differ?*

Community Clinic
Jeffrey A. Eaton, NP
Joyce D. Cappiello, NP

Name:_____ DOB_____
Address_____ Date_____

Rx

"label all unless indicated"
Refill:_____ times-- Do not refill ( )

Signed:_____
DO NOT TAKE THIS TO YOUR PHARMACIST

Community Clinic
Jeffrey A. Eaton, NP
Joyce D. Cappiello, NP

Name:_____ DOB_____
Address_____ Date_____

Rx

"label all unless indicated"
Refill:_____ times-- Do not refill ( )

Signed:_____
DO NOT TAKE THIS TO YOUR PHARMACIST

LEARNING ISSUES

In order to resolve this patient's problem, you will need to consider and address the following issues (you may generate additional issues as well):

- **Differential diagnosis of groin and testicular pain**
- **Management of office emergencies**
- **Epididymitis**
- **Cremasteric reflex**
- **Testicular torsion**
- **Torsion of testicular appendix**

INITIAL IDEAS

- Trauma
- Testicular torsion
- Infection

INTERPRETATION OF CUES, PATTERNS, AND INFORMATION (INCLUDING DIFFERENTIAL DIAGNOSIS)

Usually in the differential diagnosis process you try to cover two areas: (1) What is the most probable (common) thing this could be? and (2) What is the most serious thing this could be? In this case the answer to the first question is testicular torsion and the answer to the second question is testicular torsion.

Testicular torsion peaks at 14 years of age (Jay is 13) and usually has an abrupt onset (Jay's was a bit more gradual) with severe pain; however, it can be somewhat variable in its presentation (Jay states 6 on a scale of 1 to 10). You also do not know the status of the cremasteric reflex; if it is present, the probability of torsion drops dramatically. If there is a blue dot at the upper portion of the testicle, you have your diagnosis (torsion of the testicular appendix), but this is not always present. Torsion of the testicular appendix is similar to torsion of the entire testicle except that only a portion of the testicle is rotated.

Other Things to Consider

1. *Trauma:* Did Jay get kicked? He denies this, but he may have some reason for keeping it from you. This can still be a cause of torsion, but if the examination showed minimal tenderness of the testicle itself and bruising in the thigh area, this might explain it. Being kicked in the groin is a common problem in this age group.

2. *Incarcerated hernia:* Although he may be complaining of groin pain, on closer examination you may find that the pain is in fact more localized to the abdomen; you will still make a referral but to a general surgeon rather than a urologist. This might be more consistent with the gradual onset of pain.

3. *Epididymitis:* An epididymitis is a possibility but is uncommon in this age group. Even with a red, swollen testicle, many clinicians would want a urologist's input (some more experienced clinicians might go ahead and treat). Some clinicians say that if the pain is reduced when the scrotum is moved above the symphysis pubica, then it is probably epididymitis (Saunders and Ho, 1992). At this age an epididymitis would be associated with a urinary tract infection (UTI), so a positive urinalysis might be useful. Some clinicians believe that UTIs are more common in uncircumcised males of this age group, so that could be one more piece of data to consider. Epididymitis is often related to a sexually transmitted disease (STD), so this might raise another flag for you. Remember, the area of the epididymis may be somewhat red and painful even in a patient with torsion, so redness and pain do not rule out torsion.

4. *Torsion of the testicular appendices:* This can be difficult to discriminate from torsion, although the discomfort is usually milder.

DIAGNOSTIC OPTIONS

If on examination trauma and incarcerated hernia are ruled out (10-second examination: Is the testicle actually painful?) and the testicle is not red and hot, then an immediate urological consultation will be arranged. If there is evidence of epididymitis and the cremasteric reflex is intact, then phone consultation with a urologist might be appropriate. A significant percentage of boys with testicular torsion lose their testicle, so everything should be done to preserve the testicle and also to allow the parents the comfort that every effort was made to save the testicle. If the pain was felt to be mild and physical examination was essentially negative (including an intact cremasteric reflex), then other things like a varicocele could be considered.

THERAPEUTIC OPTIONS

Pharmacological therapy would be limited to a patient with very mild pain and an intact cremasteric reflex and would include acetaminophen. Even in that patient, serious consideration of a urological consultation should be made. Epididymitis is also possible in this adolescent, but again urological input is probably helpful.

HEALTH PROMOTION/HEALTH MANAGEMENT

Health promotion would not even be considered at this visit. After Jay has gotten this episode taken care of, a well child check (WCC) could be arranged.

FOLLOW-UP

Follow-up will be per the urologist in most cases. You will want to see Jay for a routine WCC.

References

Saunders CE, Ho MT: *Current emergency diagnosis and treatment,* Norwalk, Conn, 1992, Appleton & Lange.

After Office Hours #1
Sharon Goldstein
Age 23 years

OPENING SCENARIO

It is now the end of a busy day. Your desk has a stack of charts on it that require your attention. The chart of Sharon Goldstein has two laboratory reports attached to the front (Boxes 22-1 and 22-2).

Box 22-1 Gynecological Cytology for Sharon Goldstein from 1 Week Ago

Gynecological history:
- LMP: 10 days ago
- Pregnant: No
- Postpartum: No
- Menopause: No
- Oral contraceptives: Yes
- IUD: No
- Other: None

Slides received: 1

Gynecological source: Ectocervical/endocervical smear

Statement of adequacy: Satisfactory; endocervical component present

Gynecological diagnosis: ASCUS (atypical squamous cells of undetermined significance)

Additional comments: Inflammatory smear

Gynecological follow-up recommendation: Recommend repeat cytology or colposcopy

Ann Smith MD

Box 22-2 Genprobe for Sharon Goldstein from 1 Week Ago

Genprobe: Negative

It is often difficult for clinicians to determine the appropriate level of concern with such a report and then to explain the findings effectively to a patient. You review your note of last week on Ms. Goldstein.

What is your plan for follow-up of this Pap smear report?

Note of Sharon Goldstein's Visit of Last Week

HISTORY OF PRESENT ILLNESS

This 23-year-old single female presents for an office visit for renewal of her oral contraceptive (OC) pills. She states that she is in good health. She is happy with her contraceptive choice. She states that she does not miss pills and does not have breakthrough bleeding. She denies headaches, chest pain, abdominal pain, eye changes, or shortness of breath. Current boyfriend for 6 months. Used condoms in beginning of relationship for 1 month but no longer using protection.

MEDICAL HISTORY

No history of surgery or major medical problems. Up-to-date on usual childhood immunizations except for hepatitis. Last tetanus immunization was 9 years ago.

FAMILY MEDICAL HISTORY

MGM: 68 yr (A&W)
MGF: 71 yr (hypertension)
PGM: 64 yr (rheumatoid arthritis)
PGF: 70 yr (emphysema)
Mother: 43 yr (A&W)
Father: 49 yr (A&W)
Two sisters: 17, 19 yr (A&W)

SOCIAL HISTORY

Works in retail at the mall. Lives in apartment with roommates. Smokes 1 pack per day. Walks to work six blocks each workday and is on her feet all day. Likes to go to beach and swim on day off. Eats two meals per day. Drinks three diet colas per day. No coffee or tea. No milk; usually has cheese once a day. Vegetables are usually potatoes and a daily salad. Fruits are orange juice in the morning. Alcohol: two to three beers about three times a week. Denies drug use. Denies any concerns regarding domestic violence. Uses seatbelts.

MEDICATIONS

Ortho-Novum 7-7-7: 3 years
Daily multivitamin

ALLERGIES

Penicillin (rash)

REVIEW OF SYSTEMS

General: Feels very healthy; no complaints of fatigue

HEENT: Wears contacts; routine dental care; denies history of allergies, frequent colds, sore throats; no ear pain, hearing loss

Cardiac: No history of rheumatic fever, heart murmur, or chest pain

Respiratory: Denies shortness of breath, asthma, bronchitis

Abdomen: No complaints of heartburn, stomach problems, diarrhea, constipation, or hemorrhoids

Genitourinary: Menarche at age 12; cycles (before oral contraceptive [OC] use) 27-day, regular, 4 to 5 days of moderate flow with mild cramping; no postcoital bleeding or dyspareunia; last menstrual period (LMP) 10 days ago; no complaints of vaginal discharge, itching, burning, or odor; no history of sexually transmitted diseases (STDs) including condylomata; two previous sexual partners; four annual Pap smears all within normal limits; previous Pap smear 1 year ago; history of one urinary tract infection (UTI) 2 years ago; G0P0

Extremities: No history of fractures, sprains; no joint or muscle pain

Endocrine: Good energy level; temperature tolerances good

Neurological: Only occasional stress headache; no weakness, paresthesias, depression

PHYSICAL EXAMINATION

Vital signs: Temperature: 98.0° F; *Pulse:* 88 beats/min; *Respirations:* 18 breaths/min; *BP:* 112/66 mm Hg

HEENT: No oral lesions; good dentition

Neck: No lymphadenopathy, thyromegaly

Heart: Regular rate and rhythm; no murmurs, rubs, or gallops

Lungs: Clear to auscultation

Breasts: No masses palpated

Abdomen: No masses, tenderness; no hepatosplenomegaly

Pelvic: Vulva: no redness, discharge, lesions; vagina: no redness, discharge, lesions; cervix: pink, no visible lesions; uterus: small, smooth, firm, AV/AF; adnexa: no enlargement or tenderness

ASSESSMENT

- Healthy young female in need of continued contraception

PLAN

- Continue Ortho-Novum 7-7-7: 28 days for 1 year.
- Smoking cessation plan discussed
- Calcium carbonate 600 mg per day plus increase dietary calcium
- STD risk reduction discussed
- Genprobe taken
- Pap smear taken

LEARNING ISSUES

In order to resolve this patient's problem, you will need to consider and address the following issues (you may generate additional issues as well):

- **Bethesda System**
- **Significance of an ASCUS finding**
- **Risks factors for cervical cancer**
- **How do you communicate an ASCUS reading to a client?**
- **Appropriate follow-up**

INTERPRETATION OF CUES, PATTERNS, AND INFORMATION

The Bethesda System for Pap smear classification was developed to clarify and simplify Pap smear reports. The Class 1 through 5 system was changed to the following:

- Within normal limits
- ASCUS for abnormal smears that are not precancerous but neither are they normal; approximately 5% of Pap smears are read as ASCUS
- Low-grade squamous intraepithelial lesions (LGSIL): The term lesion was chosen because many dysplasias (up to 50%) regress spontaneously and lack any predictable progression to invasive cancer. Changes consistent with the human papillomavirus (HPV) but without evidence of any dysplasia whatsoever are also included in this category. Low-grade lesions can be assessed for additional risk factors, and then the decision can be made to either schedule a follow-up Pap smear in 3 to 6 months or schedule for immediate colposcopy.
- High-grade squamous intraepithelial lesions (HGSIL): All smears termed *high grade* need immediate colposcopy.

What is significant in her history and physical examination that may have bearing on this abnormal Pap smear? The first has to do with the prevalence and incidence of cervical cancer. The National Cancer Institute's Surveillance, Epidemiology, and End Results (SEER) show that in the United States the incidence of cervical intraepithelial lesions (CILs) and invasive cervical cancer has been increasing in young women.

The increase in cervical lesions does not seem to be due to a decline in women having Pap smears because the rate of screening has significantly risen in the past 2 decades. Many researchers feel that the increase in diagnosis of cervical cancers is due to the HPV. Genital HPV is found in 95% of all cervical cancers, but this does not mean that it is the cause of the cancer since it may merely co-occur. On the other hand, in vitro studies do suggest a causative role. Because HPV is not a reportable STD, the estimates of the incidence of HPV vary widely. Possibly upwards of 45% of the population between the ages of 18 and 35 harbor the virus. Ms. Goldstein is not aware of any exposure to HPV, but if she was exposed to the virus and did not develop visible condylomata, she would have no way of knowing this.

Be mindful that this client is a smoker. Smoking is thought to be a cofactor, perhaps because smoking makes it more difficult for the immune system to clear the HPV virus.

Another significant finding is that she does not have any history of Pap smear abnormalities in her four previous pap smears. Right away you can feel somewhat relaxed because cervical cancer generally, but not always, takes years to develop. It is possible but unlikely that a patient would have a normal reading one year and an invasive cancer the following year. Her history also tells us that she is likely to return for scheduled follow-up visits.

What is the significance of the inflammation detected on her Pap smear? This can be difficult to ascertain. Often, this finding is due to chlamydia, gonorrhea, or a vaginitis, such as monilia, trichomonas, or bacterial vaginosis. In this case you essentially have ruled out chlamydia or gonorrhea with the negative Genprobe report. Vaginitis seems unlikely because Ms. Goldstein had no complaints of vaginal symptoms, nor are there any findings on physical examination to support this diagnosis. Should she be advised to return anyway for a more thorough assessment for vaginitis? It is a tough call and will depend on your level of suspicion for vaginitis during the examination 2 weeks ago. With whatever plan you choose, advise her to call you if she develops any symptoms.

Is her OC use a cofactor in the development of cervical cancer? Research has been conflicting. Some studies do not support OCs as a risk factor. Others have found an increased risk in long-term pill users. One theory is that women on the pill may be more sexually active and therefore more exposed to HPV. The increased cervical ectopy (visible transformation zone of the squamocolumnar junction) caused by OCs may provide a larger surface area susceptible to potential infection, or perhaps OCs increase the risk by causing folate deficiences or altering host immunological responses (Carson, 1997).

THERAPEUTIC OPTIONS

1. Many clinicans will suggest a repeat Pap smear in 3 to 6 months after a single ASCUS reading, especially in a woman such as Ms. Goldstein with a negative history for prior Pap smear abnormalites. Some providers may choose to schedule a colposcopy right away if the client has a history of abnormal Pap smears or if there is concern that she will have difficulty returning for follow-up. Currently there is no appropriate evidence-based research upon which to base recommendations. Rather, guidelines represent the clinical expertise based on data currently available (American Society for Colposcopy and Cervical Pathology, 1996). This society has published the following guidelines for follow-up of ASCUS Pap smears:

a. Repeat Pap smear, *or*

b. Colposcopy all women with an ASCUS Pap smear, *or*

c. Management on the basis of an adjunctive test, such as cerviography and HPV DNA testing: The drawback to this regimen is that most primary care offices are not performing these tests, so a referral is necessary and often a colposcopy is still needed, *or*

d. Management by subdividing ASCUS into low- and high-risk groups: This approach seems unworkable to many and lacks any prospective studies to determine its validity.

These guidelines have not particularly helped to clarify options in ASCUS Pap smear follow-up. Appropriate follow-up still relies on assessing the risk factors for a patient and planning future care in conjunction with a well-informed patient.

It is advisable to wait a minimum of 3 months before repeating the Pap smear. If taken sooner, there is a higher rate of false-negative findings since whenever a Pap smear is taken, cells are disrupted by the spatula and endocervical brush. Consequently, it takes time for these cells to regenerate. You can optimize the subsequent Pap smear by advising the client to avoid inserting anything in the vagina, including tampons, for 48 hours before the Pap smear. This will serve to decrease any inflammation. If possible, schedule the Pap smear for the latter half of the menstrual cycle, although this is often not feasible. Avoid sampling during the menstrual period. Also, give a history and report any clinical findings on the Pap smear slip to assist the cytologist or pathologist in interpreting the findings.

Follow-up of the abnormal smear is very important. If the smear returns with a second ASCUS reading, more aggressive follow-up is usually recommended. Colposcopy is the next step in the diagnostic process, then biopsies if indicated, and then based on these findings, an appropriate treatment plan is developed. It is important to have a thorough office system for Pap smear follow-up. If the next Pap smear returns within normal limits, then it is appropriate to repeat the Pap smear every 4 to 6 months for 2 years until there have been three consecutive negative smears (Kurman, 1994). Assuming a false-negative rate of 20% with Pap smear interpretation, this number of repeat Pap smears should reduce the risk of missed disease to acceptable levels.

Current Pap smears have a high false-negative rate ranging from 10% to 40%. New technology is being researched constantly to improve accuracy rates. One new system is a computer-assisted inspection of a slide prepared in the usual fashion. Another technique called the Thin Prep uses a new collection system that separates mucus and debris from the cervical cells, and then the computer scans the remaining cells. Both tests may help reduce the false-positive and false-negative rates but will add significantly to the cost of screening for cervical cancer. They may be more appropriate for follow-up Pap smear testing rather than for initial screening in low-risk women.

2. Reenforce a smoking cessation plan.

3. Any change of her contraceptive method seems premature at this point. The research is not clear on the role of OCs and the development of cervical cancer, and the ASCUS reading does not create a strong suspicion of serious cervical abnormalities at this time. Also, prevention of a pregnancy remains a priority in her health care plan.

4. Reenforce safe sex practices. Safe sex practices will decrease exposure to STDs, a possible risk factor in the development of cervical neoplasias.

5. Continue daily multivitamin with at least 400 mg of folate: There is speculation that low folate levels may be a risk factor in developing cervical abnormalities.

References

American Society for Colposcopy and Cervical Pathology: Management guidelines for follow-up of atypical squamous cells of undetermined significance (ASCUS)' The Colposcopist 27(1):1, 1996.

Carson S: Human papillomatous virus infection update: impact on women's health, Nurs Pract 22(4):24, 1997.

Kurman T: Interim guidelines for management of abnormal cervical cytology, JAMA 271(23):1866, 1994.

CASE
23

OPENING SCENARIO

The office staff tell you that Phil Noonan is on the phone, and he is really upset since he just "filled the toilet bowl with blood." They want to know whether you want to send him to the emergency room (ER) or talk to him on the phone?

Depending on your decision, refer to the appropriate section of the Case Discussion.

23 *Discussion*

LEARNING ISSUES

In order to resolve this patient's problem, you will need to consider and address the following issues (you may generate additional issues as well):

- **Decision making when on call**
- **Causes of rectal bleeding in a 38-year-old man**
- **Relationship and communication between primary care providers and the ER**
- **Reimbursement issues for emergencies**

ER OPTION

"Hi, this is Bill Leonard in the ER. I have Phil Noonan here, and he said that you advised him to come in. His vital signs are stable. He's pretty much asymptomatic right now and feels fine. His hemoglobin and hematocrit are fine. I did see a small- to moderate-size anal fissure, which could have caused his bleeding. I told him to make a visit to your office next week and that you could discuss further workup. Is there anything else you wanted on him?"

Things you might think about at this point are as follows:

- Will Mr. Noonan perceive that the ER visit was the right thing to do?
- Did you call the ER ahead of time to let them know Mr. Noonan was coming and why? Did the ER perceive this referral as an appropriate use of their time?
- Could you have handled things without an ER visit? What would have been the relative advantages and disadvantages?
- Will Mr. Noonan have any problems with insurance reimbursement for this visit?

There are no definite answers to these questions since most of them involve individual perceptions. The insurance issue will be based on his insurance coverage. There is value, however, in thinking about these issues and considering your options.

PHONE CALL OPTION

Your first decision will be whether something needs to be done on an emergency basis. All phone calls come down to deciding among six options:

- This is an emergency and an ambulance should be called.
- The patient should go to the emergency room to be evaluated.
- You will see the patient in the office.
- The patient needs a medication; you will call something into the pharmacy.
- The patient needs an over-the-counter medicine and/or a treatment that can be done at home.
- This is probably a variation of normal, but if the patient has other problems or concerns, have him or her call you back.

You ask Mr. Noonan how he feels in general, and then you ask some specific questions. His response is that he is feeling okay. He denies being weak, dizzy, or lightheaded. Mr. Noonan also denies a sensation of rapid pulse or palpitations. He takes his own pulse and it is 92 beats/min. In light of his anxiety, this may not be related to blood loss. He does not seem to be exceptionally unstable. What will you do now? Some reasons for rectal bleeding in a 38-year-old man would include the following:

- Diverticulosis
- Angiodysplasia
- Neoplasm
- Inflammatory bowel disease
- Ischemic colitis
- Infectious colitis
- Anorectal diseases such as internal hemorrhoids
- Anal fissure
- Foreign body trauma

Only rarely will any of these cause significant bleeding. The decision at this point will usually come down to patient and clinician comfort. If either are still quite nervous about this bleeding, then an ER visit can be suggested. An ambulance is probably not necessary however. An office visit for an examination is an option, but laboratory studies will be more limited. A complete blood count at the laboratory could be ordered without an ER visit, and this may provide enough reassurance. Some clinicians would be comfortable telling Mr. Noonan to take his own pulse in about 15 minutes and call them back. If it returns to normal and he has no further episodes of bleeding, he could be seen tomorrow.

Handling phone calls and being on call require a clinician to make decisions with very limited information. Safety issues must be balanced with the need to avoid an inappropriate level of alarm and the accompanying reimbursement issues. These issues of course involve insurance and Health Maintenance Organizations (HMOs), but the large bill that a patient may get from an inappropriate ER visit must also be considered.

There is no clear answer in Mr. Noonan's case. The clinician must make a decision on the recommended course and then be willing to live with that decision.

After Office Hours #3
Annie Littlefield
Age 2 1/2 years

OPENING SCENARIO

A phone call is received from the mother of a 2 1/2-year-old girl known to your practice. Her mother is hysterical, stating that her daughter just passed what looked like a 12-inch long strand of spaghetti in the toilet. She states that she knows food is not passed undigested and wonders what this could be. Is it a worm?

MEDICAL HISTORY

A review of the records indicates that this child has been followed since birth in your office. There is no history of any major illnesses. Annie is up-to-date on all immunizations and has had all her routine check-ups. Her last well child check was 3 months ago with normal growth and development.

MEDICATIONS

Fluoride drops

ALLERGIES

None

ASSESSMENT *Please indicate the problems or issues you have identified that will guide your care (preferably in list form):*

PLAN *Please list your plans for addressing each of the problems or issues in your assessment:*

CASE

24 Discussion

INITIAL IDEAS

The first clinical decision is how to manage this so late in the day. Does the child need to be seen? Is laboratory confirmation essential?

IDENTIFICATION OF CUES, PATTERNS, AND INFORMATION (INCLUDING DIFFERENTIAL DIAGNOSIS)

The differential diagnosis consists primarily of various parasitic infections, with roundworm at the top of the list. Pinworm can be ruled out since they are small, not 12 inches long. Trichuriases (whipworm) are identified by ova in the stool, but the actual worm is not passed. With tapeworm, the eggs or individual segments (proglottides) are passed but not an entire, intact worm. Adult roundworm *(Ascaris lumbricoides)* is the only worm that can be seen in stool.

Specific history questions need to focus on the presence of abdominal pain and cramping, loss of appetite, weight loss, diarrhea, or vomiting. Ascariasis infections are generally asymptomatic but can have rare complications. A brief history can rule out the rare complication of obstruction by focusing on bowel habits over the past few days.

If the mother has saved the worm and you are comfortable identifying roundworm, then have her bring it to you in the office. Otherwise, advise her to take the specimen directly to the laboratory for identification. Since it is so late in the day, a result may not be available until tomorrow.

If the mother can bring the worm to your office, have her bring the child along. A quick weight check will rule out weight loss, and your observational skills will rule out a listless, sick child. Remember that you have a chart in front of you of a healthy 2 1/2 year old seen regularly by you with a normal pattern of growth and development. She was last seen 3 months ago. You can focus on the nature of roundworm infections and management rather than on an extensive physical examination.

If the mother cannot bring the worm to your office, advise her to take the specimen to the hospital laboratory this evening. When the result is available tomorrow, you must decide if you can manage this over the phone or have the mother and daughter come in. Ideally, bring the mother and daughter into the office so you can sit down face to face and educate and reassure them about roundworm. However, with a negative history of present illness, you could manage this case over the phone if the mother cannot get in, provided you can reassure her about transmission, effectiveness of treatment, and the frequency with which this occurs.

THERAPEUTIC OPTIONS

The following are commonly used anthelmintic medications:

1. First choice: Mebendazole 100 mg bid x 3 days (chewable); this drug has not been well studied in children under 2 years of age

2. Second choice: Thiabendazole bid x 2 days (dose is based on weight)

3. Third choice: Pyrantel pamoate, single dose; may not be available in most pharmacies since it comes in a large quantity and is not cost effective for pharmacies to stock

If there are other young children in the family, you will need to decide if you think there is a high likelihood of concurrent infection, and if so, order stool testing or treat empirically.

Educational

Educate the mother that because roundworm eggs can be in the soil and children often put their fingers in the mouth, this is a fairly common infection. It can also be present on garden produce, so advise that all vegetables be carefully washed.

FOLLOW-UP

Generally no specific follow-up is indicated if the child continues to feel fine.

Day TWO

OPENING SCENARIO

Kerry Bailey is a 15-year-old female in your office for a sports physical examination. She went to soccer practice yesterday, and the coach told her that she could not come back until she had her physical.

HISTORY OF PRESENT ILLNESS

"I have good exercise tolerance. I have no pain, shortness of breath, dizziness, or any other symptoms associated with exercise currently or in the past." Ms. Bailey has no current illnesses. She is only here for a sports physical examination.

MEDICAL HISTORY

No hospitalizations, surgeries, or major illnesses. Does not know whether she has had chicken pox. Immunization record is shown in Table 25-1.

Table 25-1 Immunization Record for Kerry Bailey

VACCINE	DATE	INITIALS	NOTES
DPT	2 mo	MDO	
DPT	4 mo	KJ	
DPT	6 mo	SP	
DPT	18 mo	SS	
DPT	5 yr	SS	
Td			
OPV	2 mo	MDO	
OPV	4 mo	KJ	
OVP	6 mo	SP	
OPV	5 yr	SS	
MMR	15 mo	MDO	
MMR			
HBV			
HBV			
HBV			
Hib			
Hib			
Hib			
Hib			

FAMILY MEDICAL HISTORY

No history of diabetes mellitus (DM) or cardiac problems. No history of sudden death.

SOCIAL HISTORY

Ms. Bailey is a student, and she is happy in school. Feels she is doing well (B+/A- grade average). Plays soccer. Does not feel excessively stressed at home. Youngest of two children. Brother is in his first year of college. She denies alcohol or drug intake and sexual activity.

MEDICATIONS

Multivitamin qd

ALLERGIES

None

REVIEW OF SYSTEMS

General: Denies night sweats, swelling
HEENT: Denies diplopia, blurring, hearing impairment; no history of head injury, sore throats
Cardiac: Denies chest pain; no history of murmur
Respiratory: Denies shortness of breath, dyspnea on exertion, paroxysmal nocturnal dyspnea
Gastrointestinal: Denies anorexia, nausea, vomiting, constipation, diarrhea, black or clay colored stools
Genitourinary: Denies dysuria
Hematological: Denies hematuria and excessive bruising; denies syncope
Musculoskeletal: Denies joint and back pain

PHYSICAL EXAMINATION

Vital signs: Temperature: 98.2° F; *Pulse:* 82 beats/min; *Respirations:* 20 breaths/min *BP:* 96/56 mm Hg
Height: 5' 6"; *Weight:* 133 lb; *Vision:* 20/20 uncorrected
Skin: No lesions or rashes apparent
HEENT: Head is normocephalic, atraumatic; pupils equal, round, and reactive to light; extraocular movements intact; tympanic membranes are observable without excessive cerumen; nares are patent without redness or exudate; throat is noninjected; tongue is midline; palate rises symmetrically; teeth in adequate repair
Neck: Supple without thyromegaly, adenopathy, or carotid bruits

Heart: Regular rate and rhythm; no rubs or gallops; a Grade II/VI vibratory early systolic murmur is heard at the third left ICS LSB with the patient in a sitting position; murmur is decreased with the patient supine; when Ms. Bailey performs Valsalva's maneuver, the murmur diminishes but does not disappear

Lungs: Clear to auscultation and percussion

Abdomen: Soft, nontender; no hepatosplenomegaly

Extremities: No cyanosis, clubbing, or edema; reflexes are 2+ at the biceps, triceps, brachioradialis, patellar and Achilles; no Babinski signs are present; strength and sensation are symmetrical; full range of motion is present in neck, shoulders, elbows, wrists, hands, back, hips, knees, and ankles

ASSESSMENT   *Please indicate the problems or issues you have identified that will guide your care (preferably in list form):*

PLAN   *Please list your plans for addressing each of the problems or issues in your assessment:*

Community Clinic
Jeffrey A. Eaton, NP
Joyce D. Cappiello, NP

Name:_____ DOB_____
Address_____ Date_____

Rx

"label all unless indicated"
Refill:_____ times-- Do not refill ( )

Signed:_____
DO NOT TAKE THIS TO YOUR PHARMACIST

Community Clinic
Jeffrey A. Eaton, NP
Joyce D. Cappiello, NP

Name:_____ DOB_____
Address_____ Date_____

Rx

"label all unless indicated"
Refill:_____ times-- Do not refill ( )

Signed:_____
DO NOT TAKE THIS TO YOUR PHARMACIST

CASE
25 *Discussion*

INITIAL IDEAS

One of the keys with this sports physical is remembering the setting. This may be your chance to do an evaluation of this adolescent, and since you have 1/2 hour, you should probably take advantage of the opportunity.

There are several issues for Ms. Bailey:

- Fitness for sports
- Murmur
- Immunization status
- Risk issues related to being an adolescent (can use HEADSS: Home, Education, Activities, Drugs, Sex, Suicide)
- Drugs and/or alcohol
- Sexual issues
- Depression and/or suicide
- Dietary issues

INTERPRETATION OF CUES, PATTERNS, AND INFORMATION (INCLUDING DIFFERENTIAL DIAGNOSIS)

Fitness for Sports

Sports physicals in general have a very low yield of problems. Many clinicians would do additional musculoskeletal screening, including the Two-Minute Orthopedic Examination (Table 25-2).

History questions pertaining to previous fainting or family history of sudden death are usually recognized as the most important with the current state of knowledge.

Soccer is a contact sport. Are you concerned about her Tanner stage? Many references recommend that Tanner staging be included in a preparticipation sports evaluation. The evidence that Tanner staging is an accurate predictor of injury is quite limited, and in practice, clinicians often do not exclude students from sports on the basis of Tanner stage.

Murmur

You need to decide whether this represents an innocent, functional, or pathological murmur. It has many characteristics of a Still's murmur, and additional assessment might support or dispute this.

Table **25-2** *Two-Minute Orthopedic Examination*

INSTRUCTIONS	OBSERVATIONS
Stand facing examiner	Acromioclavicular joints; general habitus
Look at ceiling, floor, over both shoulders; touch ears to shoulders	Cervical spine motion
Shrug shoulders (examiner resists)	Trapezius strength
Abduct shoulders 90° (examiner resists at 90°)	Deltoid strength
Full external rotation of arms	Shoulder motion
Flex and extend elbows	Elbow motion
Arms at sides, elbows at 90° flexed; pronate and supinate wrists	Elbow and wrist motion
Spread fingers; make fist	Hand or finger motion and deformities
Tighten (contract) quadriceps; relax quadriceps	Symmetry and knee effusion; ankle effusion
"Duck walk" four steps (away from examiner with buttocks on heels)	Hip, knee, and ankle motion
Back to examiner	Shoulder symmetry, scoliosis
Knees straight, touch toes	Scoliosis, hip motion, hamstring tightness
Raise up on toes, raise heels	Calf symmetry, leg strength

From American Academy of Pediatrics: *Sports medicine: health care for young athletes,* Elk Grove Village, Ill, 1991, American Academy of Pediatrics.

If it becomes louder in a supine position, it lacks radiation into the carotids, and the character is vibratory, some clinicians are comfortable naming this a Still's murmur. A Still's murmur is a low-pitched, systolic ejection murmur. It is best heard at about the second intercostal space on the left sternal border. It is grade II or less and is often described as vibratory in character. A Still's murmur is often identified first in toddlerhood (Algranati, 1992).

In consideration of a functional murmur (a problem that changes flow rates but is not related to cardiac structure), a further history looking for menorrhagia or other risk factors or symptoms of anemia could be done. Thyroid disease is also a possibility, and if history supported it, a thyroid-stimulating hormone (TSH) blood test would be reasonable. The most dangerous etiology of a pathological murmur in this case would be hypertrophic cardiomyopathy (HCM), also known as idiopathic hypertrophic subaortic stenosis (IHSS), although this murmur is more commonly right sternal border. HCM has been associated with sudden death in young people. Mitral valve prolapse (MVP) has also been associated with a slightly higher incidence of sudden death. The theoretical risks need to be balanced with the fact that at least half of all children (and some clinicians say all) will have a murmur at some point.

There are several choices if you decide to further evaluate this murmur.

1. *Electrocardiogram (ECG) and chest x-ray examination (CXR):* Although recommended by many pediatric texts because echocardiograms are expensive and not readily available, ECG and CXR provide limited information, and further imaging will probably be needed. Think about what you would see on an ECG or CXR that could cause a murmur. Hypertrophy of the heart might support a diagnosis of HCM, but the diagnosis could not be made on the basis of that finding.

2. *Echocardiogram:* Echocardiogram is the recommendation of most internal medicine books if evaluating adults because it gives a 95% sensitive picture of the structure of the heart.

3. *Cardiology referral:* Some cardiologists prefer this since often diagnostic testing may be avoided altogether.

In the case of Ms. Bailey, the following factors might contribute to a decision to use one of the diagnostic options previously mentioned: (1) not feeling absolutely sure that the murmur is innocent, and (2) the patient's age of 15, which means that murmurs should be becoming less frequent. An inexperienced clinician might discuss the issue with another more seasoned provider. Nurse practitioner practice will vary based on state law and clinician experience.

The issue of bacterial endocarditis prophylaxis makes things a little more complicated since there is a theoretical risk if there are any cardiac structural anomalies (thus making it more important to detect these anomalies). There has not, however, been research using placebo-controlled trials to support prophylaxis, and the risks and benefits of antibiotics have to be considered in this decision (Koda-Kimble and Young, 1995).

Informed consent may be an issue here as well. After explaining the presence of the murmur to Ms. Bailey and her parents, if your explanation that this was probably an innocent murmur seemed of concern to them, then further evaluation could be considered. Whether to clear her for sports would depend on your assessment of the murmur.

Immunization Status

Since Ms. Bailey is 15 years old, she may be due for a tetanus immunization. It is due before preschool and every 10 years. She is also reaching the age that she will be considering becoming sexually active soon, if she is not currently, thus it would be appropriate to let her know that the hepatitis B vaccine is available. She may also face a remote risk of exposure to blood or body fluids related to sports. She could also be informed that the varicella zoster virus (VZV) vaccine is available, although she would need two doses, and the cost would be about $100. A VZV titer would give you her current immunity status. She may need another measles vaccine before going back to school, but this varies from state to state.

The issue of the influenza vaccine in children is somewhat controversial. The American Academy of Pediatrics makes recommendations only for children who are at high risk for complications, such as from chronic illnesses. There are other sources that recommend a more liberal approach. In fact the Centers for Disease Control and Prevention (1996) say that anyone who wishes to lessen his or her chance of acquiring influenza vaccine may be vaccinated. At this age, loss of school time and sports activities can be very problematic, so the influenza vaccine may be appropriate.

Risk Issues Related to Being an Adolescent

Most state laws provide confidentiality in your relationships with adolescents for sexually transmitted diseases (STDs), pregnancy, and contraception issues. There is a variation, however, among clinicians in their communication with the adolescent and his or her parents regarding other aspects of the adolescent's health status. Some clinicians consider the relationship with the adolescent confidential for all issues and will not discuss anything with the parents without the adolescent's consent. Other clinicians feel that since the adolescent is a minor and parents are responsible for them that all health issues (except STDs, pregnancy, and contraception) should be discussed with the parents. A clinician must let the parents and the adolescent know what his or her practices are at the beginning of the relationship. Parents may still need to provide consent for treatment, but if the parents have agreed that the adolescent may discuss things with you confidentially, this may open up communication.

1. *Drugs and/or alcohol:* There are many ways to approach this, and each provider must find an approach that fits that individual. One approach is to ask adolescents if they have tried drugs or alcohol. If they say yes, then current usage can be explored. If they say no, asking whether a lot of their friends do and how they feel about drug and alcohol use can provide an insight into their ideas. The risks associated with being around others who are drinking (such as riding in a car) can also be discussed.

2. *Sexual issues:* Adolescents can be asked if they have questions about sexual issues and if they know about condoms and safer sex. You must make decisions at this point about how much you feel you need to "pry." An empathetic statement like, "It is really hard to decide what to do about sexual issues when you are 16" may provide an opening for discussion. This is an area where the relationship and beliefs of the provider and patient will make a world of difference in the character of the discussion. Adolescents often provide a response that either implicitly or explicitly gives some idea whether they are sexually active. One other question would be to ask is, "Do you have

any questions about how to prevent pregnancy?" If you deem it appropriate, then a statement such as, "I do not know if you need to know this now, but someday you may, and there are things we can do the next day to prevent pregnancy even if you did not use contraception or if a condom breaks." You can direct the adolescent to call and tell her that medication can be prescribed.

3. *Depression and/or suicide:* This is again an area where the individual clinician will find an approach with which he or she is comfortable. One approach would be to ask, "Do you feel depressed or sad a lot?" You should not hesitate to bring up suicide, but it may not seem appropriate in every case.

4. *Dietary issues:* Based on Ms. Bailey's height and weight, you do not have to be concerned about anorexia, but of course bulimia needs to be considered since bulimic patients are often in the normal weight range. History could provide clues, and a question about her level of satisfaction with her weight may give some insight.

FOLLOW-UP

Ms. Bailey should return when she is sexually active or when she needs her next screening examination for sports or college entry.

References

American Academy of Pediatrics: *Sports medicine: health care for young athletes,* Elk Grove Village, Ill, 1991, American Academy of Pediatrics.

Algranati PS: *The pediatric patient: an approach to history and physical examination,* Baltimore, 1992, Williams & Wilkins.

Centers for Disease Control and Prevention: *Epidemiology and prevention of vaccine preventable diseases,* ed 3, Atlanta, Ga, 1996, Centers for Disease Control and Prevention.

Koda-Kimble MA, Young L: *Applied therapeutics: the clinical use of drugs,* Vancouver, Wash, 1995, Applied Therapeutics.

C A S E
26

9:00 AM
Deborah Pierce
Age 39 years

OPENING SCENARIO

Deborah Pierce is a 39-year-old female in your office with a 3-week history of back pain.

HISTORY OF PRESENT ILLNESS

"My back pain has been bothering me for about 3 weeks. I don't remember a specific episode initiating the onset. I work as toll taker on the turnpike, and this aggravates the pain. The pain is across my entire low back and right buttock, going down into the back of my right thigh. I have no numbness or tingling." Ms. Pierce has tried Motrin 800 mg q6h that she had at home for dysmenorrhea, and "it has not done anything." There is some relief with lying down and putting ice on her back; then it is just a dull ache. Pain is a 7 on a scale of 1 to 10 when she is moving around. Pain is at its worst later in the day after she works. Never had back pain like this before.

MEDICAL HISTORY

Kidney stone 2 years ago. Treated with lithotripsy.

SOCIAL HISTORY

Lives with boyfriend. One glass of wine each day. Smokes 1/2 pack per day.

MEDICATIONS

Motrin: 800 mg q6h

ALLERGIES

Percocet makes her sick to her stomach.

REVIEW OF SYSTEMS

Gastrointestinal: Denies nausea, vomiting
Genitourinary: Denies dysuria, hematuria

PHYSICAL EXAMINATION

Vital signs: Temperature: 98.4° F; *Pulse:* 88 beats/min; *Respirations:* 22 breaths/min; *BP:* 142/84 mm Hg

Height: 5' 6"; *Weight:* 224 lb
Painful area: No external lesions or masses; tension of paraspinal muscles palpable; no excessive warmth; generally tender over low back; no tenderness specific to costovertebral angle
Gross sensory testing: Sensation present and normal along the L_4, L_5, and S_1 dermatomes
Straight leg raises (SLRs): Pain occurs in low back on right at 30 degrees, but there is no pain in the legs; pain occurs on left at 45 degrees with some pain in the posterior thigh; no shooting pain or paresthesias into calf on raising her head during SLRs
Extremities: Reflexes 2+ at patella bilaterally, 1+ at Achilles bilaterally, no Babinski signs present; range of motion: sidebending 30 degrees bilaterally, flexion 20 degrees, extension 5 degrees, rotation 10 degrees bilaterally; strength testing: 4/5 bilaterally with foot dorsiflexion and plantar flexion; gait: antalgic (obviously painful) and slow but symmetrical and steady; able to do heel walk and toe walk
Genitourinary: Urine dip negative (SG 1.015)

ASSESSMENT   *Please indicate the problems or issues you have identified that will guide your care (preferably in list form):*

PLAN   *Please list your plans for addressing each of the problems or issues in your assessment:*

CASE
26 *Discussion*

LEARNING ISSUES

In order to resolve this patient's problem, you will need to consider and address the following issues (you may generate additional issues as well):

- How do you perform systematic analysis of the chief complaint in an episodic visit (back pain in this case)?
- What can cause low back pain (LBP)?
- What physical examination techniques are appropriate to perform in a patient with LBP?
- Is there an indication for laboratory or x-ray testing in this case? What are the criteria used in making this decision?
- What type of pain management is indicated? When should you suspect a "symptom magnifier," and how do you assess for drug seeking behavior?
- What modification of activity, if any, is indicated? If Ms. Pierce requests a note for her employer regarding modification of work, how would you address this? What are the issues involved in worker compensation cases?
- What type of follow-up care is indicated? What additional treatment modalities might be employed?

INITIAL IDEAS

- Lumbosacral strain or sprain
- Herniated nucleus pulposus (HNP)
- Nephrolithiasis or ureterolithiasis
- Greater than ideal body weight (IBW), which may contribute to lumbosacral strain or sprain

INTERPRETATION OF CUES, PATTERNS, AND INFORMATION

Are the appropriate things included in the history and physical examination? Clearly, with an episodic visit such as this, what is not included is almost as important as what is included. The usual objective then is to be focused around the presenting problem. If there are other issues that need to be addressed, they should be identified, and plans should be made for later follow-up.

The presenting problem in this case is a 3-week history of back pain. This is a first episode, and it has not been responsive to relatively high-dose nonsteroidal antiinflammatory drugs (NSAIDs) (3200 mg of ibuprofen/day). She has no real radicular signs (by definition, pain must go past the knee to be radicular since several muscles travel from the low back down the leg). She had a kidney stone before, so you should keep that in mind in planning your examination, but the probability of

169

that being the cause of her pain is lowered by the lack of nausea, vomiting, or blood in her urine. This could be drug-seeking behavior, but a complaint of intolerance to Percocet would not be common in that type of case. She probably needed Percocet when she had her kidney stone.

The treatment for LBP is essentially the same no matter what the causative agent unless the following are true:

1. It has not responded to treatment in 4 weeks.
2. There is severe and/or progressive evidence of neurological involvement (especially bowel and bladder involvement).
3. There is major evidence of cancer or systemic disease such as weight loss. Recommendations from the Agency for Health Care Policy and Research (AHCPR, 1994) are for history findings to rule out this area.

The objective of the history and physical examination then is to try to determine if treatment other than the usual is needed and to establish a baseline for evaluation of treatment effectiveness. The following should always be included as part of your examination:

1. *Inspection:* Inspection is necessary to rule out a herpetic or other origin to the pain as well as to more accurately describe the affected area. If skin lesions are present, the differential diagnosis will be quite different.

2. *Palpation:* Palpation is necessary to determine the exact location of the pain and identify any trigger points (or areas of "somatic dysfunction" as defined by osteopathic medicine). In addition, especially with this patient's history, palpation may be helpful to determine whether her history of kidney stones is a factor. A costovertebral angle (CVA) "punch" may be too much for a patient with this level of pain, but the CVA area should be palpated or gently percussed to determine whether the area of pain is consistent with kidney origin.

3. *SLRs:* This is a very helpful test in patients with LBP, but caution must be exercised to not overinterpret this test. An SLR positive at less than 45 degrees can be indicative of a disc problem (HNP), but muscular pain in the back of the leg can give an artifactual result. The dura must then be stressed by dorsiflexing the foot or raising the head. Part of the issue here is to understand what is meant by a positive SLR test. Jarvis (1992) and Goroll, May, and Mulley (1995) define it as reproducing radicular pain. Hoppenfeld (1976) says that it can be positive with LBP, and then dorsiflexion or some other maneuver to stretch the dura (such as raising the head) should be carried out to determine whether the problem is radicular or muscular.

4. *Range of motion testing:* Range of motion testing is very helpful in relation to determining progress. In addition, patients with altered range of motion in sidebending are more apt to be "symptom magnifiers," although this can occur in patients with "real" back pain as well.

5. *Reflexes:* If there is an impairment of reflexes, then the case for neurological involvement is strengthened. Again, caution of overinterpretation must be exercised. Achilles reflexes often require augmentation to be normal (2+), and Ms. Pierce's level of pain would probably preclude that. Symmetry is a key factor.

6. *Strength and sensory testing:* This is an excellent indicator of neurological involvement, but pain may limit strength somewhat. Symmetry is a key factor here as well. One of your most important rule-outs is cauda equina syndrome. This is characterized by saddle numbness and bladder and/or bowel changes. Thus your history should include these areas.

7. Other areas that are appropriate to include are as follows:
   a. *Gait:* Gait is helpful to determine the level of function. You can also use toe walking (S1) and heel walking (L5) to assess strength in specific dermatomes.
   b. *Abdominal examination:* Although it is somewhat unlikely, abdominal aortic aneurysm can present with LBP.
   c. *Dip urine:* Since there was no blood in the urine, this decreases the probability of kidney infection or stone.

d. *Patrick's test, or fabere (flexion, abduction, external rotation) sign:* This is also a test that can help point toward sacroiliac (SI) or piriformis muscle problems. SI range of motion could also be tested.

8. The following tests are usually low-yield tests, and you should evaluate the need for them carefully before taking the time to do them.

a. *Peripheral pulses* are quick to check, and you can do them while checking lower-extremity sensation. The probability of detecting occlusive disease in this patient is not high.

b. Although Goroll, May, and Mulley (1995) and Kelley (1994) recommend a *rectal, groin, and pelvic examination* on every patient with low back pain, in practice many practitioners do not find these to be helpful in this population. If cauda equina syndrome is suspected, doing a rectal examination to check for tone or specific sensory testing in the pelvic area could be helpful, but history is often enough to point you away from this problem (especially with no real lower extremity symptoms). Thus each clinician must make a decision regarding the extent of examination needed.

c. *Thigh or calf circumferences* in a person with a 3-week history of back pain are not apt to have changed. In a long-term back pain patient, muscle atrophy may occur, so some clinicians will check these for baseline.

DIFFERENTIAL DIAGNOSIS

1. *Cauda equina syndrome:* If bowel or bladder changes or saddle paresthesias are present, cauda equina syndrome should be suspected.

2. *LBP:* This is probably due to lumbosacral sprain and/or strain.

3. For those who interpreted the *SLR test* as reproducing radicular pain (although Ms. Pierce really did not have it before), the assessment could be LBP, probably caused by HNP.

4. *Spinal stenosis* is also a possibility with bilateral lower extremity symptoms. If 1+ ankle jerks and 4/5 strength were interpreted as decreased, this should have been a diagnostic consideration.

5. *Nephrolithiasis or ureterolithiasis* are not high probabilities based on the quality of the pain and the lack of hematuria, but if the pain persisted or the patient became febrile, this could be revisited.

DIAGNOSTIC OPTIONS

Since she is only 39 years old and there is no history of trauma, there is not an indication for any imaging at this point including plain films based on AHCPR guidelines.

THERAPEUTIC OPTIONS

Pharmacological

The following pharmacological plan is based on the diagnosis of lumbosacral strain and/or sprain, stable HNP without cauda equina symptoms, or spinal stenosis. The AHCPR guidelines suggest a similar approach in these three diagnoses. If spinal fracture or a systemic disease was suspected or if the neurological impairments were severe or progressive, then clearly a different approach would be warranted. Some references suggest a different approach for patients with HNP, but this is predominantly in the nonpharmacological approach.

A change of NSAID could be appropriate, but based on Ms. Pierce's lack of response to ibuprofen, it may not completely control her pain. Naproxen 550 mg bid on a scheduled basis for 4 to 7 days would probably be a good approach. Pregnancy status and risk should be assessed. It could be changed to a prn status after 7 days if the pain has diminished.

Alhough there is little research evidence currently to support it, there are some clinicians who would try a course of oral steroids. This woman is not responding to NSAIDs at home, and she might respond to the steroids. There are other clinicians who would try another NSAID first and impress upon her the importance of taking them on a scheduled basis.

The use of muscle relaxants is very controversial, and although there is little research evidence that use of a muscle relaxant and NSAID is more helpful than the NSAID alone, it is a common practice to prescribe them. Since most muscle relaxants are in the benzodiazepine family, patients should be cautioned about possible sedating side effects if they are prescribed. Cyclobenzaprine (Flexeril) 10 mg po tid or diazepam (Valium) 2 mg tid would be common approaches. Again, pregnancy status and risk should be assessed.

Prescription of narcotics, although controversial in these cases, might be a reasonable approach for short- term management of her pain. She has not responded to Motrin, so she may not get adequate relief from Naproxen. Codeine, Tylenol #3, or hydrocodone/acetaminophen (Vicodin, Lortabs) would not be unreasonable as long as given for a short course. A supply for 2 or 3 days usually gets a patient through the acute phase.

There is very limited clinical support for injecting facet joints, although this is done.

Educational

Possibly the most important thing to do is to reassure her that she is going to get better and that the majority of people suffering with this problem recover completely. This reassurance may actually produce a better outcome.

If Ms. Pierce believes that her back pain is work related, she should file the necessary paperwork with the Turnpike Authority. It is often a difficult decision for clinicians to make regarding the work-relatedness of an injury. Often, patients will not have the onset of pain until well after the stress or strain that caused the problem. These decisions must be made on a case by case basis.

Other Nonpharmacological Options

Most current recommendations regarding activity are that she continue to do things to her tolerance. Bedrest, if recommended, is usually limited, and most recommendations are that it not be used at all unless absolutely necessary. Some recommendations are that if HNP is suspected, then bedrest should be recommended for 1 to 3 weeks.

If exercises are recommended, they should just be gentle range of motion exercises until the acute back spasm passes. Some clinicians recommend walking, and if this is not excessively painful, it is reasonable.

Although there is no research supporting the use of heat or cold, many patients find that they help with the pain, so recommendation of these would not be unreasonable.

Spinal manipulation or mobilization by a physical therapist, chiropractor, or osteopathic physician is helpful (Eaton, Bates, and Willard, 1991). Use of techniques such as counterstrain would probably be used in the acute phase. The practitioner would have to determine the actual risk of it being an HNP, but that in itself is not a contraindication to manipulative therapy. If you were going to recommend this, then a physical therapy referral would be one option.

Ms. Pierce should avoid things that aggravate her pain, and a decision would need to be made about work since it has been identified as an aggravating factor. The preference would be to return her to work as soon as possible. Give her a work note for 2 to 3 days, and then ask her if she can modify her job in any way for the short term.

You may also think about things that may decrease the probability of recurrence. Losing weight would put less strain on her back. "Back schools" are recommended by some clinicians, but evidence is not conclusive on their value.

FOLLOW-UP

Ms. Pierce should be asked to return to the office in 2 weeks or less. If she is getting no relief at all, she should call back in the next couple of days. At the follow-up visit, assessment of progress or lack thereof can be made. Also, if she is progressing, long-term prevention can be addressed including weight loss and job modifications. If she has not improved in 4 weeks of treatment or she starts to show neurological decline, a further workup would be indicated.

You could also discuss a plan for her long-term primary care, including appropriate screenings and health promotion, at that time.

References

Agency for Health Care Policy and Reasearch: *Acute low back problems,* AHCPR Publication No 95-0642, 1994.

Eaton JA, Bates BP, Willard FW: Osteopathic medicine, *Orthopaedic Nurs* 10(1):51, 1991.

Goroll AH, May LA, Mulley AG: *Primary care medicine,* Philadelphia, 1995, JB Lippincott.

Hoppenfeld S: *Physical examination of the spine and extremities,* Norwalk, Conn, 1976, Appleton-Century-Crofts.

Jarvis C: *Physical examination and health assessment,* Philadelphia, 1992, WB Saunders.

Kelley WN: *Essentials of internal medicine,* Philadelphia, 1994, JB Lippincott.

CASE
27

9:15 AM
Mimi Murray
Age 54 years

OPENING SCENARIO

Mimi Murray is a 54-year-old female who came to your office to establish care with a new primary care provider since her provider retired about 1 year ago. Her primary concern is that she noticed some chest tightness for a couple of days last week. She brought her records from her gynecologist. Medical records have also been requested from her prior primary care provider.

HISTORY OF PRESENT ILLNESS

"The chest tightness was just noticeable, not truly uncomfortable. It happened during the daytime last week. I was not doing anything physical, just sitting. It was not a sharp pain or burning, just a tight feeling that lasted for a few seconds but then stayed constant over several days as I went about my daily routine. I have not had symptoms this week. I went to see my gynecologist yesterday for my regularly scheduled visit. She thought I should have this evaluated and referred me here."

The patient denies pain radiation to her jaw, neck, shoulders, arms, back, or upper abdomen. No numbness of the arms, pain with movement, or diaphoresis. No palpitations, lightheadedness, dizziness. No pain with deep breathing or coughing. No recent upper respiratory infection (URI). The discomfort did not keep her awake. No nausea or symptoms related to eating. Has no history of reflux disease, cholecystitis, or peptic ulcer disease. No history of trauma to the chest, heavy lifting, or change of exercise regimen at the gym. Has not noticed any tenderness on the chest wall.

She has been on metoprolol 25 mg bid for 5 years. When she developed this discomfort last week, she increased her metoprolol to 50 mg in the morning and 25 mg in the evening. She did not notice any change in the discomfort. When she was first put on metoprolol, she used this dose but felt better on the 25 mg bid, so the dose was reduced.

She usually exercises regularly, but in the last 3 weeks she has been too busy and has not been doing any exercise.

MEDICAL HISTORY

Hypertension for 5 years. Left breast cyst removed 6 years ago. Cryosurgery for abnormal Paps (atypical cells of undetermined significance [ASCUS]) 4 years ago. No history of myocardial infarction (MI), cerebrovascular accident, or diabetes mellitus (DM).

FAMILY MEDICAL HISTORY

Mother: Deceased at 78 yr (ovarian cancer)
Father: Deceased at 71 yr (lung cancer)
10 siblings: one sister with hypertension; others healthy as far as she knows; Ms. Murray is the oldest

SOCIAL HISTORY

Smoking for 30 years at 1 1/2 packs per day. Has tried to quit on numerous occasions but always relapses. Alcohol use: 3 to 4 glasses of wine per day. Caffeine: 2 cups of tea per day. Lives with husband. Two grown sons are both married. Adopted a 14-year-old child with special needs 6 years ago. Much stress with him over the past 6 months, although he now lives on his own. Joined a meditation group 6 months ago, meditates three times a week for 30 minutes. She is a writer and owns a marketing agency with her husband.

MEDICATIONS

Metoprolol: 50 mg in morning, 25 mg in evening
Daily multivitamin
Chinese herbs

ALLERGIES

None

REVIEW OF SYSTEMS

General: Usually feels very healthy; weight slowly increasing, approximately 40 pounds over the past 10 years; no recent changes; sleeps 7 to 8 hours per night and feels rested during the day
Skin: Has not noticed any rashes, lesions
HEENT: Denies problems with allergies; no visual changes other than wears reading glasses; denies tinnitus, vertigo, pain, discharge; no nosebleeds, discharge, sinus problems; gum surgery for gingivitis 1 year ago; no hoarseness, sore throat, pain; states she has not had a cold in 15 years because she uses high doses of vitamin C, 1500 to 2000 mg per day if she feels symptomatic

174

Cardiac: Denies chest pain; just tightness as described under History of Present Illness

Respiratory: Denies asthma, shortness of breath

Breasts: Yearly mammograms since breast biopsy 6 years ago; does self breast examination

Gastrointestinal: Denies heartburn, stomach, epigastric, or abdominal pain; no constipation, diarrhea, hemorrhoids, or recent bowel changes

Genitourinary: Review of gynecological records: G2P2; menopause began 4 years ago; 2 years ago had light bleeding for 1 week after 2 years without menses; endometrial biopsy showed scant tissue; no bleeding since and did not have the endometrial biopsy repeated; takes Chinese herbs daily (prescribed by an Oriental acupuncturist) that have controlled hot flashes to an infrequent basis at this point; is still taking a daily maintenance dose; has a yearly pelvic sonogram because of her mother's history of ovarian cancer; refuses hormone replacement therapy (HRT) because of mother's history of ovarian cancer; Pap smears within normal limits since cryosurgery 4 years ago; most recent Pap smear 6 months ago

Extremities: Fracture of right ankle 4 years ago; bone density testing 2 years ago

Endocrine: Rare headaches; temperature tolerances good; no arthralgias or myalgias

Neurological: Headaches rarely

PHYSICAL EXAMINATION

Vital signs: Temperature: 98.0° F; *Pulse:* 70 beats/min; *Respirations:* 16 breaths/min; *BP:* 140/90 mm Hg
Ht: 5' 9"; *Wt:* 185; *BMI:* 27

General: Healthy, alert, calm 54-year-old female who looks her stated age

Skin: No rashes, lesions, bruising

HEENT: Pupils equal and reactive to light; fundoscopic examination: normal arteries and veins bilaterally with no arteriovenous nicking or focal constrictions; extraocular movements intact; ears: no discharge, crisp cone of light, landmarks visualized; nose: no discharge, polyps; oropharynx is moist without lesions

Neck: Supple without adenopathy, thyromegaly, jugular venous distention (JVD), or bruits

Heart: Regular rate and rhythm; no murmurs, rubs, or gallops; no discomfort elicited with pressure on costochondral joint

Lungs: Clear to auscultation bilaterally

Breast: Deferred

Abdomen: Soft, nontender, without masses; no hepatosplenomegaly or bruit; no epigastric or RUQ tenderness; negative costovertebral angle tenderness

Genitourinary: Pelvic deferred

Extremities: Negative for cyanosis, clubbing, or edema; no redness, phlebitis; pedal pulses palpable and equal bilaterally

Neurological: Normal gait; cranial nerves 2 to 12 intact; Biceps, triceps, patellar, ankle deep tendon reflexes: 2+

Office electrocardiogram (ECG) performed today (Fig. 27-1). The laboratory tests shown in Tables 27-1 to 27-4 and Box 27-1 were ordered by her gynecologist this week and faxed to you.

Table **27-1** *Chemistry Panel CP-12 for Mimi Murray*

TEST	RESULT	REFERENCE VALUE
Glucose	104 mg/dl	65-115
BUN	12 mg/dl	16-26
Creatinine	0.7 mg/dl	0.5-1.3
Calcium	9.4 mg/dl	8.2-10.2
Uric acid	6.1 mg/dl	2.5-6.6
Total protein	7.2 g/dl	6.2-8.3
Albumin	4.4 g/dl	3.4-5.2
Bilirubin, total	0.4 mg/dl	0.0-1.2
Alkaline phosphatase	100 U/L	0-125
SGOT (AST)	25 U/L	0-40
LDH	144 U/L	0-230
Cholesterol, total	314 mg/dl	<200

Table **27-2** *Cardiac Risk/Lipid Profile for Mimi Murray*

TEST	RESULT	REFERENCE VALUE
Cholesterol, total	314 mg/dl	<200
Triglycerides	195 mg/dl	<200
Cholesterol, HDL	54 mg/dl	>35
Cholesterol, LDL	221 mg/dl	<130
Chol/HDL ratio	5.8	<4.44
CHD relative risk ratio	1.6 x average	Average risk = 1.0
LDL/HDL risk	4.1	<3.22
CHD relative risk ratio	1.4 x average	Average risk = 1.0

Table 27-3 Complete Blood Count for Mimi Murray

TEST	RESULT	REFERENCE VALUE
WBC	5.2 x 1000/μl	3.9-9.9
RBC	4.56 million/μl	4.2-5.4
Hemoglobin	14.9 g/dl	12.0-16.0
Hematocrit	44.7 %	37.0-47.0
MCV	98.1 fl	81.0-99.0
MCH	32.7 pg	27.0-31.0
MCHC	33.3 g/dl	33.0-37.0
RDW	12.5 %	11.5-14.5
Platelet count	207 x 1000/μl	130-451
MPV	8.5 fl	7.0-12.0
Lymphocyte %	40.4 %	20.0-45.0
Monocyte %	4.5 %	0.2-8.0
Granulocyte %	55.1 %	42.0-80.0
Lymphocytes	2.1 x 1000/μl	1.2-4.5
Monocytes	0.2 x 1000 /μl	0.1-0.6
Granulocytes	2.9 x 1000/μl	1.4-9.9
Eosinophils	<.7 x 1000/μl	0.0-0.7
Basophils	<.2 x 1000/μl	0.0-0.2

Table 27-4 Urinalysis for Mimi Murray

TEST	RESULT	REFERENCE VALUE
Color	Yellow	
Appearance	Clear	
Specific gravity	1.015	0.003-029
pH	5.5	4.5-8.0
Protein	Negative	
Glucose	Negative	
Ketones	Negative	
Nitrite	Negative	
Bilirubin	Negative	
Urobilinogen	1.0	0.2-1.0
Leukocytes	Negative	

Box 27-1 Bone Densitometry Report

Ms. Murray is a 54-year-old White female who appears to eat calcium products regularly and does regular aerobics. She does, however, smoke 2 packs of cigarettes per day, and she apparently is on no medications except a beta blocker and various herbs and vitamins. She takes no specific calcium supplement. She has lost no height and has had three pregnancies. She stopped menstruating 2 years ago, and she had a chip fracture of her foot at age 50. There is no family history of osteoporosis.

Bone density report at this time is approximately 2 years after menopause and shows her hip to be about average for a patient in her age group and to be on the average 0.8 standard deviation (SD) below patients at peak bone mass throughout the hip. However, at the femoral neck, the most critical area for fracture, she is 1.42 SD below peak bone mass.

As far as her vertebral spine is concerned, on the average she is 110% of what you would expect to see in her age group and 101% of what you would expect to see at peak bone mass.

IMPRESSION: The patient's bone mass at her femoral neck is somewhat worrisome in that it is greater than 1 SD below someone at peak bone mass, suggesting mild osteopenia. She also has a mildly enlarged hip axis of 11.143 cm, which also increases her risk of hip fracture supposedly on just a structural basis.

My own personal feeling would be that, based on the patient's hip structure and her mild osteoporosis at the femoral neck, estrogen replacement therapy should be considered since she is still in the accelerated phase of bone loss. If I was not anxious to treat her with estrogen, then I would suggest that she be reevaluated in 2 years.

Thank you for allowing me to read the bone densitometry report on Ms. Murray.

Sincerely,
Harold Xavier, MD

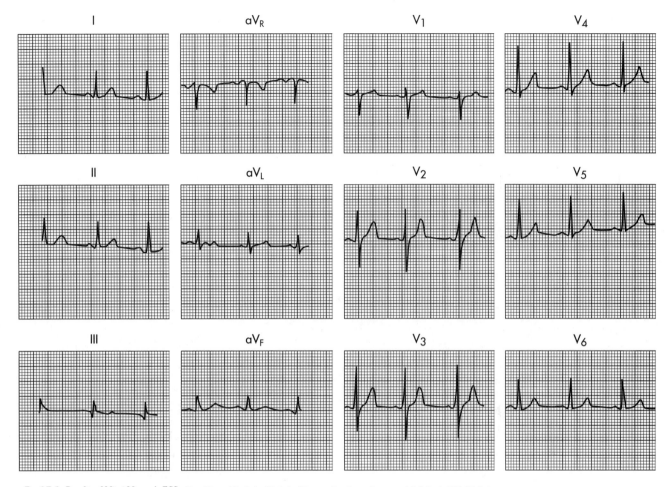

Fig. **27-1** Results of Mimi Murray's ECG. *(From Kinney MR, Packa DR: Andreoli's comprehensive cardiac care, ed 8, St Louis, 1996, Mosby.)*

ASSESSMENT   *Please indicate the problems or issues you have identified that will guide your care (preferably in list form):*

PLAN   *Please list your plans for addressing each of the problems or issues in your assessment*

Community Clinic
Jeffrey A. Eaton, NP
Joyce D. Cappiello, NP

Name:_____ DOB_____
Address_____ Date_____

Rx

"label all unless indicated"
Refill:_____ times-- Do not refill ( )

Signed:_____
DO NOT TAKE THIS TO YOUR PHARMACIST

Community Clinic
Jeffrey A. Eaton, NP
Joyce D. Cappiello, NP

Name:_____ DOB_____
Address_____ Date_____

Rx

"label all unless indicated"
Refill:_____ times-- Do not refill ( )

Signed:_____
DO NOT TAKE THIS TO YOUR PHARMACIST

LEARNING ISSUES

In order to resolve this patient's problem, you will need to consider and address the following issues (you may generate additional issues as well):

- **Pertinent history questions with a patient with potential cardiac problems**
- **Appropriate physical examination techniques**
- **ECG readings**
- **Significant laboratory findings**
- **Bone density screening**
- **Definition of osteoporosis and osteopenia**
- **Management of abnormal lipids; What is the pertinent research on this issue?**
- **Advantages and disadvantages of HRT in post-menopausal women**
- **Pertinent lifestyle changes**

INITIAL IDEAS

The first and most important issue to resolve is the origin of her chest discomfort. Is this of cardiac origin or of musculoskeletal origin? Other issues include her risk factors for cardiovascular disease, osteoporosis, and the current stress in her life. Prevention of disease is the focus with these issues.

INTERPRETATION OF CUES, PATTERNS, AND INFORMATION

This presentation of chest discomfort is not typical for cardiac pain, but the presentation of chest pain itself is often atypical in women. Ms. Murray has significant cardiac risk factors including heavy smoking, elevated lipid profile, hypertension, and menopausal status. You do not want to miss an impending MI in this patient.

The general location of the discomfort described by Ms. Murray is not specific to the costochondral juncture, a common site for irritation and inflammation; however, this condition does occur frequently in women. It usually resolves with nonsteroidal antiinflammatory drugs (NSAIDs) and avoidance of any offending activity. Tenderness is not elicited on examination today at the costochondral area, but Ms. Murray states that the symptoms have resolved. It is possible, although not likely, that this complaint could have been of musculoskeletal origin.

Could this chest tightness be related to esophageal reflux? Her risk factors include alcohol use, smoking, and being overweight. She does not report any history of reflux, so this seems less likely but not out of the question.

She reports an increase of stress in her life. Could an anxiety attack cause the symptoms? Typically, an anxiety attack would be accompanied by palpitations, shortness of breath, and a general sense of uneasiness, but this diagnosis is a possibility.

Cholecystitis seems less likely based on history and physical examination but can present atypically. If this tightness reoccurs, it can be kept in the differential.

A metastatic cancer to the chest wall seems unlikely based on her history of regular mammograms and her normal breast examinations with her gynecologist.

You would not want to miss a problem of cardiac origin. Further testing may be needed to rule this out.

Other areas on the problem list are as follows:
- Hypertension
- Hyperlipidemia
- Osteopenia
- Situational stress
- Menopausal status
- Smoking
- Daily alcohol intake
- Overweight
- Family history of ovarian cancer
- S/P left breast cyst excision
- S/P cryosurgery for ASCUS Pap smear
- S/P gum surgery
- S/P ankle fracture 4 years ago

DIAGNOSTIC OPTIONS

1. You would not want to miss a cardiac problem. The office ECG looks essentially normal. If ST and/or T changes are present in the ECG during an episode of pain and return to normal with spontaneous relief of pain or after administration of nitroglycerin, than the diagnosis of myocardial ischemia is confirmed. The ECG may also be helpful in excluding a prior infarction, but in this case, the pain had resolved and the ECG may not give such a clear diagnosis.

The U.S. Preventive Services Task Force (1996) states that studies have found that most coronary events occur in people without resting ECG abnormalities, thus it is not the most efficient test for detecting coronary artery disease (CAD) or for predicting future coronary events. The decision to order additional testing for Ms. Murray would be clearer if she were still symptomatic, but at this point symptoms have not been present for a week. Still, you do not want to miss a cardiac problem.

What additional testing could be considered? Not only is the decision of *whether* to order additional testing unclear, but *which* test to order is also unclear. The exercise ECG is more accurate than the resting ECG for detecting clinically important CAD, but most patients with asymptomatic CAD do not have a positive exercise ECG. ECG changes often do not become apparent until an atherosclerotic plaque has progressed to the point that it significantly impedes coronary blood flow. In addition, many asymptomatic persons with an abnormal exercise ECG do not have underlying disease (US Preventive Services Task Force, 1996).

An exercise tolerance test (ETT) enhanced by myocardial perfusion imaging agents such as thallium and sestamibi is approximately quadruple the cost of the ETT and is less commonly used for initial screening.

Clinicians make decisions based on research, their own experience, and the experience of their colleagues. In this situation you may have reviewed the research and may have little prior experience with this clinical scenario. Consulting with a colleague or a cardiologist would be very helpful. It is important to recognize when you are unsure how to proceed and solicit additional opinions. This allows you to draw on their analysis of the literature and broader clinical experience. In fact, in some facilities the clinician talks directly with the cardiologist when ordering a stress test so the appropriate type of testing and medications can be discussed in advance.

2. Other diagnostic testing for noncardiac disease could include testing for thyroid disease. A thyroid-stimulating hormone (TSH) would be helpful to rule this out since thyroid disease can elevate cholesterol levels in females. Other basic laboratory tests, such as the chemistry profile and complete blood count (CBC), were ordered last week. Other than the elevated cholesterol, the basic laboratory workup did not indicate any problems.

THERAPEUTIC OPTIONS

Pharmacological

Elevated Lipid Profile The lipid profile shows a cholesterol level of 314 (normal value <200), a low-density lipoprotein (LDL) level of 221 (normal value <130), a high-density lipoprotein (HDL) level of 54 (normal value >45 in females), and a triglyceride level of 195 (normal value <200, but the role of triglycerides in CAD in women is less clear than in men). By American Heart Association standards, Ms. Murray is at risk for coronary heart disease (CHD) based on her elevated LDL, age, hypertension, and smoking status. Recent studies have suggested that being overweight (defined as a BMI over 25) is also an important risk factor. Ms. Murray's BMI is 27. Current research is unclear on how alcohol impacts the development of CAD in females.

The American Heart Association has developed a CHD risk factor prediction chart to assist clinicians in determining risk of CAD when multiple risk factors are involved (Fig 27-2). Using this scoring system and assuming the system has validity, the probability that Ms. Murray will develop CHD is 8% in the next 5 years and 16% by 10 years. This is approximately twice the risk of the average 50 year old.

Given her increased risk of CHD, what can be done to lower this? What interventions have been studied and proven to have an impact? Many studies have looked at the effect of cholesterol-lowering interventions in men, but only a few have looked at this in women.

Do you know whether lipid abnormalities are as strongly associated with CHD in women as they are in men? Is there any basis for being concerned about cholesterol in women? There are only a handful of studies that have looked at primary prevention in women. More studies have been published on secondary prevention involving women. The Canadian Atherosclerosis Intervention Trial (CCAIT) and the Specialized Center of Research (SCOR) studies demonstrated that lipid-lowering agents work as well in women as men and did halt the progression of disease (Kane et al, 1990; Waters et al, 1994). The Cholesterol and Recurrent Events (CARE) trial showed that women have a reduction in relative risk when treated with pravastatin (Sachs et al, 1996). The Scandinavian Simvastatin Survival Study (4S) showed a decrease in major coronary events, but the overall effect on mortality was not statistically significant for women (Pedersen et al, 1994). Of all the secondary prevention trials, the 4S enrolled the most women at 18% of the total study population.

The largest study to look at the issue of primary prevention (treating individuals with risk factors but not CAD) was the West of Scotland Coronary Prevention Study (WOSCOPS). This definitive study showed significant reductions in risk in the 6500 men studied, but no women were included in the study (Shepherd et al, 1995). Although the implication from these studies is that cholesterol-lowering agents will lower the risk of CAD in a patient like Ms. Murray, conclusive evidence is lacking. It is unknown whether there are certain side effects of lipid-lowering therapies that are unique in women. The CARE study raised the concern of an increase of breast cancer in women using statins (12 cases in the pravastatin group and 1 in the placebo group), but the larger 4S study did not. Because the CARE study was small, the findings may have been a random cluster. Another unresolved issue is the possible interaction between lipid-lowering agents and HRT in menopausal women. To date, there is no study suggesting a problem, nor is there a study analyzing the interaction.

1. Find Points For Each Risk Factor

Age (If Female)				Age (If Male)				HDL-Cholesterol		Total-Cholesterol		Systolic Blood Pressure			Other	Pts.
Age	Pts.	Age	Pts.	Age	Pts.	Age	Pts.	HDL-C	Pts.	Total-C	Pts.	SBP	Pts.			
30	− 12	47-48	5	30	− 2	57-59	13	25-26	7	139-151	− 3	98-104	− 2		Cigarettes	4
31	− 11	49-50	6	31	− 1	60-61	14	27-29	6	152-166	− 2	105-112	− 1		Diabetic-male	3
32	− 9	51-52	7	32-33	0	62-64	15	30-32	5	167-182	− 1	113-120	0		Diabetic-female	6
33	− 8	53-55	8	34	1	65-67	16	33-35	4	183-199	0	121-129	1		ECG-LVH	9
34	− 6	56-60	9	35-36	2	68-70	17	36-38	3	200-219	1	130-139	2			
35	− 5	61-67	10	37-38	3	71-73	18	39-42	2	220-239	2	140-149	3		0 pts for each NO	
36	− 4	68-74	11	39	4	74	19	43-46	1	240-262	3	150-160	4			
37	− 3			40-41	5			47-50	0	263-288	4	161-172	5			
38	− 2			42-43	6			51-55	− 1	289-315	5	173-185	6			
39	− 1			44-45	7			56-60	− 2	316-330	6					
40	0			46-47	8			61-66	− 3							
41	1			48-49	9			67-73	− 4							
42-43	2			50-51	10			74-80	− 5							
44	3			52-54	11			81-87	− 6							
45-46	4			55-56	12			88-96	− 7							

2. Sum Points for All Risk Factors

____ + ____ + ____ + ____ + ____ + ____ + ____ = ____
Age   HDL-C   Total-C   SBP   Smoker   Diabetes   ECG-LVH   Point Total

NOTE: *Minus Points Subtract From Total.*

3. Look Up Risk Corresponding To Point Total

	Probability			Probability			Probability			Probability	
Pts.	5 Yr.	10 Yr.	Pts.	5 Yr.	10 Yr.	Pts.	5 Yr.	10 Yr.	Pts.	5 Yr.	10 Yr.
≤ 1	< 1%	< 2%	10	2%	6%	19	8%	16%	28	19%	33%
2	1%	2%	11	3%	6%	20	8%	18%	29	20%	36%
3	1%	2%	12	3%	7%	21	9%	19%	30	22%	38%
4	1%	2%	13	3%	8%	22	11%	21%	31	24%	40%
5	1%	3%	14	4%	9%	23	12%	23%	32	25%	42%
6	1%	3%	15	5%	10%	24	13%	25%			
7	1%	4%	16	5%	12%	25	14%	27%			
8	2%	4%	17	6%	13%	26	16%	29%			
9	2%	5%	18	7%	14%	27	17%	31%			

4. Compare To Average 10 Year Risk

	Probability	
Age	Women	Men
30-34	< 1%	3%
35-39	< 1%	5%
40-44	2%	6%
45-49	5%	10%
50-54	8%	14%
55-59	12%	16%
60-64	13%	21%
65-69	9%	30%
70-74	12%	24%

These charts were prepared with the help of William B. Kannel, M.D., Professor of Medicine and Public Health and Ralph D'Agostino, Ph.D., Head, Department of Mathematics, both at Boston University; Keaven Anderson, Ph.D., Statistician, NHLBI, Framingham Study; Daniel McGee, Ph.D., Associate Professor, University of Arizona. Framingham Heart Study

Fig. **27-2** Coronary heart disease risk factor prediction chart. ©American Heart Association.

Although conclusive evidence is lacking, clinicians need to make decisions on the management of patients like Ms. Murray now rather than years down the road when additional research is available. The existing data suggest more benefit than harm. It may well be more problematic to leave a patient with abnormal cholesterol and LDL levels untreated than to institute treatment based on limited data. Clinical decision making can be challenging!

The National Cholesterol Education Program (NCEP) has issued guidelines for the management of elevated lipids. Despite the fact that they were developed by an expert panel that relied heavily on analysis of secondary epidemiological data without the benefit of randomized, controlled clinical trials and did not explicitly address cost effectiveness, they appear to be reasonable guidelines both from clinical and cost-effective points of view (Schwartz, 1996), although not specifically tailored to women.

Current studies have focused on the statins rather than on niacin or bile acid sequestrants. Since little data is available on the latter two, many clinicians would choose to prescribe a statin.

You may decide that it is reasonable to first suggest a concerted effort of dietary modifications, increased exercise, reduction of alcohol, and smoking cessation over the next 3 months. A referral to a dietitian to review an American Heart Association Step II diet and a reducing diet would be very beneficial. If her LDLs are not <160 mg by the next visit, it is reasonable to begin pharmacological therapy. Start with a low dose and titrate upward until her LDL is <130 mg.

If Ms. Murray reconsiders her decision to use HRT, she may be able to delay or avoid the use of lipid-lowering agents.

Hypertension Management Some beta blockers have been known to increase cholesterol levels. Could this possibly be a factor in her elevated lipids? Generally, cardioselective beta blockers affect lipid levels less than nonselective agents, but agents with intrinsic sympathomimetic activity (ISA) or alpha-blocking properties are lipid neutral. The nonselective agents with ISA, such as pindolol (Visken), carteolol (Cartrol), and penbutolol (Levatol) do not affect lipids. Selective beta blockers such as metoprolol (Lopressor) and atenolol have little effect on lipids (Koda-Kimble and Young, 1995). Since beta blockers clearly have been shown to lower morbidity and mortality, it is felt that effects on lipids have little clinical significance (Koda-Kimble and Young, 1995).

Nonprescription Medications for Reduction of Cardiovascular Risk Vitamin E has been studied in some large studies looking at its potential for cardiovascular protection. The studies have not been done with large numbers of women but have suggested a benefit for men. Vitamin E at the common dose of 400 IU has few side effects, although at high doses an elevation of blood pressure has been noted. It may be helpful and does not appear to be harmful.

Would daily aspirin be protective in reducing Ms. Murray's potential for CAD and stroke? Again, there are no randomized controlled trials that assess the role of aspirin prophylaxis in the primary prevention of cardiovascular disease in women. Currently the Women's Health Initiative is doing such a study in women over age 45. Recent research suggests that aspirin works not only by its blood thinning ability but by its antiinflammatory effects as well. One adult or baby aspirin per day is inexpensive and generally well tolerated, although it may have the ability to induce gastrointestinal problems, especially in someone with a daily alcohol intake.

Osteopenia Therapy What is the significance of the bone densitometry report? Does Ms. Murray have osteoporosis? The definition established by the World Health Organization (WHO) is based primarily on bone mineral density (BMD), not on a history of fractures. The WHO definitions are as follows:

1. Low bone mass (osteopenia) is >1 standard deviation (SD) below the young adult mean.
2. Osteoporosis is >2.5 SD below the young adult mean.
3. Severe, established osteoporosis is >2.5 SD below the young adult mean in the presence of one or more fractures.

Ms. Murray's values included >1.42 SD below the reference mean at the femoral neck and 101% at the vertebral spine compared with the young adult mean. Some experts suggest taking the average of the site measurements when discrepancies occur. By this definition, Ms. Murray has low bone mass, or osteopenia.

Biochemical markers including serum markers of bone formation and serum and urine markers of bone resorption are on the market. Biochemical assays do not reflect bone density but are an assessment of bone turnover rate. Bone densitometry provides a current value but does not predict the rate of bone loss. You can hypothesize that this bone loss will continue based on your knowledge of accelerated bone loss after menopause. Serial BMD testing would give information about the rate of bone loss. Bone densitometry is expensive, not always covered by insurance plans, and has limitations, but to date it is the better test for establishing a diagnosis. The recommendation of a repeat test in 2 years seems reasonable.

In addition to the low BMD, Ms. Murray's risk factors include her age, female gender, White race, smoking status, and alcohol use. She reports an adequate calcium intake, but that has not been reviewed. Many individuals are not aware of the newly revised recommended daily allowance (RDA) of 1200 mg of calcium for postmenopausal women. This is about the equivalent of 4 cups of milk per day, an amount difficult for many to achieve without supplementation.

Vitamin D supplementation is less studied. One study with elderly women in a nursing home suggests that 800 mg of vitamin D in conjunction with calcium helped reduce fractures. Most over-the-counter (OTC) multivitamins have 400 mg, so if Ms. Murray continues her multivitamins she will at least have this amount daily plus the supplementation in milk.

The only current treatment approved for prevention of osteoporosis is estrogen. It is thought that long-term, continued use after menopause is needed to prevent osteoporosis, although some recent studies suggest that starting therapy many years after menopause may still confer benefits. You would need to further explore Ms. Murray's concerns about HRT. HRT would confer significant benefits to Ms. Murray in the prevention of both osteoporosis and heart disease. Current research does not identify any increased risk of ovarian cancer in women who use HRT. The impact of HRT on the development of breast cancer is less clear with conflicting studies. It does appear that a modest increase may begin after 5 years of use. Many women are more fearful about the potential for developing cancer over the risk of developing cardiovascular disease or osteoporosis.

It is not clear whether there is an ideal, cost-effective, disease-preventing point to institute drug therapy in someone with osteopenia. Calcitonin and the biphosphonates, such as etidronate and alendronate, can prevent bone loss. The parathyroid hormone, which has the potential to build new bone, is being studied currently. A discussion of osteoporosis prevention and current drug therapies is important if Ms. Murray continues to decline HRT and if subsequent testing shows significant bone loss. Most likely she has already had this discussion with her gynecologist, so the information may be somewhat familiar to her.

Nonpharmacological Regular weight-bearing exercise has been shown to preserve bone health. Ms. Murray reported a history of regular exercise except over the past 3 weeks. You would want to explore her concept of regular exercise and encourage such efforts. A minimum of 30 minutes, three to four times a week of structured activity or the broader view of incorporating regular physical activity into daily routines is recommended. Exercise is protective against cardiovascular disease, the more pressing issue for Ms. Murray. It is also an integral part of any weight loss program.

Encourage weight loss, stressing the positive impact this will have on her hypertension and lipids. A thorough discussion of dietary habits and exercise habits and a referral to a dietitian would be helpful.

Smoking cessation needs to be thoroughly discussed and facilitated.

Alcohol intake needs review. Is her level of intake a problem? Daily red wine consumption may be protective for CAD, yet Ms. Murray's intake of 3 to 4 drinks per day is a risk factor for osteoporosis and possibly for breast cancer. From the substance abuse literature, a definition of excess alcohol intake for women has been defined as follows (Bradley, Donovan, and Larson, 1993; Sanchez and Craig, 1985):

- No more than 1 to 2 drinks a day (any 24-hour period) no more than 3 days a week, or 1 drink per day with no more than 9 drinks per week.
- One drink equals 4 oz of wine, 12 oz of beer, or 1.5 oz of 80 proof beverage.

This definition of alcohol intake seems very strict given health providers' frequent advice to have a glass of wine each day to decrease the risk of cardiovascular disease. It seems reasonable to suggest that she reduce her intake to 1 to 2 drinks per day.

Caffeine intake of 2 cups of tea per day is reasonable. There is no evidence that moderate caffeine intake is a risk factor for cardiovascular disease, breast cancer, or ovarian cancer. Caffeine intake causes an increase in calcium loss, which can be offset by adequate calcium consumption. There is no research to suggest that Ms. Murray change her intake of tea.

Counseling can be suggested to help Ms. Murray with the situational stress in her life.

Cancer screening: Colon and rectal cancer screening in the form of three tests of stools for occult blood is recommended. Flexible sigmoidoscopy can be discussed. She is having a yearly Pap smear, pelvic sonogram, and mammogram with her gynecologist.

She has regular dental care.

Eye care: Is glaucoma screening useful or necessary in this patient? The Guide to Clinical Preventive Services states that there is insufficient evidence to recommend for or against routine screening by primary care clinicians for elevated intraocular pressure or early glaucoma. Patients with a family history of glaucoma, patients with diabetes, and patients with severe myopia, as well as Blacks over the age of 40 and Whites over the age of 65, may be at increased risk and benefit from screening.

Inquire if she knows the types of Chinese herbs that she is taking. Documentation of all products that she is using is important.

Lifestyle changes can make a major impact on disease prevention for this patient. The development of realistic, mutually agreed-upon risk-modification goals is essential. There are many issues to address here. Ms. Murray may decide to approach these changes slowly to avoid frustration. As the provider, you want to encourage her efforts at achieving these goals.

FOLLOW-UP

A follow-up visit or phone call is important to discuss test results. Also schedule a visit in 4 to 6 weeks to monitor liver function tests (LFTs) if she starts a statin.

References

Bradley KA, Donovan DM, Larson EB: How much is too much? *Arch Intern Med* 152:2734, 1993.

Kane J et al: Regression of coronary atherosclerosis during treatment of familial hypercholesterolemia with combined drug regimens, *JAMA* 264:3007, 1990.

Koda-Kimble MA, Young L: *Applied therapeutics: the clinical use of drugs,* Vancouver, Wash, 1995, Applied Therapeutics.

Pedersen T et al: Randomized trial of cholesterol lowering in 4444 patients with coronary heart disease: the Scandinavian Simvastin Survival Study (4S) *Lancet* 344:1383, 1994.

Sachs FM et al: The effect of pravastatin on coronary events after myocardial infarction in patients with average cholesterol levels, *N Engl J Med* 335:1001, 1996.

Sanchez-Craig M, Israel Y: Patterns of alcohol use associated with self-identified problem drinking, *Am J Public Health* 75:178, 1985.

Schwartz J: The cost-effectiveness of cholesterol-lowering therapy: a guide for the perplexed, *J Clin Outcome Manage* 3(6):48, 1996.

Shepherd J et al: Prevention of coronary heart disease with pravastatin in men with hypercholesterolemia, *N Engl J Med* 333:1301, 1995.

US Preventive Services Task Force: *Guide to clinical preventive services,* ed 2, Washington, DC, 1996, US Preventive Services.

Waters D et al: Effects of monotherapy with an HMG-CoA reductase inhibitor on the progression of coronary atherosclerosis as assessed by serial quantitive arteriography: the Canadian Coronary Atherosclerosis Intervention Trial (CCAIT), *Circulation* 89:959, 1994.

OPENING SCENARIO

Mr. Olsson is a 55-year-old male scheduled for an episodic visit for pain in his left big toe. He was seen once previously for a physical in your office 3 1/2 years ago.

HISTORY OF PRESENT ILLNESS

"Yesterday I awoke with pain in my left big toe. I don't remember injuring my foot in any way. I have not had anything like this previously. It bothers my toe to wear shoes. The pain is intense and has not improved since yesterday except when I took two extra strength acetaminophen, which gave me some relief." The patient denies fever or chills.

MEDICAL HISTORY

Was told 3 1/2 years ago that his cholesterol was borderline at 210, to watch his diet, and to increase his exercise. No hospitalizations or surgeries. No history of hypertension, diabetes mellitus (DM), cardiovascular disease, arthritis, or other joint disorders.

FAMILY MEDICAL HISTORY

Mother: 79 yr (Type II DM, onset age 70 yr)
Father: Deceased at 84 yr (myocardial infarction [MI])
Sister: 50 yr (A&W)
Brother: 57 yr (hypertension)

SOCIAL HISTORY

Happily married with two grown sons. Works long hours as an insurance agent. Nonsmoker for 3 years, previously smoked 3/4 packs per day. Drinks one glass of wine with dinner each night. Walks 1/2 mile each day on his lunch hour. Has not made any significant diet changes since last visit when his cholesterol was slightly elevated.

MEDICATIONS

None

ALLERGIES

None

REVIEW OF SYSTEMS

General: Often tired from long days of working but rests on the weekends and feels better; weight up 20 pounds in past 5 years
Skin: Denies any skin problems such as rashes, bruising, skin discoloration
HEENT: No upper respiratory infection (URI) or bronchitis since stopped smoking; wears reading glasses; regular dental care
Cardiac: No chest pain or history of cardiac problems
Respiratory: Denies cough, shortness of breath
Gastrointestinal: No nausea, vomiting, constipation, diarrhea, blood in stools
Genitourinary: Occasional nocturia and loss of force of stream
Endocrine: Denies change of skin or hair; temperature tolerances good
Extremities: No arthritis, myalgias, history of fractures; occasional low backaches if sitting all day; does not take any medication for this since it is mild; sprained right ankle 10 years ago; no problems with it since; no history of gout
Neurological: Denies weakness, paresthesias

PHYSICAL EXAMINATION

Vital signs: Temperature: 98.4° F; *Pulse:* 74 beats/min; *Respirations:* 20 breaths/min; *BP:* 142/86 mm Hg
Height: 5' 10"; *Weight:* 205 lb; *BMI:* 29
Left foot: No redness, swelling, or pain to palpation; no bony deformities noted
Right foot: First metatarsophalangeal joint is erythematous, edematous, tender to palpation; no crepitus; ankle range of motion limited because of pain; no bony deformity noted; no pain palpated in midfoot, ankle, knee

ASSESSMENT   *Please indicate the problems or issues you have identified that will guide your care (preferably in list form):*

PLAN   *Please list your plans for addressing each of the problems or issues in your assessment:*

Community Clinic
Jeffrey A. Eaton, NP
Joyce D. Cappiello, NP

Name:_____ DOB_____
Address_____ Date_____

Rx

"label all unless indicated"
Refill:_____ times-- Do not refill ( )

Signed:_____
DO NOT TAKE THIS TO YOUR PHARMACIST

Community Clinic
Jeffrey A. Eaton, NP
Joyce D. Cappiello, NP

Name:_____ DOB_____
Address_____ Date_____

Rx

"label all unless indicated"
Refill:_____ times-- Do not refill ( )

Signed:_____
DO NOT TAKE THIS TO YOUR PHARMACIST

INITIAL IDEAS

This is probably a straightforward case of gout. Gout occurs more frequently in men, usually with the first attack occurring in the fifth decade, typically monoarticular, abrupt in onset, and often occuring at night. Mr. Olsson is experiencing all of these symptoms, but be sure to consider other possibilities. If this is gout, what other health issues are of concern with this gentlemen?

INTERPRETATION OF CUES, PATTERNS, AND INFORMATION

Consider the differential diagnosis for an acute monoarticular joint problem. The diagnoses you do not want to miss are trauma and infection.

Rheumatoid arthritis and degenerative joint disease (DJD) usually have a slow, gradual onset and involve multiple joints. DJD is worse after activity and improves with rest, whereas rheumatoid arthritis presents with stiffness and pain in the morning, which improves as the day progresses. Rarely would an acute onset occur with either of these conditions.

Almost all cases of septic arthritis are febrile. Most patients with gout have no fever or a very low-grade fever. Mr. Olsson seems at low risk for disseminated gonorrhea or nongonococcal septic arthritis based on his stated happy marriage. However, a few questions about any recent new sexual partners would help to rule this out.

Pseudogout resembles gout in a pathophysiological manner but differs in its clinical presentation. Knees and wrists are more commonly involved. It also tends to occur in older patients and is often associated with hyperparathyroidism, hemochromatosis, and severe DJD. Based on the clinical presentation, pseudogout is low on the differential list, but the initial treatment is the same as for gout. Hyperparathyroidism can be screened for with an analysis of his calcium level, and hemochromatosis can be screened for with a serum iron. Severe DJD seems unlikely based on the history and physical examination.

Mr. Olsson denies any direct trauma to the foot.

A bunion is caused by a hypermobile first metatarsal bone of the great toe and not by poorly fitting shoes as generally thought (although the shoes may aggravate the condition). The presentation is of a painful great toe similar to a presentation of gout. A bunion deformity can cause enlargement of the first metatarsophalangeal joint and lateral deviation of the great toe. Crepitus can often be felt in the joint. The bursa becomes tender and inflamed, although the onset is usually gradual. The difficulty in diagnosis lies in the fact that an individual can have a bunion and a concurrent gouty attack at the same time.

It can be difficult to distinguish between a cellulitis and an attack of acute gout in this gentlemen with no history of a gouty attack. His temperature may be elevated with a cellulitis and generally is not with gout. From an epidemiological point of view, he fits the profile for a patient presenting with gout.

Physical Examination Techniques

This will be dictated by history findings. A history of multiple joint involvement necessitates a thorough musculoskeletal examination to assess for rheumatoid arthritis and DJD. A history of exposure to sexually transmitted diseases (STDs) would cause you to look for necrotic lesions on the extremities indicative of gonococcemia, human immunodeficiency virus (HIV) skin manifestations, the urethritis and conjunctivitis of Reiter's syndrome, and other oral and genital manifestations of STDs. Since Mr. Olsson's history was negative for all of the above, you can examine just his feet unless other indications arise.

Laboratory Assessment

The gold standard test to confirm the diagnosis of gout is a joint tap to identify urate crystals in the synovial fluid and may be necessary if the diagnosis is unclear. The aspiration of an acutely painful joint can be very uncomfortable and is often deferred if the diagnosis seems fairly straightforward. More commonly, a trial of therapy is done, and then if there is no improvement, additional tests are considered. In this case, Mr. Olsson is uncomfortable but not ill or appearing septic. A course of trial therapy is not unreasonable.

X-ray examination is generally normal in the early course of gout. It can identify fractures, osteomyelitis, osteoarthritic changes, and other nongouty changes. X-ray examination at this point seems to offer little to the diagnostic picture.

A complete blood count (CBC) looking for leukocytosis and an elevated sedimentation rate can be moderately helpful in distinguishing inflammatory from noninflammatory disease. The serum uric acid level (a measurement of urate) is helpful only if extreme since normal levels of serum uric acid vary widely in the normal population.

There is no specific diagnostic test other than the analysis of synovial fluid. You may decide to order a chemistry panel for information on his general health status.

THERAPEUTIC OPTIONS

Colchicine has been the old standard for treatment of gout, but because of its side effects of diarrhea, nausea, and/or vomiting, it has been replaced by nonsteroidal antiinflammatory drugs (NSAIDs). Colchicine can less commonly cause bone marrow suppression, myopathy, and neuropathy. Full-dose NSAIDs seem to be as effective and have fewer side effects (Goroll, May, and Mulley, 1995). Indomethacin and naproxen have been studied, but probably any NSAID would be effective. Indomethacin (Indocin) has been studied at 50 mg every 6 hours for 6 to 8 doses and then reduced to 25 mg every 6 hours for 5 to 7 days since higher doses should be given for the first few days and then tapered down for 3 to 5 days. Alternatively, naproxen has been used at 750 mg initially followed by 250 mg for the remainder of therapy.

Rest, immobility of the joint, and ice packs may help decrease discomfort. Advise him to call you if there is no relief in 24 to 48 hours.

HEALTH PROMOTION/HEALTH MAINTENANCE

Gout is more common in obese or hypertensive individuals, especially those treated with thiazide diuretics (Barker, Burton, and Zieve, 1995). Gout is also more common in patients with a chronically high alcohol intake, especially if they are obese or have mildly impaired renal function. Mr. Olsson's reported alcohol intake of one glass of wine per day does not qualify as a high alcohol intake and is thought to be protective for cardiovascular disease. More detailed questions about his alcohol intake may be necessary to ascertain if this level is accurate.

The Framingham study confirmed a suspicion of an increased incidence of coronary heart disease in men with gout. This was independent of other measured risk factors such as DM and hypercholesterolemia. Association of gout with hypertriglyceridemia has been noted, but it is unclear if this is related to diet, alcohol intake, obesity, or genetic factors (Abbott et al, 1988).

Based on this evidence, Mr. Olsson may be at an increased risk for cardiovascular disease. Also, his cholesterol was identified as borderline 3 1/2 years ago, lifestyle is sedentary, blood pressure is slightly elevated today, BMI is high, and his family history is positive for cardiovascular disease. The good news is that he stopped smoking.

FOLLOW-UP

Mr. Olsson is in need of a follow-up visit for a complete history and physical with a fasting lipid profile. A chemistry panel ordered today would give you general health status information on renal function, calcium, cholesterol, glucose, and uric acid.

Further history needs to clarify his mild changes in urinary habits. Some degree of benign prostatic hyperplasia is common in males over age 50 but may be amenable to therapy.

References

Abbott R et al: Gout and coronary heart disease: the Framingham study, *J Clin Epidemiol* 41:237, 1988.

Barker L, Burton J, Zieve P: *Principles of ambulatory medicine,* ed 4, Baltimore, 1995, Williams & Wilkins.

Goroll A, May L, Mulley AG: *Primary care medicine,* Philadelphia, 1995, JB Lippincott.

OPENING SCENARIO

Rose D'Angelo is a 78-year-old female on your schedule for a complete physical examination.

HISTORY OF PRESENT ILLNESS

"My granddaughter thought I should have a physical. My back aches a lot, and my right hip has been bothering me too. My back has been bothering me for years. It's worse if I do a lot during the day. Tylenol makes it a little better but not much. I'd rate it a 6 on a scale of 1 to 10. It's mostly an ache, but it feels kind of sharp sometimes. It's in my back and deep in my right hip. The back pain came on first about 15 years ago. It has gradually been getting worse over the years. The hip pain started last year, and it has also gradually been getting worse." Ms. D'Angelo denies radiation down the leg, other associated symptoms, saddle paresthesias, bowel and bladder changes, and trauma.

MEDICAL HISTORY

Has not been to a doctor in about 20 years. Only problems before that were coughs and colds. Obstetrical history: one child, now 60 years old; two miscarriages after that.

FAMILY MEDICAL HISTORY

Mother and Father: Died years ago (both over 80 years old of natural causes); does not remember the years that they died
Father's sister: Died young (possible diabetes mellitus [DM])
Brother: 83 yr (stroke; is aphasic)
Sister: 80 yr (hypertension)
Brother: 77 yr (high cholesterol)
Sister: 76 yr (Type II DM and hypertension)
Daughter: 60 yr (A&W)
Three granddaughters: 30, 35, 37 yr (A&W)

SOCIAL HISTORY

Husband died about 5 years ago of sudden cardiac event.

He stayed active until his death. He was 80 years old. She never worked other than at the chicken farm that she and her husband owned. They sold it and moved near the ocean 35 years ago (100+ miles from here). About 6 months ago, her granddaughters talked her into moving into an apartment near here. One lives here in town, one about 1/2 hour away, and one about 45 minutes away. Never smoked. Alcohol: wine whenever the family gets together (about once a month).
Economic: has insurance as well as Medicare; has investments that provide for her; collects social security from her husband; reticent about discussing. Not currently active sexually.

Functional Assessment

Lives in an apartment with three steps at the entrance. Has a handrail. Apartment is all on one floor. No bathtub rail or toilet bars. Continues to drive her car. Does her own shopping. Has a washer and dryer in her apartment. Goes on trips with the Senior Center, takes a ceramics class weekly, gets hair done weekly. Sleeps about 7 1/2 hours per night and takes a 1 hour nap in the afternoon most days. Nutrition: 24-hour recall; fruit and coffee for breakfast, a sandwich for lunch, meat and vegetables for dinner, snack in the evening. Culture: First generation Italian; husband was born in Italy; he came over to the United States at age 13. Religion: Roman Catholic; attends mass sometimes, other times watches on television. Education: Finished elementary school, then worked in her parents store until she got married. Smoke detectors in her apartment. Does not use her seatbelt very often.

MEDICATIONS

Vitamin C: 2000 mg per day
Vitamin E: 400 IU per day
Zinc: one tablet (unknown mg)

ALLERGIES

A little hayfever sometimes
NKDA

REVIEW OF SYSTEMS

General: Denies night sweats, swelling; says energy level is good

HEENT: Denies diplopia; notes occasional blurring; some hearing impairment; denies sore throats
Cardiac: Denies chest pain; no peripheral edema
Respiratory: Denies shortness of breath, dyspnea on exertion, and paroxysmal nocturnal dyspnea
Gastrointestinal: Denies anorexia, nausea, vomiting; occasional constipation (takes a laxative about twice a week and takes Metamucil every day to stay regular); denies diarrhea, black or clay colored stools; sometimes a little bright red blood on the toilet paper
Genitourinary: Denies dysuria, hematuria; leaks a little urine rarely when she coughs or sneezes
Hematological: Denies excessive bruising; no history of transfusion

PHYSICAL EXAMINATION

Vital signs: Temperature: 97.1° F; *Pulse:* 88 beats/min; *Respirations:* 22 breaths/min; *BP:* 148/84 mm Hg
Height: 5' 3"; *Weight:* 170 lb
HEENT: Head is normocephalic, atraumatic; pupils equal, round, and reactive to light; extraocular movements intact; tympanic membranes observable without excessive cerumen; nares patent without redness or exudate; throat is noninjected; tongue is midline; palate rises symmetrically; teeth in adequate repair
Neck: Supple without thyromegaly, adenopathy, or carotid bruits
Heart: Regular rate and rhythm; no murmurs, rubs, or gallops
Lungs: Clear to auscultation and percussion
Breasts: Without dimpling, discharge, or masses
Abdomen: Soft, nontender; no hepatosplenomegaly
Gastrointestinal: Brown stool, no masses
Genitourinary: Normal externally; pelvic exam refused
Extremities: Without cyanosis, clubbing or edema
Neurological: Reflexes are 2+ at the biceps, triceps, brachioradialis, patellar; Achilles reflexes are absent bilaterally; Babinski signs are not present; strength and sensation are symmetrical; Folstein administered: loss of point for county, loss of one point for recall; no other deductions: 28/30

See Tables 29-1 to 29-3 and Box 29-1 for laboratory results for Ms. D'Angelo.

Table **29-1** *Complete Blood Count for Rose D'Angelo*

CBC	RESULT	NORMAL RANGE
WBC	8.2 × 1000/μl	4.5-10.8
RBC	4.45 million/μl	4.20-5.40
Hgb	13.9 g/dl	12.0-16.0
Hct	38.2%	37.0-47.0
MCV	98.3 fl	81.0-99.0
MCH	31.2 pg	27.0-32.0
MCHC	33.4 g/dl	32.0-36.0
RDW	15.2%	11.0-16.0
Platelets	221 × 1000/μl	150-450
Segs	64%	50-65
Lymphocytes	23%	25-45
Monocytes	9%	0-10
Eosinophils	4%	0-4

Table **29-2** *Chemistry Profile for Rose D'Angelo*

TEST	RESULT	NORMAL RANGE
FBS	100	60-110
BUN	20 mg/dl	18-28
Creatinine	1.0 mg/dl	0.5-1.5
Sodium	137	135-145
Potassium	4.3	3.5-5.5
Chloride	104	95-105
Albumin	4.2 g/dl	4.0-6.0
Total protein	6.6 g/dl	6.5-8.0
Alkaline phosphate	100 U/L	30-120
ALT (SGPT)	22	0-40
AST (SGOT)	28 U/L	0-40
LDH	134 U/L	50-150
Cholesterol	220 mg/dl	110-200
Calcium	9.0 mg/dl	8.8-10.2
GGT	29	0-30
Magnesium	2.1	1.6-2.4
Bilirubin	0.7 mg/dl	0.1-1.0
Conjugated bilirubin	0.1	0.0-0.2
Iron	61	60-160
Uric acid	6.3 mg/dl	2.0-7.0

Table **29-3** *Urinalysis for Rose D'Angelo*

Color	Yellow
Character	Clear
SG	1.015
Urine pH	5.5
Glucose	Negative
Nitrite	Negative
WBCs	0-2
RBCs	0-1
Epithelial Cells	0-5
Crystals	None

Box **29-1** *Chest X-ray Examination for Rose D'Angelo*

The lung fields are clear of infiltrates. The pulmonary vasculature and markings are normal. The heart size is within normal limits.

Impression: Normal chest x-ray

Boyd Bates, DO

ASSESSMENT   *Please indicate the problems or issues you have identified that will guide your care (preferably in list form):*

PLAN   *Please list your plans for addressing each of the problems or issues in your assessment:*

Community Clinic
Jeffrey A. Eaton, NP
Joyce D. Cappiello, NP

Name:_____ DOB_____
Address_____ Date_____

Rx

"label all unless indicated"
Refill:_____ times-- Do not refill ( )

Signed:_____
DO NOT TAKE THIS TO YOUR PHARMACIST

Community Clinic
Jeffrey A. Eaton, NP
Joyce D. Cappiello, NP

Name:_____ DOB_____
Address_____ Date_____

Rx

"label all unless indicated"
Refill:_____ times-- Do not refill ( )

Signed:_____
DO NOT TAKE THIS TO YOUR PHARMACIST

Community Clinic
Jeffrey A. Eaton, NP
Joyce D. Cappiello, NP

Name:_____ DOB_____
Address_____ Date_____

Rx

"label all unless indicated"
Refill:_____ times-- Do not refill ( )

Signed:_____
DO NOT TAKE THIS TO YOUR PHARMACIST

Community Clinic
Jeffrey A. Eaton, NP
Joyce D. Cappiello, NP

Name:_____ DOB_____
Address_____ Date_____

Rx

"label all unless indicated"
Refill:_____ times-- Do not refill ( )

Signed:_____
DO NOT TAKE THIS TO YOUR PHARMACIST

LEARNING ISSUES

In order to resolve this patient's problem, you will need to consider and address the following issues (you may generate additional issues as well). Not all learning issues are addressed in the Case Discussion, but they are provided for the opportunity to consider the issues that can be generated in an encounter such as this:

- Appropriate health examination for a 78-year-old woman
- Obesity in an elderly woman
- Differential diagnosis of back pain
- Differential diagnosis of hip pain
- Rh incompatibility
- Family history as a predictor of Type II DM
- Models of functional assessment
- Health promotion issues in a 78-year-old woman
- Differential diagnosis of blurred vision including cataracts as a potential etiology
- Hearing impairment and options for evaluation
- Constipation management
- Urinary incontinence (UI)
- Vitamin supplementation
- Zinc as a dietary supplement
- Diagnosis of hypertension
- Issues of pelvic examination refusal in an elderly woman
- Laboratory evaluation
- Mental status testing
- Differential diagnosis of loss of Achilles reflex in an elderly woman
- Evaluation of rectal bleeding
- Approach to hayfever

INITIAL IDEAS

- She is here under someone else's agenda (her granddaughter's)
- Back pain
- Hip pain
- Possible cataracts
- Possible hearing impairment
- Obesity
- Family history of DM
- Mild constipation
- Rectal bleeding (probable hemorrhoids)
- UI
- Possible mild hypertension
- Intact cognition
- Mildly decreased lymphocyte count
- Mildly elevated cholesterol level

INTERPRETATION OF CUES, PATTERNS, AND INFORMATION (INCLUDING DIFFERENTIAL DIAGNOSIS)

Since Ms. D'Angelo has so many issues, it may be best to look at the information you have in the context of the current ideas.

1. *Someone else's agenda:* This may be quite important in her willingness to make behavioral alterations. It may be dangerous to make any assumptions in this area, but each issue will have to be explored with this factor in mind. She clearly has some definite ideas, and (as almost always) establishing a collaborative relationship may be the best thing.

2. *Back pain:* Many things can cause back pain. Additional examination of the back and hip including straight leg raises (SLRs), Patrick's (fabere) test, and palpation and observation of the entire spine may help you establish a better diagnosis. A more extensive neurological review, including asking specifically about numbness and tingling, may be helpful. Sensory testing may be helpful for baseline, but as long as you have ruled out saddle numbness (and thus cauda equina syndrome) it probably will not change your treatment. No cranial nerve examination is documented, and this could give you valuable information. Asking specifically about dizziness or symptoms similar to those of transient ishemic attack (TIA) (weakness, speech difficulties, bowel and/or bladder changes) may be appropriate, but there is no reason for a high suspicion in this patient.

Plain films of her lumbosacral spine (assuming this is confirmed as the site of her back pain on physical examination) are indicated based on Agency for Health Care Policy and Research (AHCPR) guidelines (1994). These guidelines suggest an x-ray examination in patients over 50 years old with back pain. The x-ray examination may show osteoporosis (although a significant amount of bone loss is necessary before it will show up on x-ray examination) or findings such as myeloma. Some clinicians might consider single or dual absorptiometry or quantitative computerized tomography (CT) to look for osteoporosis, although this is quite variable among clinicians.

3. *Hip pain:* An x-ray examination could be done at this point, or it could be deferred until the initial workup of the back pain is completed since this may be a referred pain.

4. *Possible cataracts:* A quick screen of visual acuity will give you an idea of safety issues as well as how quickly you need to get her in to see ophthalmology. A Snellen or Rosenbaum test would be adequate for this or even reading the newspaper for a gross screen.

You also need to think about nonophthalmological causes before referring since the eye doctor may assume that these have already been ruled out. Is there any chance of multiple sclerosis (MS) or other neurological problems? These are low probability with current history, but it is worth a brief thought.

Can you refer her to an optometrist rather than an ophthalmologist? If you are suspicious of cataracts that will require surgery, you can keep the number of changes down by referring her directly to an ophthalmologist.

5. *Possible hearing impairment:* With these complaints, a referral to an audiologist to see whether hearing aids are appropriate is reasonable.

6. *Obesity:* Ms. D'Angelo clearly meets the criteria for obesity, but you would need to explore the significance of this to her and her willingness and/or interest in changing. There is much talk about promoting independence in this age group, yet health providers often tell older people what to do. Her apparently low lymphocyte count and low normal albumin level are of concern as well since these may be indicative of nutritional deficiencies. Efforts should be made to help her eat better rather than eat less, and a dietitian might be helpful.

You may also want to assess her previous height since some of the extra weight may actually be appropriate when considered in light of height loss. Arm span can be used as a gross estimate of previous height, but she probably knows what her height was before. A loss of height may indicate osteoporosis or some other metabolic problems.

An assessment of current activity level may be helpful both to see current trends and for planning. Maintaining her activity level may have benefits beyond weight loss as well.

7. *Family history of DM:* This was fairly late onset, but obviously you might be more vigilant in looking for signs in Ms. D'Angelo. Her aunt's early demise is probably not of real concern at this point. There is no current evidence to indicate that Ms. D'Angelo has DM now.

8. *Mild constipation:* This is very common in this age group and may reflect a functional constipation. Consideration of other problems such as thyroid disease may also be appropriate. Ms. D'Angelo's extra weight and age in general make thyroid testing appropriate.

9. *Rectal bleeding (probable hemorrhoids):* A flexible sigmoidoscopy and/or fecal occult blood test (FOBT) might be considered just on the basis of her age and lack of a full family history. An external examination specifically looking for hemorrhoids (and/or anoscopy) is a simple quick first step and may provide an indication to the most probable cause of her bleeding. If the FOBT is positive, then it would be necessary to progress to endoscopic evaluations.

10. *Urinary incontinence:* Although she has a UI that is very suspicious of stress incontinence, you cannot rule out an overflow incontinence without catheterization for postvoid residual (PVR). Treating this problem symptomatically at this point and then exploring it further later might be an option since there are so many issues with Ms. D'Angelo. You need to explore the significance of this problem with Ms. D'Angelo and let her know that the majority of patients with UI can be cured or improved (Ham and Sloane, 1997).

11. *Possible mild hypertension:* You cannot make a diagnosis on the basis of a single reading, but if she stays consistently at this level she will meet the criteria for stage I isolated systolic hypertension. The Systolic Hypertension in the Elderly Project (SHEP) has shown improved outcomes in elderly people treated for systolic hypertension. A low-salt diet may be helpful if she has salt-sensitive hypertension, but the benefits of a low-salt diet regarding long-term survival are unproven as well.

12. *Intact cognition:* Ms. D'Angelo had a Folstein minimental status examination (MMSE) score of 28 out of a possible 30, which indicates a very low probability of dementia. Deciding whether to do this kind of testing on an asymptomatic elder is a decision each clinician must make. The Folstein takes about 10 minutes but provides a good screen for dementia. Lower scores correlate with a higher probability of dementia. There may also be enough depression in this age group to consider screening for this problem. The Yesavage Geriatric Depression Scale (GDS) or a similar tool could be used. Ms. D'Angelo has no gross signs of depression, but since depression can present without sadness in the elderly, it is more difficult to diagnose.

13. *Mildly decreased lymphocyte count:* The first thing to consider is whether this represents measurement error or real pathology? Repeating in a month or so may be the best course. Another issue to consider is that a change in one type of white blood cell (WBC) may cause what appears to be a change in another WBC. To compute an actual lymphocyte count, all you need to do is multiply the percentage of those cells (in this case 23%) by the total WBC count (in this

case 8200). This results in a product of 1886. The normal is 1500 to 3500 (Liu, 1986), so this may not represent a true decrease in the lymphocyte count.

14. *Mildly elevated cholesterol level:* The current data regarding cholesterol as a risk factor in older women is difficult to interpret, and the most appropriate thing is to review the data and come to your own conclusion. There was not an improved overall mortality in women in the Scandinavian Simvastatin Survival Study (4S) (1994), although there was a decrease in cardiovascular mortality. The lack of conclusive studies in this area requires that the clinician review the data available and then determine what recommendations to make.

REVISED IDEAS

- Back pain
- Hip pain
- Occasional bright red blood per rectum: rule out hemorrhoids
- Blurring of vision: rule out cataracts
- Function-impairing hearing loss
- Mild constipation
- Health promotion/health maintenance

THERAPEUTIC OPTIONS

Since this a very complex situation, a single approach is described. You may have different approaches, but the following represents one reasonable approach.

Pharmacological

- Pneumococcal vaccine today
- Tetanus-diphtheria (Td) immunization today
- Influenza shot if the season
- Tylenol: 1000 mg po q4h prn for pain
- Metamucil: 1 tablespoon per day
- Continue current vitamins

Educational

- Talk with Ms. D'Angelo about the importance of seatbelts and the advances that have been made in comfort.
- Begin simple dietary instructions regarding foods that are high in fat.
- Discuss options for increasing activities that do not increase back pain.
- Provide information regarding living wills and durable power of attorney (DPOA) for health care
- If she has concerns about her UI, suggest that she maintain a continence diary so that further evaluation can be facilitated.

Other Nonpharmacological Options

- FOBT: 3 to 6 cards
- Ophthalmology examination
- Audiology consult
- Thyroid-stimulating hormone (TSH), complete blood count (CBC), and fasting lipid profile in about 2 weeks
- Mammogram
- Lumbosacral spine x-ray examination

HEALTH PROMOTION/HEALTH MAINTENANCE

Disease Prevention

Immunizations Has Ms. D'Angelo had the pneumococcal pneumonia vaccine (current recommendation is every 6 years)? Has she had a primary series of tetanus immunization, or does she need a booster? Do you think she has any risk of hepatitis B infection? Is it the season for the influenza vaccine? Does she need one?

Screening *Mildly elevated cholesterol level:* See under Interpretation of Cues, Patterns, and Information.

Colon cancer: This may be a case where you will need to negotiate with her. Many clinicians with a case of this age and history would want her to have at least a flexible sigmoidoscopy. The American Cancer Society recommends this every 5 years for people of average risk, although the U.S. Preventive Services Task Force (1996) feels that there is not enough evidence to make a recommendation. FOBT may be an alternative, although she needs to be willing and able to do this. She may have hemorrhoids, but you do not have information to say conclusively that this is the only site of bleeding.

Glaucoma: She needs testing.

Cervical cancer: This is somewhat controversial in this age group and possibly not significantly able to affect the length of her life since a cervical cancer might not have time to develop to a lethal degree. You cannot really screen anyway since she has refused a pelvic examination. Why is she refusing her pelvic examination? How much will you encourage her to have a pelvic examination based on your level of the assessment of risk?

Breast cancer: A mammogram is recommended.

Family history of DM: Some clinicians would do an occasional fasting blood sugar (FBS), and others would be satisfied with her current laboratory workup unless she develops symptoms.

Health Promotion

Seatbelt: She should be encouraged to use her seatbelt with realistic expectations for change.

Vitamin therapy: Explore the meaning to her, and then consider changes. She is taking well above the recommended daily allowance (RDA) of vitamins C and E, although neither are probably in doses that will be harmful. Why is she doing this? Should she save some money by cutting back? How much zinc is she taking? Would a multivitamin be easier and cheaper and still satisfy her? You may also want to consider whether you should recommend a calcium supplement. A multivitamin would also provide vitamin D.

Low dose aspirin: Some clinicicans would consider this, although there are no conclusive data.

Potential Safety Concerns

Driving: Grossly assess her response times during examination; consider testing if felt to be appropriate based on clinical impression. Has she been in a motor-vehicle accident?

Falls: Assess for throw rugs, lighting, uneven walkways, etc.

Hand rails: These may be helpful; explore why they have not been installed previously and her ideas about them.

Advance Directive

This is related to the previous discussion regarding her objectives about her health care. Encouraging her to think about a DPOA for healthcare is very desirable. A living will can be an adjunct to a DPOA.

FOLLOW-UP

Seeing her back in 1 month will allow a recheck of her blood pressure, the possibility of doing a pelvic examination, as well as possible follow-up on consultations and laboratory tests. This is a very complex case, and it may take you several visits to feel like you have a handle on things. Start the process, address the most serious problems first, and be persistent to the level appropriate.

References

Agency for Health Care Policy and Research: *Acute low back problems,* AHCPR Pub No 95-0642, 1994.

Ham RJ, Sloane PD: *Primary care geriatrics,* St Louis, 1997, Mosby.

Liu P: *Blue book of diagnostic tests,* Philadelphia, 1986, WB Saunders.

Scandinavian Simvastatin Survival Study Group: Randomized trial of cholesterol lowering in 4444 patients with coronary heart disease: the Scandinavian Simvastatin Survival Study (4S), *Lancet* 344:1383, 1994.

US Preventive Services Task Force: *Guide to clinical preventive services,* Baltimore, 1996, Williams & Wilkins.

OPENING SCENARIO

Lisa Pacheco is a 9-month-old female on your schedule for diarrhea for 5 days.

HISTORY OF PRESENT ILLNESS

(Obtained from mother)

"Lisa had a runny nose and cough about 1 week ago, and her stuffiness seems to be getting better. She started with diarrhea about 5 days ago, and that is still present. She had one episode of vomiting about 5 days ago but none since. Her stools are almost pure brown liquid, and she has about 4 to 5 per day. She seems a little uncomfortable just before she moves her bowels and seems to act like she feels better after she goes. She is feeding and drinking well. She is nursing, and I have been giving her cheese and bananas hoping it would bind her up. She is urinating about four to five times a day, which is her normal pattern. Her sister has no symptoms. She is getting a little diaper rash. She attends family daycare 5 days per week."

MEDICAL HISTORY

No accidents or hospitalizations. Immunization record is shown in Table 30-1.

SOCIAL HISTORY

Father smokes 1 pack per day, mother does not smoke. She has one 3-year-old sister.

MEDICATIONS

None

ALLERGIES

None

REVIEW OF SYSTEMS

(Obtained from mother)

General: No night sweats
Cardiac: No evidence of dyspnea, swelling

Gastrointestinal: No anorexia, nausea, vomiting, black or clay colored stools
Genitourinary: No hematuria or pain
Hematological: No excessive bruising

PHYSICAL EXAMINATION

Vital signs: Temperature: 98.6° F (tympanic); *Pulse:* 108 beats/min; *Respirations:* 24 breaths/min
Height: 28"; *Weight:* 18.5 lb (6-month check: 32", 16.5 lb)
Skin: Intact in rectal area; mild to moderate perirectal redness (about 3 cm in diameter); no satellite lesions seen; skin turgor without skin tenting
HEENT: Head is normocephalic, anterior fontanel is flat; pupils equal, round, and reactive to light; extraocular movements intact; tympanic membranes are observable without excessive cerumen or redness; nares are patent without redness or exudate; throat is noninjected; tongue is midline and moist; palate rises symmetrically; all three teeth are in adequate repair
Neck: Supple without thyromegaly or adenopathy

Table **30-1** *Immunization Record for Lisa Pacheco*

Vaccine	Date	Initials	Notes
DPT	2 mo	MDO	Tetramune
DPT	4 mo	KJ	Tetramune
DPT	6 mo	SP	Tetramune
DPT			
DPT			
Td			
OPV	2 mo	MDO	
OPV	4 mo	KJ	
OPV	6 mo	SP	
OPV			
MMR			
MMR			
HBV	2 mo	MDO	
HBV	4 mo	KJ	
HBV	6 mo	SP	
Hib	2 mo	MDO	Tetramune
Hib	4 mo	MDO	Tetramune
Hib	6 mo	MDO	Tetramune

Cardiac: Regular rate and rhythm; no murmurs, rubs, or gallops
Respiratory: Clear to auscultation and percussion
Abdomen: Soft, nontender; no hepatosplenomegaly

Extremities: Without cyanosis, clubbing, or edema
Neuromuscular: Babinski reflexes are equivocal; strength and sensation are symmetrical

---

ASSESSMENT   *Please indicate the problems or issues you have identified that will guide your care (preferably in list form):*

PLAN   *Please list your plans for addressing each of the problems or issues in your assessment:*

Community Clinic
Jeffrey A. Eaton, NP
Joyce D. Cappiello, NP

Name:_____ DOB_____
Address_____ Date_____

Rx

"label all unless indicated"
Refill:_____ times-- Do not refill ( )

Signed:_____
DO NOT TAKE THIS TO YOUR PHARMACIST

Community Clinic
Jeffrey A. Eaton, NP
Joyce D. Cappiello, NP

Name:_____ DOB_____
Address_____ Date_____

Rx

"label all unless indicated"
Refill:_____ times-- Do not refill ( )

Signed:_____
DO NOT TAKE THIS TO YOUR PHARMACIST

Community Clinic
Jeffrey A. Eaton, NP
Joyce D. Cappiello, NP

Name:_____ DOB_____
Address_____ Date_____

Rx

"label all unless indicated"
Refill:_____ times-- Do not refill ( )

Signed:_____
DO NOT TAKE THIS TO YOUR PHARMACIST

Community Clinic
Jeffrey A. Eaton, NP
Joyce D. Cappiello, NP

Name:_____ DOB_____
Address_____ Date_____

Rx

"label all unless indicated"
Refill:_____ times-- Do not refill ( )

Signed:_____
DO NOT TAKE THIS TO YOUR PHARMACIST

LEARNING ISSUES

In order to resolve this patient's problem, you will need to consider and address the following issues (you may generate additional issues as well):

- **Causes of diarrhea in an infant**
- **Diagnostic evaluation for diarrhea**
- **Signs and criteria for dehydration in an infant**
- **Care of perirectal irritation**
- **Treatment of diarrhea in an infant**
- **Oral fluid replacement**
- **Height and weight measurement issues**
- **Normal vital signs for a 9 month old**
- ***Clostridium difficile* as a cause of diarrhea**
- **Diarrhea and breast feeding**

INITIAL IDEAS

- Viral diarrhea
- Low chance of bacterial (food poisoning) or parasitic diarrhea
- Dietary or malabsorption problem
- Perirectal irritation: rule out fungal infection

INTERPRETATION OF CUES, PATTERNS, AND INFORMATION

This problem has only been present for about 5 days. There is no evidence that this has ever happened before, although you may want to ask that question specifically. There is also a history of a stuffy nose that preceded the diarrhea, so that is support for a viral etiology.

How will you decide whether she is at risk for a bacterial or parasitic diarrhea? In general, fever is more common in diarrhea of bacterial origin. Dietary history would be important. Bacterial diarrheas such as salmonella, shigella, or *E. coli* are possible, but if mild, they are usually treated similarly to viral infections. The diarrhea is not bloody, and if it was, greater concern for a problem such as enterotoxic *E. coli* would be a consideration, especially if the child had eaten meat that was not fully cooked.

If Lisa had been exposed to other children who had a bacterial or parasitic infection, she might have contracted an infection by putting soiled toys or objects into her mouths. Her sister has no symptoms, but is anyone else in the family ill? Have they been camping, or do they have well water that could potentially be contaminated with *Giardia?* These are low probabilities at this point since she has only had the diarrhea for about 5 days, but they may be worth at least brief consideration.

Dietary history would also be important to determine whether there was some new food that Lisa was not tolerating. Has she been getting excessive amounts of juice because she was not feeling well? Has that juice had an artificial sweetener that has been associated with causing diarrhea?

Another low probability but potentially serious issue is whether she has had a recent course of antibiotics. If she had an antibiotic such as a cephalosporin or amoxicillin/clavulanate then *Clostridium difficile* infection should be suspected.

Another cause of diarrhea that should be considered in a child is appendicitis. About 15% of children with appendicitis develop diarrhea (Johnson and Oski, 1997). It is quite uncommon in an infant, however, so that lowers the probability in Lisa. If she did have what appeared to be an acute surgical abdomen, immediate referral would be appropriate.

Lisa's height and weight are quite important but in this case are somewhat problematic. Do you think she really lost 4 inches of length in 3 months? The probability is that there was some sort of measurement error. Her 2-pound weight gain in the past 3 months would have her moving from the 50th percentile to about the 45th. At this point, that does not seem to be of any concern, but long-term monitoring will be done as it would in all children.

Do not forget to treat Lisa's symptoms and look after her comfort, so you also have to consider her perirectal irritation. Her physical examination showed no satellite lesions, so it appears that this is not a fungal infection. Therefore you can probably make a presumptive assessment that the redness is related to the chemical irritation of the diarrhea and that simple barrier treatment may be enough at this point.

REVISED IDEAS
- Viral diarrhea
- Perirectal irritation related to chemical irritation from diarrhea (doubtfully fungal infection)

DIFFERENTIAL DIAGNOSIS
- Viral infection
- Bacterial infection
- Parasitic infection
- Dietary intolerance
- Appendicitis (low probability)

DIAGNOSTIC OPTIONS

How precise do you need to be in this particular diagnosis? Is it enough to rule out potentially serious causes of diarrhea through history and physical findings and then provide symptomatic and supportive therapy? In general, as long as the child does not appear dehydrated, has not had diarrhea for more than 7 to 10 days, and is not having any other symptoms, knowing the exact cause of the diarrhea (viral, Campylobacter, or mild salmonella) may not change the therapy or outcome in any way.

Stool cultures and samples for ova and parasites are options, but they are probably best reserved for a later time.

THERAPEUTIC OPTIONS

Pharmacological

Medications are usually avoided in infants with diarrhea. Consultation with a pediatrician might be appropriate before starting a child in this age group on a medication therapy for diarrhea.

To treat the perirectal irritation, some simple Vaseline or a zinc oxide ointment could be helpful. Desitin has 40% zinc oxide as compared with 20% in most zinc oxide ointments, so many clinicians recommend Desitin. If satellite lesions were present, a mild antifungal would be more appropriate.

Educational

Probably the most important part of the educational approach is that the family understand the self-limiting nature of most diarrheal episodes in children. Maintenance of oral intake is key as well. Cleaning Lisa quickly and applying the barrier chosen after each stool will probably clear up the irritation quickly.

Should Lisa be sent to daycare? Clearly this is an individualized decision that varies depending on the case. In this case you do not know the parents occupations and the 'need' to go to daycare as perceived by the parents. You also do not know if Lisa has been going to daycare all along. If the parents are amenable, specifically discussing the case and helping the parents make appropriate decisions may be to the best advantage for both the child and other children at the daycare. Many clinicians would recommend that Lisa be kept at home until she has been without diarrhea for about 24 hours.

Other Nonpharmacological Options

Maintenance of hydration is essential, and yet this is an evolving area of knowledge. Traditional diarrhea therapy has included a period of bowel rest followed by clear liquids and the avoidance of milk or other potentially irritating substances. The American Academy of Pediatrics has, since 1985, recommended that bowel rest is unnecessary. Vomiting is also not a contraindication to providing fluid replacement via the oral route. Evidence seems to indicate that early feeding is beneficial and that it may reduce stool output and hasten recovery. Meyer (1995) suggests rapid, oral rehydration with a glucose or cereal-based rehydration solution and early refeeding with a mixed diet. Cessation of breast feeding is not necessary, and removal of lactose from the diet is not recommended unless the child has signs of lactose intolerance. If the diarrhea is severe or persistent, antimicrobial therapy can be considered. Clinicians need to explore their own ideas and the evidence base supporting those ideas as well as the conventional wisdom that patients and families will have learned. The World Health Organization has also provided recommendations regarding the optimal constituents of a replacement solution.

HEALTH PROMOTION/HEALTH MAINTENANCE

Lisa is up-to-date on her immunizations, so she will just need to come back at 12 months for her next immunizations. This diarrhea alone is probably not a contraindication to immunization if she was behind for any reason.

Depending on the amount of time that you have and your assessment of Lisa's illness, you may want to carry out some anticipatory guidance (AG). AG that could be given at a 9-month visit would include issues of babyproofing since she is entering a stage where she will be increasingly mobile. Ipecac should be obtained if it has not already. A review of anticipated development could include the fact that Lisa will be soon increasing babbling sounds and sitting by herself if she has not already. You may want to think about doing the AG now since you probably will not see Lisa for another 9-month check, but you will base this on how receptive the parents will be based on their current level of worry. A tuberculosis (TB) test and/or a hematocrit are also a consideration. Lead screening and testing if needed could be carried out. See what her parents are doing currently.

FOLLOW-UP

Lisa can probably be followed up at her 1 year visit unless there is a lack of resolution of the diarrhea. The parents should then call or return.

References

Johnson KJ, Oski FA: *Essential pediatrics,* Philadelphia, 1997, JB Lippincott.

Meyer A: Modern management of acute diarrhea and dehydration in children, *Am Fam Physician,* 51(5): 1103, 1995.

CASE
31

OPENING SCENARIO

Lynne Spencer is a 19-year-old, single, female college sophomore scheduled for a gynecological/physical examination. This is her first visit to your practice. She is slumped in her chair and appears tired.

HISTORY OF PRESENT ILLNESS

"I'm here for my annual gynecological examination for renewal of birth control pills. Since the beginning of the semester, I've been feeling depressed and increasingly stressed. Much of this stress is due to financial concerns because I need a job to pay tuition. Last summer I had a good work-study job that I really liked, but it did not carry over into this semester. I don't have friends other than my boyfriend, and we don't seem to have much fun anymore."

MEDICAL HISTORY

History of chronic allergies with ongoing sinus and bronchitis problems. Mononucleosis as a high school sophomore. After this she was diagnosed with chronic fatigue syndrome (CFS). Had a series of sinus infections through her junior and senior years resulting in missing a great deal of school, which was difficult socially. Sinus surgery during her senior year with fewer infections since then. History of asthma, controlled currently with cetirizine, beclomethasone dipropionate inhaler daily, and albuterol prn.

FAMILY MEDICAL HISTORY

MGM: 67 yr (hypertension)
MGF: 69 yr (emphysema)
PGM: 71 yr (A&W)
PGF: 71 yr (Alzheimer's disease)
Mother: 45 yr (A&W)
Father: 47 yr (chronically depressed)
One sister: 23 yr (A&W)

SOCIAL HISTORY

Lives in dorm with one roommate; they do not get along. Is afraid to confront her about issues. Has not made many friends; feels since she does not drink alcohol she is not popular. Only friends are her boyfriend (some distress over this relationship) and his roommate. Has recently completed a course that will enable her to teach aerobics and is hopeful that this activity will be a way to meet people and earn some money.

Usually visits her parents on the weekend; parents are supportive. Her father is a carpenter who is frequently unemployed because of the seasonal nature of his work. Her mom works in a bank. Her sister just moved to a state far away; she misses her very much. Her father has been chronically depressed since serving in the Vietnam War, and it is worse when he is out of work. There is no history of depression on her mother's side of the family.

She denies smoking, alcohol, or drug use. Doing adequately in school, getting B and C grades; had better grades as a freshman. Denies history of domestic violence. Does not use seatbelt.

Complains of difficulty sleeping; stays up late (midnight to 1 AM) because she cannot fall asleep earlier and then wakes frequently during the night. Sometimes she goes back to sleep easily but other times just lies awake feeling sad. Has low energy and feels tired during the day. Rarely takes a daytime nap.

MEDICATIONS

Cetirizine HCl (Zyrtec): 10 mg daily
Ovcon 35: Daily
Beclomethasone dipropionate (Beclovent) metered dose inhaler: 4 puffs bid
Albuterol (Proventil) inhaler: 2 puffs every 4 hours prn

ALLERGIES

None

REVIEW OF SYSTEMS

General: States that she has low energy and her mood is low; her weight has been stable for many years
HEENT: Currently no sinus problems of headache, pain, nasal discharge, or postnasal drip but was treated 3 months ago with course of cefuroxime, 500 mg bid for 10 days with good results; this was her first sinus infection in over 1 year; sees dentist yearly; no dental problems
Cardiac: No chest pain; no history of murmurs or rheumatic fever

Respiratory: No shortness of breath, difficulty breathing, wheezing, or cough; diagnosed with asthma in high school; uses Beclovent inhaler bid without fail and uses the albuterol inhaler infrequently in the fall or winter; she is bothered more in the summer months with allergies to grasses; uses protective plastic mattress and pillow to protect against dust mites; participates in aerobics without problems; peak flows average 400, which she hasn't checked since she had the sinus infection

Gastrointestinal: Denies heartburn, abdominal pain, nausea, vomiting, diarrhea, or constipation; appetite less for several weeks, but states she does eat; no weight loss

Genitourinary: Last menstrual period (LMP) was 1 week ago; on Ovcon 35 for 2 years; same sexual partner for 2 years, has known him for 5 years; denies dyspareunia or postcoital spotting; expresses concerns about lack of sex drive and not having orgasms; denies history of sexual or physical abuse; all previous Pap smears normal

Endocrine: Low energy; temperature tolerances good, denies dry skin or hair, hoarseness

Neurological: Tension headaches 1 to 2 times per week relieved by acetaminophen; saw psychiatrist for two visits during her senior year in high school for insomnia and depression after sinus surgery and slow recovery; no medications or follow-up at that time; states that she fleetingly feels suicidal with no real plans; knows she would never do it since her elementary school teacher committed suicide, and she saw what distress this caused the friends and family of the teacher; feels unhappy with self, insecure; has few close friends

Extremities: No history of fractures, sprains; denies current arthralgias, myalgias

PHYSICAL EXAMINATION

Vital signs: Temperature: 97.8° F; *Pulse:* 74 beats/min; *Respirations:* 16 breaths/min; *BP:* 120/76 mm Hg
Height: 5' 5"; *Weight:* 125 lb; *BMI:* 21
General: Flat affect; speech a bit slow; mood low
HEENT: No frontal or maxillary pain elicited; nasal mucosa slightly pale, no polyps; eardrums: no redness, landmarks visualized; good dentition; no postnasal mucus noted
Neck: No thyromegaly or lymphadenopathy noted
Heart: Regular rate and rhythm; no murmurs, rubs, or gallops
Lungs: No cough or secretions noted; slight expiratory wheezes; no other adventitious sounds
Breasts: No masses noted
Abdomen: Bowel sounds present; no masses, tenderness noted; no hepatosplenomegaly
Genitourinary: Vulva: no lesions, redness; vagina: no discharge, lesions; cervix: clear without lesions; uterus: anteverted, smooth, nontender; adnexa: nontender, no enlargement
Extremities: Normal gait
Neurological: Speech is clear but slow; thought processes appropriate; cranial nerves 2 to 12 intact

ASSESSMENT   *Please indicate the problems or issues you have identified that will guide your care (preferably in list form):*

PLAN   *Please list your plans for addressing each of the problems or issues in your assessment:*

Community Clinic
Jeffrey A. Eaton, NP
Joyce D. Cappiello, NP

Name:_____ DOB_____
Address_____ Date_____

Rx

"label all unless indicated"
Refill:_____ times-- Do not refill ( )

Signed:_____
DO NOT TAKE THIS TO YOUR PHARMACIST

Community Clinic
Jeffrey A. Eaton, NP
Joyce D. Cappiello, NP

Name:_____ DOB_____
Address_____ Date_____

Rx

"label all unless indicated"
Refill:_____ times-- Do not refill ( )

Signed:_____
DO NOT TAKE THIS TO YOUR PHARMACIST

Community Clinic
Jeffrey A. Eaton, NP
Joyce D. Cappiello, NP

Name:_____ DOB_____
Address_____ Date_____

Rx

"label all unless indicated"
Refill:_____ times-- Do not refill ( )

Signed:_____
DO NOT TAKE THIS TO YOUR PHARMACIST

Community Clinic
Jeffrey A. Eaton, NP
Joyce D. Cappiello, NP

Name:_____ DOB_____
Address_____ Date_____

Rx

"label all unless indicated"
Refill:_____ times-- Do not refill ( )

Signed:_____
DO NOT TAKE THIS TO YOUR PHARMACIST

LEARNING ISSUES

In order to resolve this patient's problem, you will need to consider and address the following issues (you may generate additional issues as well):

- **Reliability of screening tests for depression**
- **Diagnostic and Statistical Manual of Mental Disorders (DSM-IV)**
- **Screening for suicidal tendencies**
- **How do you decide on counseling and/or pharmacological approaches?**
- **Choice of an appropriate antidepressant**
- **Differential diagnosis appropriate to this patient**
- **Role of oral contraceptives (OCs), if any, in this patient's depression**

INITIAL IDEAS

In this case, depression is near the top of the differential list based on symptoms, family history, and life stresses.

INTERPRETATION OF CUES, PATTERNS, AND INFORMATION

Screening for Depression

The Guide to Clinical Preventative Services states that there is insufficient evidence to recommend for or against the routine use of standardized questionnaires to screen for depression in primary care, although depression is a common and costly illness seen in primary care. The most serious endpoint is suicide, which unfortunately has been on the increase especially among adolescents and young adults. The most common impact of major depression, however, is on the quality of life and the level of productivity. This effect is widespread and has been shown to be comparable with the effects associated with major chronic medical conditions such as diabetes, hypertension, and coronary heart disease. Moreover, individuals with undiagnosed depression often present to clinicians with somatic symptoms that lead to extensive, costly, and often unnecessary medical testing and interventions (US Preventative Services Task Force, 1996).

There are several widely used screening tools such as the Beck Depression Inventory, the Zung Self-Rating Depression Scale, and the Center for Epidemiological Studies Depression Scale with sensitivities of 90% to 100% and specificity's of 60% to 90% when used in primary care settings. Other tools have been developed for children and adolescents. Whooley et al (1997) found that two simple clinical questions are a sensitive method for detecting depression:

- "During the past month, have you been bothered by feeling down, depressed, or hopeless?"
- "During the past month, have you been bothered by little interest or no pleasure in doing things?"

A positive response to one or both questions indicates the need for a more thorough assessment, whereas negative responses to both questions were shown to rule out depression.

The diagnosis of depression seems quite clear in Ms. Spencer's case, even without the use of a screening tool. Use of the screening tool may provide a helpful comparison during subsequent visits in evaluating response to treatment.

Some providers find it easier to ask first about physical symptoms of depression, such as appetite, sleep, and energy level. The mnemonic SIG E CAPS is used by some providers and is listed in Box 31-1.

The current criteria for the diagnosis of depression as described in the DSM-IV for a dysthymic disorder (mild depression) is as follows (American Psychiatric Association, 1994):

A. Depressed mood for at least 2 years

B. Presence, while depressed, of at least two of the following:
   1. Poor appetite or eating
   2. Insomnia or hypersomnia
   3. Low energy or fatigue
   4. Low self-esteem
   5. Poor concentration
   6. Feelings of hopelessness

C. During the 2 years of the disturbance, never without the symptoms for more than 2 months at a time

D. Not due to drugs, recent major depression, or schizophrenia

Screening for Suicide

Anyone who is identified as having symptoms of depression must be asked about their potential for suicide. A direct question such as, "Have you considered committing suicide?" is appropriate. If the response is positive, ask how the individual plans to do so. This individual then needs an immediate referral to a mental health provider. Asking about suicide will not put the idea into someone's head. Patients who are serious about suicide may be relieved to be asked the question. If not suicidal as of this visit, a contract for safety can be discussed whereby the patient agrees to call you if feeling suicidal in the future.

OTHER IDEAS

- Rheumatoid disease
- Substance abuse

Box 31-1 SIG E CAPS

S: Is your SLEEP disturbed?
I: Have you noted a loss of libido or INTEREST in your usual activities?
G: Are you feeling GUILTY or having self-deprecating thoughts?
E: Have you noticed a decrease in your ENERGY level?
C: Have you been having trouble CONCENTRATING?
A: Have you experienced changes in your APPETITE and weight?
P: Have you been physically slowed down or sped up (PSYCHOMOTOR abnormalities)?
S: Have you thought of SUICIDE, feelings of hopelessness, or preoccupation with issues related to death?

- Lyme disease
- Fibromyalgia
- Thyroid disease
- CFS

DIAGNOSTIC OPTIONS

Most of the other ideas can be ruled out by history. Rheumatoid disease can be ruled out since she has no joint pain. It is unlikely that antihistamines or inhaled corticosteroids would cause a depression. Depression can be related to OC use, although the incidence is less today since the amount of hormones in pills has decreased. Ask if the depression began or became worse after starting the pill. In Ms. Spencer's case, the symptoms became acute over the past few months, but you question whether she has struggled with a chronic, low-level depression for many years. The symptoms do not seem to coincide with initiation of OC use 2 years ago.

She denies substance abuse, which is encouraging since there is a clear association between alcohol abuse and depression in women (Carlson and Eisenstat, 1995).

Lyme disease seems low on the differential list. She has no history of a skin reaction, severe headaches, or serious fatigue. Although there are some complaints of fatigue, they do not seem to be debilitating. Her musculoskeletal and neurological examinations do not indicate any problems associated with Lyme disease.

Trigger points were not found to suggest fibromyalgia.

Thyroid disease could be a concern. Accordingly, a thyroid-stimulating hormone (TSH), a cost-effective and accurate test, could be ordered.

CFS is still a possibility, especially since she was diagnosed with this in high school. It may also be that the symptoms she was experiencing in high school were somatic complaints secondary to an undiagnosed depression. The common symptoms in patients with CFS are easy fatigueability, difficulty concentrating, headache, sore throat, tender lymph nodes, muscles aches, joint aches, fever, difficulty sleeping, and psychiatric problems. Ms. Spencer is complaining of few of these physical symptoms. Depression may be a component of CFS, thus treating the depression would be helpful.

An anemia could cause fatigue. A complete blood count (CBC) or hemoglobin and hematocrit in the office would give information on anemia.

Environmental Allergies and Asthma

It appears that these problems are fairly well controlled. She can participate in aerobics and rarely uses her albuterol inhaler. Sinusitis, bronchitis, and asthmatic attacks seem to occur less frequently than during her high school years. At least from her point of view, daily use of medication seems to control symptoms, but mild wheezing was noted on examination, which indicates that her asthma is not totally controlled. Depending on the season, a flu shot is indicated with a history of asthma.

Physical Examination

The usual assessment of heart and lungs was performed; HEENT was examined because of the history of asthma. Because of the need to narrow the differential list, a musculoskeletal examination is included. Testing of the cranial nerves, however, added little to the diagnostic picture but does help rule out organic disease.

WORKING DIAGNOSIS

- Depression
- Asthma

THERAPEUTIC OPTIONS

Depression

The choices are to treat her depression with medication, refer her for counseling, do both, or not treat at all. Given her symptoms and overall mood, it appears that her quality of life is affected and intervention is needed.

Counseling can add an important component to the treatment. Models of female development, unlike models of male development, suggest that women define themselves primarily through relationships with others—family, friends, lovers, and children. Thus any attempt to understand women's development, and especially depression, must place relationship issues at the center (Carlson and Eisenstat, 1995). A skilled counselor can help Ms. Spencer explore her difficulty negotiating relationships with peers and issues with her boyfriend. Most insurance providers will pay for at least a limited number of visits for psychotherapy. Usually, you or your office will have previously identified a network of mental health providers in your community to whom you can make referrals. In this case, a referral to the college mental health services will be covered under her health fee.

Antidepressants can also play a significant role in the treatment of Ms. Spencer. There are many choices of antidepressants today (Table 31-1), but keep in mind that the efficacy rate is similar in all antidepressants. The main difference between the tricyclic and monoamine oxidase (MAO) inhibitors and the newer selective serotonin reuptake inhibitors (SSRI) and selective serotonin norepinephrine inhibitors (SSNI) is the safety and side-effect profile. Even a week's worth of the tricyclic antidepressants is enough for a successful suicide overdose. This is not true with the newer drugs since they are not as toxic and have an emetic effect in large quantities. Thus prescriptions can safely be written for a longer period of time before a refill is needed.

New primary care providers would do well to familiarize themselves with the SSRI and SSNI and avoid prescribing other antidepressants to reduce any suicidal overdose potential. The newer drugs are more expensive, but most of the pharmaceutical companies offer plans to provide indigent patients with free medications. Antidepressants produce improvement in about two thirds of patients in clinical trials involving major depression. The onset of action occurs within 2 to 6 weeks after beginning the medications. Thus an adequate therapeutic trial is considered to be 6 weeks. However, many patients become impatient with this time frame. In actuality, most patients who respond to a medication will begin to do so by 3 to 4 weeks, provided that the drug is in the upper therapeutic dose range. Often, a clinical decision to switch to another antidepressant is made before 6 weeks.

Table **31-1** *Categories of Newer Antidepressants*

Drug	Trade Name	Dosage
SSRI		
Fluoxetine	Prozac	20-80 mg
Sertraline	Zoloft	50-200 mg
Paroxetine	Paxil	20-50 mg
SSNI		
Nefazodone	Serzone	100-500 mg
Venlafaxine	Effexor	75-375 mg
ATYPICAL		
Bupropion	Welbutrin	200-250 mg
Trazodone	Desyrel	150-400 mg
Mirtazapine	Remeron	15-45 mg

The choice of which drug to use is guided by the side-effect profile and the neurotransmitter action. DeWester, in the 1996 supplement to the *Journal of Family Practice,* expertly reviews prescribing issues:

"Most of the new antidepressants target serotonin, some target norepinephrine, and two drugs target dopamine. If the use of a drug targeting serotonin is unsuccessful, then try a medication targeting norepinephrine. If both of these approaches are unsuccessful, try a medication that targets dopamine, such as bupropion. Because bupropion has a unique side-effect profile of visual disturbances, nausea, appetite suppression and activation, and on rare occasions seizures, it is relegated to second line therapy."

Before prescribing these medications, it is necessary to consider the side-effect profile of each drug or category. In general, the side-effect profile of the SSRIs includes headache, nausea, sleep disturbance, and sexual dysfunction.

In addition to the recognized side effects of this class, each individual SSRI has a specific side-effect profile. Fluoxetine frequently causes anxiousness, jitteriness, restlessness, and nervousness on initiation of therapy. The latter is seen less commonly with sertraline and rarely with paroxetine. If a patient is presenting with a complaint of anxiety, there may be difficulty with the activation stage of fluoxetine. The usual dose is 20 mg daily, but fluoxetine is available in 10 mg doses to allow a slow titration upwards.

Sertraline may cause loose stools and diarrhea. Patients with irritable bowel symptoms should avoid this drug and may do better on paroxetine.

Paroxetine can cause somnolence and constipation because of the mild anticholinergic properties, which may explain the calming effect that often occurs during therapy.

All SSRIs inhibit several cytochrome P-450 enzymes. Many commonly used drugs in primary care are metabolized by these enzymes. Since it is not possible to predict the development of significant drug interactions, careful clinical monitoring of all medications is necessary.

Nefazodone is chemically related to trazodone but causes less sedation, orthostasis, and priapism. It inhibits serotonin and norepinephrine uptake but mainly acts as an antagonist of the 5-HT2 receptor. The main difference in side effects from the SSRI is the lack of early agitation, no disturbance of sleep patterns, and no sexual dysfunction. Unfortunately, because of its short half life, it must be given two to three times a day rather than once a day. Nefazodone cannot be started shortly after discontinuing a SSRI because of the drug interactions involving the cytochrome P-450 system.

Venlafaxine selectively inhibits serotonin and norepinephrine reuptake. It can cause increases in blood pressure, sexual dysfunction, sweating, and somnolence. It must be started slowly and titrated upwards to reduce nausea and vomiting. Because of its short half-life, it must be given two to three times a day. Because of these side effects, it is considered a second-line drug for depression.

Mirtazapine is a new medication that enhances transmission of norepinephrine and serotonin with the side effects of sedation and weight gain. It has few gastrointestinal side effects or associated sexual dysfunction (DeWester, 1996).

The next step to this clinical decision making is to specifically tailor medication to this individual. Ms. Spencer currently complains of difficulty falling asleep and waking frequently. Because of the sleep problems, nefazodone may be a good first choice, but it needs to be taken two to three times a day. The ease of taking the antidepressant may be a very important issue to this young woman. There is not a clear reason to prescribe a particular antidepressant to Ms. Spencer, so you may choose a medication with which you have the more extensive experience or based on a prescribing formulary. The asthma medications she routinely uses do not involve the cytochrome P-450 system, and therefore potential drug interactions are not an issue.

Improvement is usually seen primarily in the physiological areas, whereas some of the other symptoms like low self-esteem and depressed mood may not completely respond to medication.

The best barometers of early medication response include improved sleep, less daytime fatigue, and some improvement in emotional control (less frequent crying or better frustration tolerance). The clinician may need to inquire specifically about these symptoms because many depressed people will say, "I'm not better," despite the fact that there is symptomatic improvement

The length of therapy will vary for individuals. Typically, it may take 4 to 8 weeks for a major depression to subside. If medication were to be discontinued at this point, relapse would be quite high. A general rule is to continue 6 months beyond the point of symptomatic improvement and to reduce the dose gradually. This is typically 9 to 12 months.

During the first month of pharmacological treament, weekly visits will help increase compliance and provide an opportunity to adjust doses and monitor side effects. After the acute phase and the appropriate dose of the medications is determined, monthly or 6-week visits are adequate (Carlson and Eisenstat, 1995).

Give her positive reenforcement about her decision to become an aerobics instructor. This not only provides exercise but causes her to interact with new people and will help to ease her financial situation.

Finances continue to be a stressful area. She probably should return to the financial aid office for additional assistance or other work-study jobs.

Asthma

It would be helpful to obtain some current peak flow measurements on her. A baseline could be obtained at the office, and she can follow up with additional measurements at home. These can be reviewed in 1 week, and then the decision can be made regarding adjustments to her medication. Remind her to use her albuterol (2 puffs qid) if she notices any problems and, of course, to continue with the beclomethasone dipropionate as baseline therapy. A review of inhaler technique while in the office is always appropriate.

The Cetirizine HCl may contribute to her fatigue. If this symptom does not improve, a medication change can be considered.

Contraception

Continue Triphasil. If Ms. Spencer's depressive symptoms do not improve with therapy and medication use, the role of OCs in her depression can be revisited. Some authorities speculate that low vitamin B_6 levels secondary to OC use may play a role in depression. It is easy enough to suggest a low dose of 25 to 50 mg per day. Vitamin B_6 can be purchased over-the-counter. Large doses of 1 to 2 grams per day are contraindicated because of side effects of reversible peripheral neuropathy.

HEALTH PROMOTION/HEALTH MAINTENANCE

Issues of updating immunizations, screening for substance abuse, domestic violence, urging use of seatbelts, and exercise levels have been addressed. Any change in her appetite and sleep disturbances will be a barometer of her response to medication and psychotherapy.

References

American Psyciatric Association: *Diagnostic and statistical manual of mental disorders,* ed 4, Washington, DC, 1994, American Psychiatric Association.

Carlson K, Eisenstat S: *Primary care of women.* St. Louis, 1995, Mosby.

DeWester J: Recognizing and treating the patient with somatic manifestations of depression, *J Fam Pract,* 43, 6 (Suppl) S3-S13, 1996.

US Preventive Services Task Force: *Guide to clinical preventive services,* ed 2, Baltimore, 1996, Williams & Wilkins.

Wooley et al: Case-finding instruments for depression, *J Gen Intern Med* 12:439, 1997.

CASE
32

1:00 PM
Irene Anderson
Age 39 years

OPENING SCENARIO

Irene Anderson is a 39-year-old female in your office for an annual gynecological examination and Pap smear. She was last seen in your office 1 year ago. This is her second visit with you.

HISTORY OF PRESENT ILLNESS

"Last year I saw you for my Pap smear. I have been thinking about that visit for the past year. I lied to you. You asked if anyone was hurting me and I said no. (Client is now very distraught and can barely talk.) This is the second time that I have had an abusive partner. I'm so embarrassed. I have never told this to anyone. Everyone thinks we are a great couple. I work in town at the Pelican Coffee Shop, and I would never want all the townspeople to know this about me. He has hit me a few times, but lately he's constantly yelling and swearing at me. He makes me feel terrible all the time, like I'm no good."

MEDICAL HISTORY

The visit 1 year ago addressed her expressed need for contraception. She did not follow through with the plan to use depomedroxyprogesterone acetate (DMPA). Had dental surgery just before visit of last year and was using Percocet occasionally. Other surgery: bilateral reduction mammoplasty at age 20. No history of diabetes mellitus (DM), hypertension, or other chronic diseases.

FAMILY MEDICAL HISTORY

MGM: 79 yr (arthritis)
MGF: Deceased at 72 yr (myocardial infarction [MI])
PGM: 83 yr (adult onset DM diagnosed last year)
PGF: Deceased at 56 yr (auto accident)
Mother: 60 yr (A&W)
Father: 62 yr (mild hypertension)

SOCIAL HISTORY

Has never smoked. When asked, states she is drinking alcohol to block out her concerns about the relationship. Drinks 4 to 5 drinks (beers, wine, or mixed drinks) per day. The CAGE questionnaire reveals the following:
- **C:** She thinks she should cut down on her drinking.
- **A:** No one is angry about her drinking.
- **G:** She feels guilty about her drinking.
- **E:** She does not need an eye opener but sometimes feels shaky.

Ms. Anderson denies recreational or prescription drug use. Drinks 3 cups of coffee per day, no soda or tea. States she eats 3 balanced meals per day. Uses Stairmaster 3 times per week plus active job as a waitress. Sleeps 5 to 6 hours per night. Wears seatbelts. States it was difficult to get time off for this appointment. Works long hours and cannot miss work. Does not have health insurance. Requests that the office not call her house for any reason because her partner would become suspicious. Has lived with this partner for 1 1/2 years. States she does not make enough to handle the rent for living alone. No children in the household. Her family lives 2 hours away but are not supportive emotionally or financially.

MEDICATIONS

None

ALLERGIES

None

REVIEW OF SYSTEMS

General: All childhood immunizations; tetanus-diphtheria (Td) 5 year ago; no hepatitis vaccines
Skin: Uses tanning booths regularly; no changes in moles
HEENT: States chronic gum problems for which she is seeing a dentist; denies problems with vision or hearing; no history of frequent colds, seasonal allergies, sore throats
Cardiac: Denies chest pain, palpitations, elevated blood pressure
Respiratory: Chronic problems as a child (not sure if it was asthma); no shortness of breath, asthma, cough as an adult
Breast: Mammogram negative last year; ordered at visit last year since you had difficulty performing accurate examination because of multiple areas of scar tissue after reduction surgery; does not do self breast examinations

Gastrointestinal: Appetite fair; no weight loss or gain; denies heartburn, nausea or vomiting, epigastric pain, abdominal pain; no chronic problems with diarrhea, constipation, hemorrhoids, blood in stools

Genitourinary: Menarche at age 12; history of regular cycles every 28 days, lasting 4 to 6 days with moderate flow and occasional menstrual cramps; last menstrual period (LMP) 2 weeks ago; denies dyspareunia or postcoital spotting; no vaginal itching, burning, discharge; no history of sexually transmitted diseases (STDs); mild premenstrual syndrome (PMS) symptoms; contraception: condoms; G1P0Ab1 (early miscarriage 10 years ago); urinary tract infections (UTI): two about 10 and 15 years ago; denies urinary stress incontinence

Musculoskeletal: No history of sprains, fractures, joint pain; ingrown right great toenail for 2 months causing mild discomfort

Neurological: Tension headaches about once a week relieved by Tylenol; no weakness, seizures, paresthesia, memory changes; feels depressed at times over the past year; denies suicidal feelings

Endocrine: Temperature tolerances good; occasional fatigue

PHYSICAL EXAMINATION

Vital signs: Temperature: 98.0° F; *Pulse:* 74 beats/min; *Respirations:* 16 breaths/min; BP: 140/90 mm Hg
Height: 5' 3"; *Weight:* 110 lb
General: Tanned, well nourished female looking distressed

Skin: No bruising, cuts, abrasions noted; multiple small brown nevi on trunk

HEENT: Pupils equal and reactive to light; tympanic membranes: crisp cone of light, no redness; nares patent; gums reddened secondary to surgery; pharynx: no redness or exudate

Neck: Thyroid: no enlargement or nodularity noted; no supraclavicular lymphadenopathy

Cardiac: Regular rate and rhythm; no murmurs, rubs, or gallops

Respiratory: Lungs clear to auscultation

Breasts: Faint scar lines visible on each breast; on palpation, 3 cm wide prominent strip in each breast extending from nipple downward to mammary ridge; firm, very well defined scar line secondary to reduction mammoplasty

Abdomen: No hepatosplenomegaly; soft, nontender, no masses palpated

Pelvic: Vulva: no lesions, redness, discharge; vagina: scant white mucus, no lesions; cervix: no redness or lesions; uterus: anteverted, small, nontender; adnexa: no tenderness or enlargement

Extremities: Right great toe: redness, tenderness at nailbed; minimal swelling, no drainage; no bruises noted anywhere on body

Neurological: Alert with appropriate affect; muscle strength testing normal (5/5), muscle sensation equal bilaterally; biceps, triceps, patellar, ankle reflexes 2+; Babinski signs not present; cranial nerves 2 to 12 intact.

ASSESSMENT   *Please indicate the problems or issues you have identified that will guide your care (preferably in list form):*

PLAN   *Please list your plans for addressing each of the problems or issues in your assessment:*

Community Clinic
Jeffrey A. Eaton, NP
Joyce D. Cappiello, NP

Name:_____ DOB_____
Address_____ Date_____

Rx

"label all unless indicated"
Refill:_____ times-- Do not refill ( )

Signed:_____
DO NOT TAKE THIS TO YOUR PHARMACIST

Community Clinic
Jeffrey A. Eaton, NP
Joyce D. Cappiello, NP

Name:_____ DOB_____
Address_____ Date_____

Rx

"label all unless indicated"
Refill:_____ times-- Do not refill ( )

Signed:_____
DO NOT TAKE THIS TO YOUR PHARMACIST

LEARNING ISSUES

In order to resolve this patient's problem, you will need to consider and address the following issues (you may generate additional issues as well):

- Why screen for domestic violence in your practice?
- Ways to screen for domestic violence
- If a patient replies positively to your screening questions, how will you respond?
- Appropriate physical examination techniques
- Available community resources
- Health maintenance issues to be addressed now or at subsequent visits.
- Appropriate follow-up

INITIAL IDEAS

The social issues are the most pressing health needs of Ms. Anderson. How does a provider ask questions about sensitive issues? How does a provider effectively respond to these needs? What are the available community resources?

INTERPRETATION OF CUES, PATTERNS, AND INFORMATION

Possible Screening Questions for Domestic Violence

The major discomfort of most providers with this issue is how to ask appropriate questions:
1. Have you been hit, kicked, punched, or otherwise hurt by someone within the past year? If so, by whom?
2. Do you feel safe in your current relationship?
3. Is there a partner from a previous relationship who is making you feel unsafe now?
The sensitivity of these questions in detecting partner abuse was found to be 64.5% with a specificity of 80.3%. The first question was more sensitive and specific than the questions regarding safety and detected almost as many of the abused patients as all three questions (Feldhaus et al, 1997). Examples of additional questions are located in the resource section at the end of this case.

The challenge is to understand and remember the main objectives of these questions and put them in your own words. Then gently ask questions that allow a fearful woman to acknowledge abuse and begin to seek help, even if she is not ready to leave the abusive relationship. Providers often feel more comfortable with prefacing these type of questions with a statement such as, "Because many women are hurt or threatened by their partner, I've begun to ask about it routinely." Avoid using the words abuse, battered, or domestic violence since patients often do not perceive or identify themselves with these words.

Mandatory reporting is not required unless you are dealing with an individual under 18 years of age, a disabled person, or an elder. It is thought that mandatory reporting would frighten women away from seeking help rather than encouraging it.

Any time you ask questions of your patients, you need to be prepared for their responses. Will you be uncomfortable with the subject, fear offending the women, feel powerless to help, or have too little time? Look at each of these issues. These reasons for not asking about domestic violence were identified in a study of physician attitudes in a large urban Health Maintenance Organization (HMO) (Sugg and Inui, 1992). If you are uncomfortable with the subject, there are a variety of ways to work on this. The first is to read about the subject. In the past several years, articles have begun to appear regularly in the professional journals since this issue can have such a major impact on the health of women. Many published studies have shown that domestic violence is the reason for a high number of female visits to emergency rooms. The injury and trauma is usually responded to appropriately, but less emphasis has been placed on trying to understand the source of these injuries. As health professionals, historically we have not done a good job of assessing patients for domestic violence. Some 92% of women who have been physically abused by their partners did not discuss the incident with their health providers. About 57% did not discuss the abuse with anyone.

Will this line of questioning offend the patient? The experience of the author has been that gentle, concerned questioning has not offended but rather has generated positive comments. Often the response is, "This is not an issue for me, but that is a very interesting question. I think it is good that you ask."

Sometimes the response is, "This is not an issue for me, but I have a friend with this problem." This needs a thorough response with information about community resources that can be given to the friend. It may be that the "friend" is the client in front of you who is in need. This could be a more comfortable way for her to ask for help without initially admitting the problem. Unless you ask every patient, you will miss some who are experiencing domestic violence because it cuts across all races, ages, classes, socioeconomic levels and professions.

Are you powerless to help? Many communities have a variety of organizations that can provide ongoing support and assistance to this woman. You need to be familiar with these organizations and have pamphlets, business cards, or phone numbers (including 24-hour toll-free numbers) available. Visit the office of your local organization, and talk with staff about the referral process and what services are available. This may increase your confidence in your ability to successfully assess and support your patients. If you have met the staff at a local domestic violence program, you are more likely to refer a patient there. Some shelters for battered women will send a staff person to your office if you have a patient who is fearful of returning home and would like immediate shelter.

For the woman not yet ready to make this step, a follow-up visit in your office in a week may be helpful. Remember that change often occurs in small increments and may progress more slowly than clinicians would like. This can be very frustrating for the clinician, but respect the needs of your patient.

Time is a precious commodity, especially with the demands of health care today. With proper training and access to resources, domestic violence cases can be identified and addressed in an efficient and effective manner. If you feel that you do not have the time to discuss referrals and resources in depth, is there a staff nurse who can do this? Tell the client that you have other patients waiting, and ask if she would be willing to speak with a very knowledgeable nurse about this. Can the nurse work with the patient who does not need or want immediate shelter? Has an emergency escape plan been developed to be put in place if needed?

The other option is to schedule a return appointment in a few days but with the concern that she may not actually return for the visit. Be sure that you have assessed her immediate need for safety. Over half of the women murdered in the United States are killed by their male partners.

The acronym RADAR developed by the Massachusetts College of Emergency Physicians summarizes the previous paragraph:

- **R:** Routine screening
- **A:** Ask direct questions
- **D:** Document findings
- **A:** Assess patient safety
- **R:** Review patient options (e.g., help from shelters, support groups, and legal advocates)

See the resource section at the end of this case for additional information regarding the RADAR approach.

The health provider's response is key. You must clearly state that no one deserves to be abused. It is important to end any visit with an acknowledgment of the situation: "You are a very powerful woman, and I am sorry about the things that have happened to you. You are very strong and courageous. Look at all the things you do: you take care of children, you go to work everyday, and you bring a paycheck home to your partner. I want you to know that I do not have any magical prescription for what you should be doing immediately, but I want you to come back and see me over and over again. I can be a link for you in addressing this problem" (Chez, King, and Brown, 1997). Education may be your best tool.

Alcohol

Continuous domestic abuse is associated with an increased risk for alcoholism, substance abuse, mental illness, somatization, and eating disorders.

The four-question CAGE questionnaire popular in primary care has a good sensitivity (74% to 89%) and specificity (79% to 95%) and has yielded positive responses. The limitations of this screening tool are its emphasis on symptoms of dependence rather than early drinking problems, lack of information on the level and pattern of alcohol use, and failure to distinguish current from lifetime problems. There are more detailed questionnaires that can be used at this point, such as the 10-point Alcohol Use Disorders Identification Test (AUDIT) or the 25-question Michigan Alcoholism Screening Test (MAST). If you look at the entire picture, you realize that she may be at risk for alcohol or drug dependence because of the stress of the domestic violence history.

Clinicians often have difficulty screening for drug use. Time may be limited, some clients may not acknowledge drug problems because of denial, and others are reluctant to admit to using drugs for fear of discrimination by health care providers or concerns about confidentiality. There is little data to determine whether the use of standardized screening questionnaires can increase the detection of potential problems among patients. Brief alcohol screening instruments, such as the CAGE, can be modified by substituting the term drug use for alcohol use, but this has not been compared with other means of assessment.

Some offices keep sensitive information on drug abuse and sexual abuse in a separate portion of the record. Any request for records must specifically ask for this information or it will not be sent.

Depression

How should you screen for depression? There are several brief (2 to 5 minutes) questionnaires, such as the Beck Depression Inventory, the Zung Self-Rating Depression Scale, and the Center for Epidemiological Studies Depression Scale. Although the questionnaire is brief, it still may take a few minutes to discuss over 20 questions. Many clinicians put these questions in a self history form filled out at an initial visit, which may be updated in the future. With Ms. Anderson, there is a high risk of depression.

Be particularly alert to clinical signs of depression, such as inability to sleep, change of appetite, fatigue, and memory loss. Assessment of suicidal tendencies is done by a direct question of whether the patient has ever felt suicidal. In this situation, you might also assess whether she has felt that she would harm someone else (e.g., her partner). If weapons are present in the home, the potential for deadly harm may be increased.

Physical Examination Techniques

She admits to mostly verbal abuse, but you would still need to carefully screen for any signs of physical abuse. You should be concerned about acute or chronic injuries that she may be embarrassed to discuss. A careful review of symptoms and a complete physical examination are indicated. There is a higher likelihood of you or this record being subpoenaed as evidence in a court of law. Document carefully and thoroughly.

DIAGNOSTIC OPTIONS

Since she has given you a history of alcohol use, it would be appropriate to check liver function studies if the use has been long term. This can be ordered separately or as part of a chemistry profile, which would also give you a glucose and cholesterol level. Her family history of DM is somewhat low, and cholesterol screening on a 39-year-old menstruating woman is controversial. Ordering liver function tests (LFTs) would be only slightly less expensive than a chemistry profile. Some clinicians may want to order a thyroid-stimulating hormone (TSH) since thyroid disease increases with age, especially in females. A complete blood count (CBC) will give information about anemia and dietary intake. If an office hemoglobin and hematocrit is available, it would be a less expensive screening.

A discussion of the need for STD screening is advised.

REVISED IDEAS

- Domestic abuse
- Situational stress without social or financial support
- Alcohol use
- Elevated BP
- Excessive exposure to ultraviolet light
- Contraception
- Cancer screening
- Chronic gingivitis (s/p surgery 1996)
- Onychocryptosis
- Mild headaches
- Health maintenance

THERAPEUTIC OPTIONS

Refer Ms. Anderson to a domestic violence prevention program. Discuss a plan for addressing alcohol use, and refer her to a community agency such as Alcoholics Anonymous (AA). Caution her to avoid driving while drinking.

Bloodwork as discussed previously.

Check her BP in 1 week. It may be elevated in response to the situational stress.

A Pap smear can be performed at this visit along with STD screening if indicated. A mammogram (her second) can be deferred until age 40 if no changes were noted in her breast examination. Discuss contraception: Is she wanting to change to DMPA this year?

Educate her about skin damage from tanning booths.

Advise her to continue with dental treatment.

The headaches seem to be mild tension headaches. Acetaminophen (2 tabs po prn) for these seems reasonable.

An ingrown toenail, where the sides of the nailbed penetrate the flesh, is a common problem. Ingrown toenails have been attributed to factors such as improper trimming, improper shoe fit, tight socks, and trauma. However, no clear-cut etiology has been proven, and perhaps there are many factors. Usually this involves the great toe and can be diagnosed by inspection and palpating the margin of the nail to find point tenderness. Often, a small piece of nail is piercing the skin of the toe, which may be difficult to see. Unless this is removed completely, the pain will not improve. A referral to a podiatrist may be necessary for successful treatment. Once all of the nail is removed, soaking in warm water and a topical antibiotic cream may help clear the condition. Systemic antibiotics are rarely indicated.

FOLLOW-UP

Schedule a follow-up appointment in 1 week to check her BP, review laboratory results, and support her in addressing the violence in her life.

References

Chez R, King MC, Brown J: Honing in on abuse: what to ask and how to listen; *Contemp Nurs Pract* 2(1):20, 1997.

Feldhaus K et al: Accuracy of 3 brief screening questions for detecting partner violence in the emergency department, *JAMA* 277(17):1357, 1997.

Sugg NK, Inui T: Primary care physician's response to domestic violence: opening Pandora's box, *JAMA* 267(23): 3158, 1992.

Additional Resources

1. National Domestic Violence Hotline: 1-800-799-SAFE
2. National Resource Center on Domestic Violence: 1-800-537-2238
3. Department of Justice Information Center: 1-800-421-6770
4. National Council on Child Abuse and Family Violence: 1-800-222-2000
5. American Bar Association's Commission on Domestic Violence World Wide Web site: http://www.igc.apc.org/fund/the_facts/health_response.html
6. The Radar Domestic Violence Training Project for Health Care Providers: Overview and Evaluation by The Philadelphia Family Violence Working Group, 8/1/96. For more information: Philadelphia Physicians for Social Responsibility, 704 N 23rd Street, Philadelphia, PA 19130.

Additional Examples of Questions to Assess for Abuse

1. McFarland et al: Assessing for abuse during pregnancy, *JAMA* 267(23):3176, 1992.

This 5-question tool has been validated against more comprehensive tools in increasing the detection of abuse. The following is a summary of the questions:
a. Have you ever been emotionally or physically abused by your partner or someone important to you?
b. Within the last year, have you been hit, slapped, kicked, or otherwise physically hurt by someone?
c. Since you have been pregnant, have you been hit, slapped, kicked, or otherwise physically hurt by someone?
d. Within the last year, has anyone forced you to have sexual relations?
e. Are you afraid of your partner?

2. Carlson K, Eisenstat S: *Primary care of women,* St Louis, 1995, Mosby.

The following are examples of screening questions:
a. Is anyone hitting you?
b. Is anyone threatening you?
c. Does your partner prevent you from leaving the house?
d. Does your partner threaten to hurt you when you disagree with him?

3. American Medical Association Guidelines issued in 1992 to encourage clinicians to screen for abuse:
a. Are you in a relationship in which you have been physically hurt or threatened by your partner? Have you ever been in such a relationship?
b. Are you in a relationship in which you feel you have been treated badly? In what ways?
c. Has your partner ever destroyed things that you cared about?
d. Has your partner ever threatened or abused your children?

e. Has your partner ever forced you to have sex when you did not want to? Does he force you to engage in sex that makes you feel uncomfortable?

f. We all argue at home. What happens when you and your partner fight or disagree?

g. Do you ever feel afraid of your partner?

h. Has your partner ever prevented you from leaving the house, seeing friends, getting a job, or continuing your education?

i. You mentioned that your partner uses drugs and/or alcohol. How does he act when he is drinking or on drugs? Is he ever verbally or physically abusive?

j. Do you have guns in your home? Has your partner ever threatened to use them when he gets angry?

CASE
33

Lunchtime Follow-up
Donna Downing
Age 40 years

OPENING SCENARIO

You find a mammogram report on your desk of a patient you saw 2 weeks ago (Box 33-1).

You review her record from 2 weeks ago (see note).

Record for Donna Downing from 2 Weeks Ago

HISTORY OF PRESENT ILLNESS

"I am here for my annual Pap smear. I have just moved to the area. My last examination was 3 years ago. Generally my health is good but I have been tired lately. I'd like to have my cholesterol checked since heart disease runs in my family."

MEDICAL HISTORY

Severe headaches since childhood, diagnosed in her teens as probable migraines. History of depression for 2 years. Currently on sertraline (Zoloft), 100 mg daily through a mental health provider whom she sees every 2 to 4 weeks.

FAMILY MEDICAL HISTORY

MGM: 78 yr (diabetic for 1 year)
MGF: 79 yr (hypertension)
PGF: Deceased at 70 yr (myocardial infarction [MI])
Mother: 65 yr (hypertension, varicose veins that required surgery)

Father: 66 yr (A&W)
Paternal uncle: 70 yr (cancer, type unknown)
Paternal uncle: 77 yr (arthritis)

SOCIAL HISTORY

Single, no current significant other. Lives in apartment with one roommate. Nonsmoker. Office worker. No caffeine use. Two beers per night. Denies recreational drug use. Sleeps 8 to 9 hours per night. Exercises three times per week. States diet is high in sweets, low in calcium; does not really prepare meals for herself, so she compensates by taking vitamin pills. Snacks on healthy foods.

MEDICATIONS

Sertraline 100 mg daily
Multivitamins: 4 or 5 multivitamins per day
Metamucil daily

ALLERGIES

NKDA
Environmental: Cats

REVIEW OF SYSTEMS

General: States she feels healthy overall
HEENT: Denies history of sinus pain or problems; no current nasal problems or rhinitis; no ear or dental problems; wisdom teeth extraction under general anesthesia as a teenager
Cardiac: No chest pain, palpitations
Respiratory: No shortness of breath, dyspnea
Breast: No masses or pain; performs self breast examination every few months; has not had a mammogram

---

Box 33-1 Mammography Report for Donna Downing

Mammography/bilateral screening:
Moderate density because of fibroglandular tissue is present without a dominant mass or suspicious calcification. There is a fairly well-circumscribed focal area of increased density in the inferior aspect of the right breast. This most likely represents asymmetric fibroglandular tissue, but a follow-up examination of the right breast in 6 months to exclude an active lesion is suggested.
Harold Xavier, MD
Radiologist

227

Gastrointestinal: Denies heartburn, nausea and vomiting, abdominal pain, rectal bleeding; has had problems with diarrhea and constipation for many years; uses Metamucil daily, which controls symptoms

Genitourinary: Last menstual period (LMP) 1 week ago; regular 28-day cycles; denies cramping, intermenstrual bleeding, premenstrual syndrome (PMS); heterosexual; no current contraceptive needs but has diaphragm that she brought with her; G1P0AB1

Musculoskeletal: No history of fracture, sprains, joint pain

Endocrine: Fatigue over the past 1 to 2 years; sleeping 8 to 9 hours per night, less when on fluoxetine; no dryness of skin or hair; temperature tolerances good; weight stable

Neurological: Severe headaches since childhood diagnosed as migraines by previous primary care provider; occur approximately six times per year, more often premenstrually; has nausea and dizziness, then headaches occur; no vomiting; has tried various preparations that have helped for a while; currently using ibuprofen 800 mg at onset of headache; sometimes this upsets her stomach and makes the nausea worse, but it helps the headache; sleep helps; depression diagnosed 2 years ago; on fluoxetine 20 mg, which caused insomnia, plus alprazolam 0.25 mg prn, then switched to sertraline 100 mg.per day about 8 weeks ago, which seems to be working well

PHYSICAL EXAMINATION

Vital signs: Temperature: 98.4° F; *Pulse:* 70 beats/min; *Respirations:* 16 breaths/min; *BP:* 134/82 mm Hg

Height: 5' 7"; *Weight:* 150 lb

General: Slightly fatigued 40 year old who appears her stated age

HEENT: Pupils equal and reactive to light; extraocular movements intact; no facial pain, nasal discharge; good dentition; Ears: no cerumen, crisp cone of light; Pharynx: no redness or exudate

Neck: No thyromegaly or supraclavicular lymphadenopathy

Heart: Regular rate and rhythm; no murmurs, rubs, or gallops

Lungs: Clear to auscultation

Breasts: No tenderness, skin changes, or masses; no palpable axillary nodes

Abdomen: Soft, no tenderness; no hepatosplenomegaly

Genitourinary: Vulva: no redness, lesions; vagina: scant, clear discharge; uterus: anteverted, anteflexed, nontender; adnexa: no enlargement, no tenderness, # 75 diaphragm fits adequately; diaphragm itself in good shape; does not need replacement

Neurological: Cranial nerves 2 to 12 intact

LABORATORY RESULTS

Hematocrit (from fingerstick): 41 (range 37 to 45)

ASSESSMENT

- Fatigue
- Depression
- Migraine headaches
- History of diarrhea and constipation
- Family history of cardiac disease

PLAN

- Thyroid-stimulating hormone (TSH)
- Lipid profile
- Bilateral screening mammogram
- Pap smear
- Continuation of sertaline and counseling with mental health provider
- Continuation of ibuprofen 800 mg for headaches with addition of metoclopramide (Reglan) 10 mg with ibuprofen at onset of headaches
- Continuation of daily Metamucil
- Request of records from her previous primary care provider
- Advice to decrease to one multivitamin per day
- Dietary counseling

ASSESSMENT   *Please indicate your level of concern regarding this report:*

PLAN   *Please list your plan for addressing this report:*

LEARNING ISSUES

In order to resolve this patient's problem, you will need to consider and address the following issues (you may generate additional issues as well):

- **Follow-up of laboratory and other tests**
- **Utilization of recommendations of specialists in clinical decision making**
- **Issues involved in referring a breast complaint to a surgeon**
- **Differential diagnoses for the complaint of fatigue**

INITIAL IDEAS

The issue here is follow-up of the mammogram report. The options are to repeat the mammogram in 6 months or refer for a surgical consult.

INTERPRETATION OF CUES, PATTERNS, AND INFORMATION

How high risk is Ms. Downing for breast cancer? She has a negative family history, is a nonsmoker (smoking may be a risk factor in women with certain types of genetic predispositions), and exercises regularly, which may be protective. Nulliparity and the history of 2 drinks per night may be risk factors, although her major risk factor is being female and growing older. The highest prevalence occurs postmenopausal. Her risk is similar to most women in the North American population at age 40.

What are the advantages of a surgical consult? Surgeons are the specialists in the United States who follow breast problems. A surgeon will review the mammography films, so this means another opinion on the actual reading of the films. The surgeon will perform another breast examination and provide an informed discussion of the pros and cons of mammography follow-up compared with various types of biopsy. Usually the surgeon will also review future follow-up films.

Is this worth the additional expense and time for the patient? It may be more anxiety-producing for Ms. Downing to have this visit, although in the long run she may actually be relieved by another opinion. You will need to discuss this fully with her.

What are the advantages for the provider? The obvious is that you no longer bear the full brunt of the decision making and are less vulnerable from a medical/legal viewpoint. Also, you have decreased the likelihood of missing an atypical-presenting carcinoma of the breast.

It is important to know your referral surgeon. Obviously you do not want to send her to someone who automatically biopsies all patients but to someone who will give a balanced discussion of the risks of cancer based on this individual patient's profile.

Some clinicians may question the value of even ordering mammography testing in this 40 year old. A national expert panel convened in late 1996 by the U.S. government could not determine the value of mammography screening in women ages 40 to 49 after reviewing extensive literature and research. Since that time, various organizations have been reanalyzing and/or developing their own guidelines. Additionally, long-term studies may be necessary to shed light on this debate. In the meantime, clinicians must weigh the issue of cancer detection versus the adverse effects of a false-positive test both from a financial and emotional well-being point of view.

If you do refer, most surgeons want the patient to bring the actual films with them to the visit. As a courtesy and to provide an accurate transfer of information, send a referral note to the surgeon.

FOLLOW-UP

After the mammogram is performed, follow-up is completed, and her past medical records arrive, discuss the fatigue issue with her again. Is this a component of her depression? Are the longstanding constipation and diarrhea actually irritable bowel syndrome (IBS)?

CASE
34

OPENING SCENARIO

Emma Thurlow is a 68-year-old female who vacations in this area. She called ahead and was assured by the office staff that you would see her and take care of her allergy shots for the summer. The physician assistant who works with you gave her the shots last week. She came in with a letter and instructions from her allergist. These instructions give a gradually increasing dosage of her allergy solutions.

PART I

Today she is to get 0.5 ml SC for dust mites and molds and 0.5 ml for cats. How will you proceed? Take a few minutes to consider this before you go on to Part II. You may want to review the Case Discussion for Part I before going on to Part II.

PART II

About 15 minutes after the injections, Ms. Thurlow comes to the desk and says that her neck feels itchy. What, if anything, will you do at this point?

PART III

About 10 minutes later, Ms. Thurlow says that she is having a hard time breathing. You examine her and find that she is red over most of her torso. You listen to her lungs and hear significant inspiratory and expiratory wheezes. How will you proceed?

ASSESSMENT   *Please indicate the problems or issues you have identified that will guide your care (preferably in list form):*

PLAN   *Please list your plans for addressing each of the problems or issues in your assessment:*

Community Clinic

Jeffrey A. Eaton, NP
Joyce D. Cappiello, NP

Name:_____ DOB_____
Address_____ Date_____

Rx

"label all unless indicated"
Refill:_____ times-- Do not refill ( )

Signed:_____

DO NOT TAKE THIS TO YOUR PHARMACIST

Community Clinic

Jeffrey A. Eaton, NP
Joyce D. Cappiello, NP

Name:_____ DOB_____
Address_____ Date_____

Rx

"label all unless indicated"
Refill:_____ times-- Do not refill ( )

Signed:_____

DO NOT TAKE THIS TO YOUR PHARMACIST

Community Clinic

Jeffrey A. Eaton, NP
Joyce D. Cappiello, NP

Name:_____ DOB_____
Address_____ Date_____

Rx

"label all unless indicated"
Refill:_____ times-- Do not refill ( )

Signed:_____

DO NOT TAKE THIS TO YOUR PHARMACIST

Community Clinic

Jeffrey A. Eaton, NP
Joyce D. Cappiello, NP

Name:_____ DOB_____
Address_____ Date_____

Rx

"label all unless indicated"
Refill:_____ times-- Do not refill ( )

Signed:_____

DO NOT TAKE THIS TO YOUR PHARMACIST

CASE
34 Discussion

PART I

If you are uncomfortable at all with giving the allergy shots and you say no, there will be political issues to deal with. Questions will be asked: Why did you turn this patient away? We already told her she could come here. Unfortunately, her allergist's office is too far away to send her there. Most clinicians would agree to give the allergy shots even if not fully familiar with the process.

There are two things to consider in your decision on whether to give these injections: (1) What is the risk? and (2) What will you do if something goes wrong? Obviously the worst risk is that of anaphylaxis. Before you give these injections (or allow your office staff to give them) you need to decide what you need for an emergency situation and then make sure that equipment and/or medication is available. Then you might tell your staff to go ahead and administer the injection and keep Ms. Thurlow in the waiting room for at least 20 minutes after.

Should you take the time to get a medical history on Ms. Thurlow? If something goes wrong, a basic medical history, medications, and allergies could be helpful. A set of baseline vital signs would also be a good idea.

PART II

Ms. Thurlow says that her neck is a bit itchy. This could be the result of an allergic reaction, or she could have been bitten by a mosquito in the waiting room. You need to examine her and see whether she has a good reason for the itching, and determine whether she has other symptoms. If the itching neck was the only symptom, some clinicians would continue to watch her. Others would try a dose of epinephrine or some diphenhydramine (Benadryl). Her medical history and overall medical state may help in this determination.

PART III

Although your treatment for anaphylaxis will vary somewhat based on what you have available in your office, the following would be ideal (although some clinicians are comfortable treating anaphylaxis in the office, many would consider this initial treatment and would be making appropriate arrangements for transfer to an inpatient facility before or during this process):

1. Oxygen: 5 to 10 liters
2. IV if available
3. Epinephrine: 0.3 to 0.5 ml SC or IM (repeat every 10 minutes if symptoms continue)
4. Diphenhydramine (Benadryl): 50 mg IM (po if IM not available)

5. Hydrocortisone: 100 mg IM (or IV) if available (some would leave this decision for the inpatient setting, but if available, a single dose will not do any harm)
6. Beta agonist aerosol if available
7. IV H_2 blocker (this would usually be reserved for the inpatient setting, although oral H_2 blockers could be given)
8. Observation for about 6 hours
(Ewald and McKenzie, 1995)

You should also put an item on the agenda at the next provider meeting to discuss allergy shot administration in the office.

References

Ewald GA, McKenzie CR: *The Washington manual: manual of medical therapeutics,* Boston, 1995, Little, Brown.

CASE
35

OPENING SCENARIO

Albert Steinberg is a 44-year-old male on your schedule for a cough and fever.

HISTORY OF PRESENT ILLNESS

"I have been sick for about a week. I've felt like I have been running a low-grade fever, but when I took my temperature 2 days ago, it was just a little over 100° F. I have been coughing up some reddish brown sputum, but not all that much of it. I cough fairly frequently, but I didn't have any cough medicine in the house. I really hope that you can do something for me because I haven't been this sick in a long time. I feel like I've been run over by a truck. I've had bronchitis a couple of times before, but it's never been this bad. I had a tuberculosis test 4 or 5 years ago and it was negative." Mr. Steinberg has no known exposures, although he is exposed to a lot of people through his police work. He denies sweats and chills. His appetite is decreased but still "okay". He denies shortness of breath but does note that he gets winded much more quickly lately. His wife had some Sudafed from the last time she was sick, and she wanted him to try that, so he has been taking it for about 3 days.

MEDICAL HISTORY

Tonsillectomy and adenoidectomy as a child. Denies other surgeries or hospitalizations. No history of diabetes mellitus (DM), cancer, or heart disease.

FAMILY MEDICAL HISTORY

MGM: Died at 82 yr (breast cancer)
MGF: Died at 77 yr (heart attack)
PGM: Died at 80 yr (complications of Type II DM)
PGF: Died at 74 yr (stroke)
Mother: 81 yr (A&W)
Father: Died at 80 yr (stroke)
Son: 22 yr (A&W)

SOCIAL HISTORY

Police sergeant. Married. Wife works as an office manager for an oil company. One grown son who lives on his own. Smokes 1 1/2 packs per day. Alcohol: a few drinks on the weekend; never more than 2 to 3 beers in an evening; goes all week without alcohol.

MEDICATIONS

Vitamin C: 2000 mg per day
Sudafed SA: 120 mg bid for the past 3 days

ALLERGIES

None

REVIEW OF SYSTEMS

General: Good energy level usually
Skin: No itching or rashes
HEENT: No history of head injury; no corrective lenses; denies eye pain, excessive tearing, blurring, or change in vision; no tinnitus or vertigo; denies frequent colds, hay fever, or sinus problems
Neck: no lumps, goiters, or pain
Thorax: denies shortness of breath (usually); no recent nocturnal dyspnea, mild shortness of breath with activity
Cardiac: No chest pain; usually no shortness of breath with normal activity, but he feels his energy is lower and stamina is less than usual
Abdominal/Gastrointestinal: No nausea, vomiting, constipation, or diarrhea; denies belching, bloating, and black or clay colored stools.
Geniturinary: No dysuria; no difficulty starting stream
Extremities: Mild joint pain with significant activity
Neurological: No headaches, seizures
Endocrine: No polyuria, polyphagia, polydipsia; temperature tolerances good
Circulatory: No excessive bruising; no history of transfusions

PHYSICAL EXAMINATION

Vital signs: Temperature: 98.4° F; *Pulse:* 86 beats/min; *Respirations:* 22 breaths/min; *BP:* 126/82 mm Hg
Height: 5' 10"; *Weight:* 172 lb
General: Well developed, well nourished; in no acute distress; appears stated age

HEENT: Normocephalic without masses or lesions; pupils equal, round, and reactive to light; extraocular movements intact; fundi benign, nares patent and non-injected; throat without redness or lesions

Neck: Supple without thyromegaly or adenopathy

Thorax: Coarse breath sounds scattered throughout both lungs; no wheezes or crackles; symmetrical resonant percussion notes; lung sounds do not change with cough

Heart: Regular rate and rhythm; no murmurs, rubs, or gallops

Abdomen/Gastointestinal: No hepatosplenomegaly; abdomen soft, nontender; bowel sounds normoactive

Genitourinary: Normal male, circumcised, both testicles descended

Extremities: Range of motion functionally intact; no cyanosis, clubbing, or edema

Neurological: Reflexes 2+ at Achilles, patellar, biceps, triceps, and brachioradialis; no Babinski signs present

---

ASSESSMENT   *Please indicate the problems or issues you have identified that will guide your care (preferably in list form):*

PLAN   *Please list your plans for addressing each of the problems or issues in your assessment:*

Community Clinic
Jeffrey A. Eaton, NP
Joyce D. Cappiello, NP

Name:_____ DOB_____
Address_____ Date_____

Rx

"label all unless indicated"
Refill:_____ times-- Do not refill ( )

Signed:_____
DO NOT TAKE THIS TO YOUR PHARMACIST

Community Clinic
Jeffrey A. Eaton, NP
Joyce D. Cappiello, NP

Name:_____ DOB_____
Address_____ Date_____

Rx

"label all unless indicated"
Refill:_____ times-- Do not refill ( )

Signed:_____
DO NOT TAKE THIS TO YOUR PHARMACIST

Community Clinic
Jeffrey A. Eaton, NP
Joyce D. Cappiello, NP

Name:_____ DOB_____
Address_____ Date_____

Rx

"label all unless indicated"
Refill:_____ times-- Do not refill ( )

Signed:_____
DO NOT TAKE THIS TO YOUR PHARMACIST

Community Clinic
Jeffrey A. Eaton, NP
Joyce D. Cappiello, NP

Name:_____ DOB_____
Address_____ Date_____

Rx

"label all unless indicated"
Refill:_____ times-- Do not refill ( )

Signed:_____
DO NOT TAKE THIS TO YOUR PHARMACIST

CASE
35 *Discussion*

LEARNING ISSUES

In order to resolve this patient's problem, you will need to consider and address the following issues (you may generate additional issues as well):

- **Differential diagnosis of lower respiratory infection (LRI)**
- **Diagnostic criteria for pneumonia**
- **Criteria for and choice of antibiotics for LRI**
- **Choice of antibiotics in a smoker**
- **Appropriate use of chest x-ray (CXR) examination in diagnosis of LRI**
- **Criteria for relieving patients of work responsibilities**
- **Use of pneumonia vaccine**
- **Health maintenance in a 44-year-old man**
- **Vitamin C supplementation**

INITIAL IDEAS
- Bronchitis
- Pneumonia

INTERPRETATION OF CUES, PATTERNS, AND INFORMATION

In Mr. Steinberg's case the clinician must determine what is causing his LRI and the severity of that infection. Mr. Steinberg is a smoker, so that plus the reddish-brown sputum would increase the probability of a bacterial origin to his infection. These factors also raise the suspicion of bacterial pneumonia. Arguing against a pneumonia are his lack of fever and the lack of adventitious sounds. His respiratory rate is also only 22 breaths/min.

He is also a police officer, so you have to be somewhat concerned about his occupational exposure to certain at-risk populations. Further history should be obtained, and the differential diagnosis would then be broadened appropriately.

REVISED IDEAS
- Bronchitis
- Pneumonia
- Viral
- Bacterial
- Mycoplasmal
- Protozoal (such as *Pneumocystis carinii*)

DIFFERENTIAL DIAGNOSIS

In evaluating the various possibilities on the differential, the following should be considered:

1. *Viral etiology of bronchitis or pneumonia:* Viruses are common causes of LRI symptoms, and if viral in etiology, the infection will not usually be significantly affected by antibiotics.

2. *Mycoplasmal etiology:* Often called *walking pneumonia,* mycoplasmal pneumonia is often of a longer duration but with less severe symptoms than a bacterial pneumonia. Its course can be affected by antibiotics, so it may be worth considering when choosing antibiotic coverage.

3. *Bacterial etiology:* Consider whether this is a bacterial infection, and also consider the various types of bacterial origins that may occur. A bacterial infection will usually cause greater symptoms than a viral infection.

The most common organisms that cause a community-acquired pneumonia are *Streptococcus pneumoniae, Mycoplasma pneumoniae,* respiratory viruses, *Chlamydia pneumoniae,* and *Haemophilus influenzae.* Other less common causes include staphylococcus species, legionella, mycobacterium tuberculosis, and other gram-negative bacteriae. In smokers such as Mr. Steinberg the environment created is conducive to the growth of other bacteria. Thus the organisms that cause LRIs in smokers most commonly also include *Branhamella catarrhalis. Branhamella catarrhalis* would usually not include the myalgias and degree of symptoms that Mr. Steinberg is experiencing and is possibly related to the co-morbidities of smoking, such as chronic obstructive pulmonary disease (COPD), rather than the smoking itself.

Another organism that needs to be considered is *Legionella. Legionella* often presents with a more severe onset than Mr. Steinberg's, but if the history indicated possible exposure to other infected individuals or risk factors, then this could be a consideration.

4. *Protozoal etiology:* Does Mr. Steinberg have any evidence of immunosuppression? Does he have any risk factors for human immunodeficiency virus (HIV) or acquired immunodeficiency syndrome (AIDS)? Pneumocystis would usually present with a nonproductive cough. Even if you decided on another diagnosis and went ahead with antibiotics, it would not make diagnosis of *Pneumocystis carinii* pneumonia (PCP) any more difficult at a later time since the cysts will persist.

5. *Mycobacterial etiology:* Does Mr. Steinberg have tuberculosis or mycobacterium avium complex?

Can lung cancer present this way? This would be a way for a bronchogenic carcinoma to present. In a smoker, this factors into the decision on obtaining a CXR.

Because the difference between pneumonia and bronchitis is not a sharp distinction based on current information, some clinicians would diagnose this a bronchitis and others would diagnose it a "mild" pneumonia. The treatment may be similar in either case.

DIAGNOSTIC OPTIONS

Does Mr. Steinberg need a CXR? Based on the fact that he is a smoker and is over 40 years old argues in favor of a CXR. In some cases with a younger nonsmoker, clinicians will make the diagnosis of pneumonia on the basis of clinical findings. Whether the CXR reveals evidence of bacterial pneumonia may not change treatment at this point. If there was a pleural effusion, evidence of PCP, or greater than expected involvement, the CXR will have proved helpful.

Sanford, Gilbert, and Sande (1996) suggest the following criteria for a CXR: Respiratory symptoms plus temperature greater than 37.8° C, pulse greater than 100 beats/min, abnormal lung examination, and the absence of asthma. These guidelines may provide some guidance, but the decision will still come down to the individual clinician.

If a CXR is positive the clinician should consider repeating it in 4 to 6 weeks. Mr. Steinberg is a smoker, and since a bronchogenic cancer may have a similar radiological appearance to that of pneumonia, it is appropriate to ensure that the x-ray changes in fact clear after treatment. Lack of resolution would of course make the clinician suspicious of the original diagnosis of pneumonia.

A sputum culture is often recommended in cases such as this, but the decision to obtain one is usually based on the perceived difficulty in obtaining the specimen in a manner that allows meaningful analysis. If certain etiological agents are suspected, most notably *M. tuberculosis* or *Legionella,* then Gram's stain and specific cultures may be very worthwhile.

Will a complete blood count (CBC) be helpful? It may give you some evidence regarding viral versus bacterial etiology. Many clinicians will have made the choice, based on symptoms, whether to give antibiotics and thus may not order a CBC. If there were more comorbidities or Mr. Steinberg appeared sicker and hospitalization was being considered, a CBC would add valuable information.

THERAPEUTIC OPTIONS

Pharmacological

With his reddish-brown sputum, feeling as lousy as he does, and being a smoker, Mr. Steinberg probably meets the criteria for antibiotics. Erythromycin will cover most of the most common etiologies of community-acquired pneumonia. Azithromycin and clarithromycin have greater effect against H. *influenzae* and thus might be the best choice in a smoker. Of the most common organisms causing lower respiratory infections, Erythromycin will cover *S. pneumoniae, M. pneumoniae, C. pneumoniae, B. catarrhalis,* and *Legionella.* As noted, *H. influenzae* coverage is less predictable.

If Mr. Steinberg had COPD, trimethoprim sulfamethoxazole (TMP/SMX) or doxycycline would have been reasonable choices.

If a cough was keeping Mr. Steinberg from resting, a cough suppressant could be ordered for limited use. Most clinicians believe that it is better for secretions to be raised and do not use cough suppressants. Bedtime use may allow sleep, and if use is limited, should not cause problems.

Analgesics may make him more comfortable. Acetaminophen or ibuprofen should be adequate.

He can continue the pseudoephedrine if he is getting symptomatic relief from it, although it will probably have no effect on his chest symptoms. Discontinuing it will simplify his drug regimen, and thus a case can be made for stopping it on that basis.

His vitamin C intake is far greater than the recommended daily allowance (RDA), but this is a common approach that patients will take for infection based on their reading in the lay literature and talking to friends. It is probably doing no harm, may be helping, and thus continuing the dose should do no harm other than financial cost to Mr. Steinberg.

Educational

Mr. Steinberg needs to rest and stay out of work until his symptoms are much better. Nutritional intake (especially fluids) should be adequate.

HEALTH PROMOTION/HEALTH MAINTENANCE

At 44 years old the following health promotion could also be considered, although it is probably best left for a follow-up visit:
- Smoking cessation
- Tetanus-diphtheria immunization (Td); check hepatitis B vaccine status
- Serum cholesterol level
- Regular physical activity
- Dental review
- Influenza vaccine in the fall
- Purified protein derivative (PPD) if not done through occupational environment
- Some clinicians would consider baseline peak flow test in a smoker

One question that should be raised is whether Mr. Steinberg should receive the pneumonia vaccine after he has recovered. There are multiple strains of pneumococcus (Streptococcus pneumoniae), and vaccines include over 20 strains of the bacteria. Since he is a smoker and has already proven to be susceptible to this type of pneumonia, administering the vaccine a few weeks to a few months after this episode would be the option chosen by most clinicians. Insurance coverage could be investigated if that was a concern since preventive services such as vaccines are not covered by many insurance companies.

FOLLOW-UP

Mr. Steinberg will probably need to return to be cleared for work. A follow-up visit could be scheduled based on your assessment. This most probably will be in the 3- to 7-day range. He, of course, would be counseled to return for any worsening or failure to improve.

References

Sanford JP, Gilbert DN, Sande MA: *The Sanford guide to antimicrobial therapy*, Dallas, 1996, Antimicrobial Therapy.

1:30 PM
Betty Hackett
Age 33 years

OPENING SCENARIO

Betty Hackett is a 33-year-old female on your schedule for a 20 week prenatal check. You have her initial database (see note) and her pregnancy flow chart (Table 36-1). Her laboratory workup is documented in the flow chart.

Betty Hackett's Initial Database from 15 Weeks Ago
(First Prenatal Visit)

MEDICAL HISTORY

Ms. Hackett is a 33-year-old female who is new to this practice. She is about 1 week late for her period and has tested positive for pregnancy on a home pregnancy test. This pregnancy is planned and wanted. She and her husband have been trying to conceive for about 1 year. They own their own home and state that finances are not a big issue for them. Pregnancy history: therapeutic abortion (TAB) at age 19. No other pregnancies. On oral contraceptives (OCs) until about 1 year ago.

FAMILY MEDICAL HISTORY

MGM: 82 yr (mild arthritis)
MGF: Died at 71 yr (heart attack)
PGM: Died at 64 yr (Alzheimer's disease)
PGF: Died at 79 yr (stroke)
Mother: 63 yr (breast cancer at age 44)
Father: 65 yr (glaucoma)
Brother: Died at age 12 yr (leukemia)

SOCIAL HISTORY

Married for 10 years. Works as a bank loan officer. Never smoked. Alcohol: very rare glass of wine. No pets.

MEDICATIONS

None

ALLERGIES

None

REVIEW OF SYSTEMS

General: Good energy level
Skin: No itching or rashes
HEENT: No history of head injury; no corrective lenses; denies eye pain, excessive tearing, blurring, or change in vision; no tinnitus or vertigo; denies frequent colds, hay fever, or sinus problems; occasional headaches since pregnancy began
Neck: no lumps, goiters, or pain
Thorax: denies shortness of breath, paroxysmal nocturnal dyspnea
Breast: No breast pain or discharge
Cardiac: No chest pain; no shortness of breath with normal activity
Abdominal/Gastrointestinal: Mild nausea, rare vomiting, no constipation or diarrhea; denies belching, bloating, and black or clay colored stools
Genitourinary: No difficulty starting stream; denies dysuria but it does not really feel like she is emptying her bladder; no discharge or bleeding since last period
Extremities: No joint pains or swelling
Neurological: No seizures
Endocrine: No polyuria, polyphagia, polydipsia; temperature tolerances good
Circulatory: No excessive bruising; no history of transfusions
Other: Denies history of physical abuse
Diet: No red meat; drinks 1.5 liters of Diet Coke per day; otherwise uses food pyramid approach

PHYSICAL EXAMINATION

Vital signs: Temperature: 98.4° F; *Pulse:* 78 beats/min; *Respirations:* 18 breaths/min; *BP:* 106/64 mm Hg
Height: 5' 3"; *Weight:* 127 lb
General: Well developed, well nourished; in no acute distress; appears stated age
HEENT: Normocephalic without masses or lesions; pupils equal, round, and reactive to light; extraocular movements intact; fundi benign; nares patent and noninjected; throat without redness or lesions
Neck: Supple without thyromegaly or adenopathy
Thorax: Clear to auscultation and percussion
Breast: No asymmetry, masses, or discharge
Heart: Regular rate and rhythm; no murmurs, rubs, or gallops

Abdomen/Gastrointestinal: No hepatosplenomegaly; abdomen soft, nontender; bowel sounds normoactive; rectal without masses; stool brown; guaiac negative

Genitourinary: External without lesions; vaginal mucosa pink; cervix without gross lesions; no discharge noted; uterus anteroflexed; no adnexal tenderness

Extremities: Range of motion functionally intact; no cyanosis, clubbing, or edema.

Neurological: Reflexes 2+ at Achilles, patellar, biceps, triceps, and brachioradialis; no Babinski signs present; cranial nerves 2 through 12 intact

You are seeing her today for her 20 week visit. Please indicate what you will do in today's visit. Note that the blood pressure (BP), urine dip, and fetal heart rate (FHR) have been done already by your office staff.

As you are closing the interview, when you ask if she has any other questions or concerns, she responds that she has been talking with her husband about the issue of whether to circumcise a boy if she has one. She asks if you have any recommendations. What will you tell her?

She also asks when she will have to stop sexual activity. How will you respond?

Table **36-1** *Pregnancy Flow Chart for Betty Hackett*

	WEEK OF PREGNANCY				
TYPE OF DATA	5	9	13	17	20
BP (mm Hg)	106/64	110/74	116/80	114/80	118/82
Urine protein	Negative	Negative	Negative	Negative	Trace
Urine sugar	Negative	Negative	Negative	Negative	Negative
Height	5' 3"				
Weight (lb)	127	126	128	131	132
Fundal height				2f ↓ u	
Movement					
Blood type		B+			
FHR				144	144
Pelvic examination	Done				
AFP				Done	
Hematocrit	37%				
US					
GC/Chlamydia	Negative				
RPR	Negative				
HBsAg	Negative				

EDC (dates) _____
EDC (US) _____
LMP: 20 weeks ago
Notes:
5 weeks: Declined HIV test; started on prenatal vitamins; moderate morning sickness already
9 weeks: Morning sickness about the same; behavioral approaches seem to be working
13 weeks: Morning sickness still improving but not totally gone
17 weeks: Alpha fetoprotein (AFP) done; morning sickness only occasionally now
18 1/2 weeks: Laboratory report back; AFP 15.4 (not elevated)

Community Clinic

Jeffrey A. Eaton, NP

Joyce D. Cappiello, NP

Name:_____ DOB_____

Address_____ Date_____

Rx

"label all unless indicated"

Refill:_____ times-- Do not refill ( )

Signed:_____

DO NOT TAKE THIS TO YOUR PHARMACIST

Community Clinic

Jeffrey A. Eaton, NP

Joyce D. Cappiello, NP

Name:_____ DOB_____

Address_____ Date_____

Rx

"label all unless indicated"

Refill:_____ times-- Do not refill ( )

Signed:_____

DO NOT TAKE THIS TO YOUR PHARMACIST

LEARNING ISSUES

In order to resolve this patient's problem, you will need to consider and address the following issues (you may generate additional issues as well):

- Components of a prenatal visit
- Alpha fetoprotein (AFP) testing
- Caffeine intake during pregnancy
- Artificial sweetener intake during pregnancy
- Proteinuria during pregnancy
- Pregnancy-induced hypertension (PIH)
- Weight gain patterns during pregnancy
- Ultrasonography during pregnancy
- Circumcision
- Sexual activity during pregnancy
- Breast cancer family history and pregnancy

INITIAL IDEAS

Assume that Ms. Hackett has a normal pregnancy, but you need to be vigilant for potential problems. Assess her for general health, nutrition (including weight gain), signs and symptoms of preterm labor, fetal movement, and psychosocial problems.

INTERPRETATION OF CUES, PATTERNS, AND INFORMATION

Her estimated date of confinement (EDC) should be calculated using a wheel or Nagele's rule (count back 3 months and add 7 days). This assumes a regular 28-day cycle. Women who have more irregular cycles may vary more from their EDC.

Review of Missing Data

The prenatal laboratory package drawn on her first visit would usually include complete blood count (CBC), rapid plasma reagin (RPR), blood type and Rh, antibody screen, rubella titer, screening for hepatitis B, and urinalysis. A Pap smear and genprobe are often done at the first visit. If a woman is not rubella immune, then she is instructed to notify you of any possible exposure so that you can give gamma globulin (rubella immune globulin). The vaccine is probably safe (and there has not been evidence to the contrary in women who were vaccinated and did not know they were pregnant), but most clinicians do not give the vaccine during pregnancy.

Varicella is another issue that you may want to consider. Varicella zoster immune globulin (VZIG) can be given to a woman who is exposed to chicken pox who has not been documented to be immune. If you wait until after a woman has been exposed to draw a varicella titer, then it will not have returned from the laboratory in time to avoid the need for VZIG. Thus a titer should be done early in pregnancy. Knowing that she is immune may also give her reassurance, or it may encourage her to be more careful if she is not immune.

Breast examination would be part of her initial physical examination, especially in view of her mother's history of breast cancer. She is 33 years old now. When would you get a mammogram considering that her mother had breast cancer at age 44? Should you repeat a clinical breast examination later in her pregnancy?

Do you need records from her TAB? Current research reports that a single first trimester TAB with suction aspiration technique (which is the current technique) has no effect on subsequent pregnancies. If she knows the length of gestation of that terminated pregnancy (she is Rh+ so she would not need RhoGAM), the records will offer little useful information.

Pelvimetry is not indicated since it does not adequately predict who can give birth vaginally. A trial of labor will be the best judge of this. You can attempt these measurements during the pelvic examination, but remember that the information is not very useful.

Other Issues from Her History

AFP tests should be drawn ideally between 16 and 18 weeks' gestation, but laboratories will accept them between 15 and 20 weeks. If Ms. Hackett's blood was drawn at 17 weeks' gestation, it should be fine. This is her first visit since having the AFP done, so you will want to review the results with her.

Is her history of Diet Coke consumption significant? If your concern is with the caffeine intake, it is important to know that while some studies have shown conflicting results, most scientific research continues to indicate that moderate caffeine consumption does not affect fertility or cause adverse health effects in the mother or child (Caffeine and Women's Health, 1994). Switching to a caffeine-free diet is an option if she is willing. She may want to gradually taper her caffeine intake to avoid symptoms.

Aspartame is currently under research with varying reports. Moderation is always prudent.

Targeted questions regarding drug use and HIV risk are appropriate. Fundal height of 20 cm is appropriate for 20 weeks' gestation. You will not usually be able to assess fetal lie and presentation with Leopold maneuvers until 28 to 30 weeks. Even if you were, what helpful information would it provide at this point?

FHR is in the normal range of 120 to 160.

Fetal movement: Most clients would feel movement by the accepted parameter of 20 weeks' gestation. If she has not, most clinicians would give her another 1 to 2 weeks before being alarmed since the uterus is enlarging appropriately and you hear a fetal heartbeat.

Her BP shows an 18-point increase of diastolic pressure, which should be rechecked and bears close monitoring if it continues to be elevated on recheck.

Her urine dipstick shows a trace protein. You need to ask open ended questions regarding urinary symptoms and specifically ask regarding dysuria and urgency. Check for costovertebral angle (CVA) tenderness. Keep in mind that asymptomatic urinary tract infections (UTIs) are more common in pregnancy. If any of these are present, a dipstick for leukocytes and nitrites would be a logical next step, and if positive, a full culture should be obtained. A trace of protein can also be vaginal discharge contamination in the urine. Remember that UTIs can be a factor in premature labor. Urine testing for protein is also a way to check for preeclampsia. The positive predictive value of dip urines in the prediction of abnormal 24-hour urines is not very high, so interpret with caution but underinterpret at your own peril as well.

The most disturbing problem that could occur if the above symptoms (elevated BP and urine protein) progress is pregnancy-induced hypertension (PIH). PIH is traditionally defined as hypertension of 140/90 mm Hg or greater, 3+ protein in the urine on two occasions, and generalized (nondependent) edema. Checking for generalized edema (not just hands and feet) would be an important part of the physical examination. A recheck of her BP in the left lateral position and urine in a few days or a week at the most might be an option. Other signs of PIH could be a change in reflexes. They should be checked for baseline at the very least. In PIH they can become 3+ or even 4+ (clonus present). Fundoscopic examination would also be appropriate. Laboratory tests that could be considered would be a CBC, liver function tests (LFTs), blood urea nitrogen (BUN), and creatinine, although not all clinicians would draw at this point. These tests are helpful because they can identify the woman with HELLP (hypertension, elevated liver functions, low platelets) syndrome.

The development of a headache in pregnancy is not an unusual occurrence, but it needs to be addressed with a targeted history, and if indicated, a neurological examination. Generally, you would expect her headaches to decrease in frequency and severity as the pregnancy progresses. Headache can also be a symptom associated with PIH, so monitoring its progress is appropriate for several reasons. If a patient complains of epigastric pain, that may also be a sign of liver effects.

The other major issue noted at this visit is her suboptimal weight gain. The current accepted standards of weight gain suggest 22 to 27 lb with 0.7 lb/wk from 8 to 20 weeks' gestation and 1 lb/wk from 20 weeks' gestation to birth. Ms. Hackett notes nausea and rare vomiting. A quick 24-hour dietary recall may be enlightening. If you are concerned about poor intake, you can dip her urine for ketones to verify this. Referral to a nutritionist would be very helpful at this point. You can also explore whether some of her lack of weight gain is intentional. If so, education about the baby's nutritional needs may cause her to choose a better diet. Another possibility that could be considered (if there were cues to support it) is that Ms. Hackett may have an eating disorder. Her weight loss is probably related to the usual nausea and vomiting associated with early pregnancy.

You can reassure Ms. Hackett that the nausea of pregnancy usually resolves at this point. Is she taking her daily prenatal vitamins? Although the American College of Obstetricians and Gynecologists (ACOG) recommendations do not include prenatal vitamins for all women, Ms. Hackett should probably be taking them because of her questionable nutritional intake. The most remarkable findings about weight gain in pregnancy are that a wide range is compatible with good clinical outcomes and that departures from "normality" are very nonspecific for any adverse outcome in a given individual (Cunningham et al, 1993).

A review of her current symptoms, or lack thereof, may allow for opportunities to make her pregnancy more comfortable. Constipation, backaches, and false labor are all areas for education. As always, she should be instructed to report vision changes, chills or fever, bleeding more than a spot after intercourse, or basically anything that is of concern to her or her husband. She should continue to use her seatbelt, and the lap belt should go under her abdomen with the shoulder belt placed between her breasts.

What are her plans for childbirth? Does she need to take Lamaze classes or some other childbirth preparation course? Will she be breast feeding? Are there written or live resources that can be provided?

DIFFERENTIAL DIAGNOSIS
- Normal pregnancy
- Pregnancy with PIH
- Pregnancy with HELLP

DIAGNOSTIC OPTIONS
Some clinicians might want to order an ultrasound. Generally, if insurance is to pay, there are certain criteria that must be met, such as uncertain LMP, large for dates, small for dates, fetal heart not heard, etc. Curiosity about the sex of the fetus does not meet insurance criteria. There is always the option for parents to pay out of pocket, but charges are in the $150 to $250 range. When an indication for the test is given, make sure the case is well made and documented.

THERAPEUTIC OPTIONS

Pharmacological

Ms. Hackett has not really identified any issues that would require medication at this point. Nausea of this degree is usually managed with behavioral and dietary interventions. If she had a UTI, then amoxicillin would be a common empiric choice since it is well tolerated in pregnancy. Sensitivities of course might not allow this option, and then Table 7 in the *Sanford Guide* (Sanford, Gilbert, and Sande, 1996) or a reference on medications in pregnancy and lactation would provide guidance regarding the appropriate use of a particular medication during pregnancy.

Educational

Of course the usual education concerning the development of the fetus would be included. Several other areas of potential education have been included under Interpretation of Cues, Patterns, and Information. Ongoing education regarding the need for dental care, exercise, rest periods, and measures for addressing the discomforts of pregnancy would of course be included.

FOLLOW-UP

A routine follow-up visit would be in 4 weeks, but you may have her back sooner for a BP and urine check. You may also schedule her for a 1-hour glucose tolerance test (GTT) at one of her next visits. A common practice is to obtain the GTT at 28 weeks' gestation or at 20 to 24 weeks if a woman has risk factors, which Ms. Hackett does not.

ADDITIONAL QUESTIONS

How will you respond to her concerns about whether to circumcise the baby?

Exploring her and her husband's attitudes is appropriate.

Many health professionals are not clear on how to address this issue, so it is no wonder that parents are confused. In 1971 and 1975, the Committee on the Fetus and Newborn of the American Academy of Pediatrics (AAP) recommended that routine circumcision of newborn males not be done. This same position was reaffirmed along with the AAP and the ACOG in their 1983 publication *Guidelines for Perinatal Care*. In the late 1980s there was a significant decline in the number of males circumcised with only about 2/3 of boys being circumcised.

In the 1992 *Guidelines for Perinatal Care* (American Academy of Pediatrics and ACOG), circumcision was no longer condemned, but it also was not recommended. This change likely resulted from the American Academy of Pediatrics Report of the Task Force on Circumcision (1989). The Task Force concluded that properly performed newborn circumcision prevented phimosis, paraphimosis, and balanoposthitis, and it decreased the incidence of penile cancer. (There is no current evidence to indicate that it has any effect on prostate cancer). The committee could not agree that circumcision resulted in a decreased incidence of urinary infections in babies because of the lack of well-designed prospective studies. They also agreed that an increased incidence of cancer of the cervix had been reported in sexual partners of uncircumcised men infected with the human papilloma virus. Finally, the Task Force could not agree on whether circumcision resulted in a decreased incidence of sexually transmitted diseases (STDs). Contrary to these findings, Laumann, Masi, and Zuckerman (1997) found no association with STDs, although they did note that uncircumcised men did have a slightly greater incidence of sexual dysfunction. The reasons for this are currently unclear however.

The Task Force concluded (without a recommendation) that newborn circumcision was generally a safe procedure when performed by an experienced provider, and circumcision should be an elective surgery performed in a healthy, stable neonate. Local anesthetic (dorsal penile nerve block) appeared to reduce the pain of the procedure, but the anesthetic was not without its own complications. In a noncommittal last paragraph, the Task Force stated: "Newborn circumcision has potential medical benefits and advantages as well as disadvantages and risks. When circumcision is being considered, the benefits and risks should be explained to the parents and informed consent obtained" (Cunningham et al, 1993).

Dorsal penile nerve blocks or other local anesthetics have been found to be effective in reducing behavioral distress and adrenocortical stress response in neonates undergoing circumcision. Newborn pain is often a factor in parent's decision making about circumcision, and the fact that anesthetics decrease this response seems to indicate that without anesthetic the baby does feel some pain. It is important to know the policies of the pediatrician or obstetrician who would be doing the procedures to help parents make an appropriate choice.

The issue of looking similar to other boys is probably less of an issue now that the number of uncircumcised males has increased. Thus they may be the same as some of their friends and different than others no matter what. The issue of looking similar to the father may be of some concern, although there is no real evidence that boys care.

Insurance coverage may also be a factor in the decision-making process for some parents.

How will you respond to her question regarding sexual activity?

Your client can be instructed that sexual activity will pose no risk to her or the fetus provided she has no bleeding, premature cramping, or ruptured membranes. Also, she and her partner should be cautioned to avoid orogenital sexual practices that blow air into the vagina. There have been reports of fatal and near fatal cases caused by air embolism with this practice.

Changes in position may be required to accommodate the enlarging abdomen. By the third trimester it is advisable to avoid the supine position because the weight of the uterus compresses the vena cava producing low BP and dizziness. Remind the couple that the fetus is well protected in the amniotic sac and is not injured by coitus. Comfort issues may also be addressed by utilizing alternatives to intercourse. You may also want to let her know that that woman's level of desire may be very different from her usual as well as different during the times within the pregnancy.

At term, if the cervix is favorable, nipple stimulation or sexual activity may actually stimulate the onset of labor.

References

American Academy of Pediatrics and American College of Obstetricians and Gynecologists: *Guidelines for perinatal care,* ed 2, Washington, DC, 1983, AAP/ACOG.

American Academy of Pediatrics and American College of Obstetricians and Gynecologists: *Guidelines for perinatal care,* ed 3, Washington, DC, 1992, AAP/ACOG.

American Academy of Pediatrics: Report of the task force on circumcision, *Pediatrics* 84:388, 1989.

Caffeine and women's health, *AWHONN,* 1994.

Cunningham FG et al: *Williams obstetrics,* ed 19, Norwalk, Conn, 1993, Appleton & Lange.

Laumann EO, Masi CM, Zuckerman EW: Circumcision in the United States: prevalence, prophylactic effects, and sexual practices, *JAMA* 277:1052, 1997.

Sanford JP, Gilbert DN, Sande MA: *The Sanford guide to antimicrobial therapy,* Dallas, 1996, Antimicrobial Therapy.

1:45 PM
Olga Manjakhina
Age 54 years

OPENING SCENARIO

Olga Manjakhina is a 54-year-old female of Russian heritage on your schedule for urinary incontinence (UI). She has not been to your practice before.

HISTORY OF PRESENT ILLNESS

"I have been having problems over the past 3 to 4 months with losing my urine. I have leaked a small amount of urine when I laugh or when I sneeze for quite some time, but over the past few months it seems to be getting worse. There are also times more recently, for about the past month, when I am just sitting quietly and I get an uncontrollable urge to urinate. When I urinate at that time it is in fairly large amounts. I have been using incontinence pads with good success in keeping my clothing dry." Patient denies dysuria and difficulty starting stream. She loses her urine whenever she coughs and at times when she is lifting or carrying things. Also at rest at times as noted. No known history of urinary tract infections (UTIs). Menopause at age 49. Up once each night to void. Voids about every 1 1/2 hours during the day in moderate amounts.

MEDICAL HISTORY

She has been quite healthy all of her life. The delivery of one of her children was "traumatic." The doctor had a hard time delivering the baby and had to use forceps; she describes it as very painful. "The doctors thought he might die, but he did fine."

FAMILY MEDICAL HISTORY

Mother: 84 yr (mild arthritis)
Father: 86 yr (mild lung problems)
Four sisters: Range from 40 to 61 yr (A&W)
Two brothers: 52, 57 yr (A&W)
Two children: 30, 34 yr (A&W)

SOCIAL HISTORY

Lives with husband who is an engineer. Came to the United States with family from Leningrad, Russia (now St. Petersburg) 14 years ago. Smokes 1 pack per day. One alcoholic drink per evening. Does not work outside of the home. Limits her social activities to about 2 hours because of urine leakage.

MEDICATIONS

None

ALLERGIES

None

REVIEW OF SYSTEMS

General: Good energy level
Skin: No itching or rashes
HEENT: No history of head injury or headaches; no corrective lenses; denies eye pain; no excessive tearing, blurring, or change in vision; no tinnitus or vertigo; denies frequent colds, hay fever, or sinus problems
Neck: No lumps, goiters, or pain
Thorax: Denies shortness of breath, paroxysmal nocturnal dyspnea
Cardiac: No chest pain, no shortness of breath with normal activity
Abdominal/Gastrointestinal: No nausea, vomiting, constipation, or diarrhea; denies belching, bloating, and black or clay colored stools
Genitourinary: See History of Present Illness
Extremities: No joint pain or swelling
Neurological: No seizures; denies numbness, paresthesias, or weakness
Endocrine: No polyuria, polyphagia, polydipsia; temperature tolerances good
Hematological: No excessive bruising; no history of transfusions

PHYSICAL EXAMINATON

Vital signs: Temperature: 98° F; *Pulse:* 76 beats/min; *Respirations:* 18 breaths/min; *BP:* 120/74 mm Hg
Height: 5' 6"; *Weight:* 167 lb
General: Well developed, well nourished; in no acute distress; appears stated age
HEENT: Normocephalic without masses or lesions; pupils equal, round, and reactive to light; extraocular movements intact; fundi benign; nares patent and noninjected; throat without redness or lesions

Neck: Supple without thyromegaly or adenopathy
Thorax: Clear to auscultation and percussion
Heart: Regular rate and rhythm; no murmurs, rubs, or gallops
Abdomen/Gastrointestinal: No hepatosplenomegaly; abdomen soft, nontender; bowel sounds normoactive; rectal without masses; stool brown; guaiac negative; normal sphincter tone
Genitourinary: External without lesions; vaginal mucosa pink with mild atrophy; cervix without gross lesions; no discharge noted; uterus is anteroflexed; no adnexal tenderness; Pap smear sent; Grade 1 cystocele; no rectocele; Dip urine: SG 1.010, negative for glucose and protein, positive for nitrites and leukocytes
Extremities: Range of motion functionally intact; no cyanosis, clubbing, or edema
Neurological: Reflexes 2+ at Achilles, patellar, biceps, triceps, and brachioradialis; no Babinski signs present

ASSESSMENT   *Please indicate the problems or issues you have identified that will guide your care (preferably in list form):*

PLAN   *Please list your plans for addressing each of the problems or issues in your assessment:*

Community Clinic

Jeffrey A. Eaton, NP
Joyce D. Cappiello, NP

Name:_____ DOB_____
Address_____ Date_____

Rx

"label all unless indicated"
Refill:_____ times-- Do not refill ( )

Signed:_____
DO NOT TAKE THIS TO YOUR PHARMACIST

Community Clinic

Jeffrey A. Eaton, NP
Joyce D. Cappiello, NP

Name:_____ DOB_____
Address_____ Date_____

Rx

"label all unless indicated"
Refill:_____ times-- Do not refill ( )

Signed:_____
DO NOT TAKE THIS TO YOUR PHARMACIST

LEARNING ISSUES

In order to resolve this patient's problem, you will need to consider and address the following issues (you may generate additional issues as well):

- Types of UI
- Cultural issues in caring for a person of Russian heritage
- Diagnostic evaluation for UI
- Hormone replacement therapy (HRT)
- Health maintenance in a 54-year-old woman
- Immunizations in an adult immigrant
- Cystocele

INITIAL IDEAS

- Stress incontinence
- Urge incontinence
- Mixed incontinence
- Overflow incontinence

INTERPRETATION OF CUES, PATTERNS, AND INFORMATION

This problem is obviously bothering Mrs. Manjakhina or she would not be in your office. A good place to start is to verbalize that you recognize how difficult and embarrassing that this must be, but that in most cases of incontinence a cure or significant improvement can be obtained.

UI is a problem that many women inappropriately accept as a normal change of aging. It has social, financial, and psychological outcomes that can be very negative for an older woman. UI is more common in women who have had multiple children, are overweight, smoke, are postmenopausal, are not on estrogen supplementation, or have mobility problems. Ms. Manjakhina has four of these risk factors.

When taking a UI history, there are several key elements. The abruptness of onset, the amount voided, the circumstances surrounding the UI episode, and any other urinary symptoms can provide clues to the cause of the UI. You should also ask questions regarding sexual issues, prescription medications, over-the-counter (OTC) medications, and habits such as nicotine, alcohol, and caffeine intake.

Ms. Manjakhina's history is consistent with both leaking a small amount of urine with increases in intraabdominal pressure (which would be consistent with stress incontinence) and voiding large amounts after an uncontrollable urge to void (which would be consistent with urge incontinence). The stress incontinence symptoms have been present for some time, but the urge incontinence symptoms may represent a transient incontinence related to a more short-term problem. A common cause

of an urge incontinence like this would be a UTI. Ms. Manjakhina has a dip urine with positive nitrites, which is highly suspicious of a UTI. Negative nitrites does not rule out a UTI, since if a
woman is voiding frequently, there may not be time for the bacteria to convert nitrates to nitrites
in the bladder.

How does Ms. Manjakhina's cultural heritage make a difference in her care? She may have very
specific ideas about health care consistent with her previous culture, or those ideas may have
changed in her 14 years here. In Russia a nonphysician primary care provider would be quite unusual. In rural areas a *felshur* might provide health care advice and treatment, but traditionally in
Russia, physicians are the recognized primary care providers. A woman such a Ms. Manjakhina
might have a difficult time taking advice from a nurse practitioner or physician assistant. Also the
clinician must remember that the environmental risk factors that are assumed in the United States
for a patient may be very different for Ms. Manjakhina. She may have come from a particularly in-
dustrialized section of St. Petersburg and had environmental exposure to very different substances
than she would have in the United States.

She also may have lifestyle issues that are different. She does smoke, and she should be encouraged to stop. Her alcohol intake appears to be moderate. Dietary intake could be assessed to
determine whether she is at risk for other problems.

REVISED IDEAS

- Mixed incontinence: A combination of stress incontinence and urge incontinence

DIFFERENTIAL DIAGNOSIS

1. *Stress incontinence:* Stress incontinence is incontinence that is caused by a rapid rise in intraabdominal pressure, which then exceeds the pressure of the urethral sphincter and results in a leakage of urine. As noted, her history is consistent with stress incontinence. Stress incontinence may
be worsened by structural problems, although her Grade 1 cystocele is probably not a major issue.
Hutt (1995) says that a cystocele must be Grade 3 or larger to contribute significantly to UI.
2. *Urge incontinence:* Urge incontinence is characterized by an urgent desire to void followed by
involuntary loss of urine (Merck Manual, 1992). Urge incontinence can be transient (often related
to UTIs) or chronic (usually related to neurological problems). If treatment of the UTI did not resolve the urge component, diagnostics to determine whether detrusor instability was present could
be conducted.
3. *Mixed incontinence:* This is a combination of stress incontinence and urge incontinence.
4. *Overflow incontinence:* In a patient with diabetes or some other reason for bladder neuropathy,
a more flaccid bladder can result. These people have large amounts of urine in the bladder and void
small amounts. Thus the symptoms may be similar to those of stress incontinence. Outflow resistance can also cause this problem, although this is more common in men related to prostatic enlargement.

A search for transient causes of UI can use an approach that rules out those things shown in
Box 37-1.

DIAGNOSTIC OPTIONS

A urine culture will allow accurate treatment of the suspected UTI. A case could be made for empiric treatment if this was felt to be her first UTI, but with the level of symptoms that it is causing,
a full urine culture may be defensible. A full urinalysis should also be carried out to screen for other
problems such as an occult bladder cancer.

A catheterization for postvoid residual (PVR) can rule out overflow incontinence, although not
all clinicians would do it at this point. A PVR of over 100 ml would be very suspicious of an overflow incontinence.

A urinary diary will also give valuable information about the current voiding patterns.

Box 37-1 *Common Causes of Transient Incontinence*

Delirium or confusional state
Infection, urinary (symptomatic)
Atrophic urethritis or vaginitis
Drugs
- Sedatives or hypnotics, especially long-acting agents
- Loop diuretics
- Anticholinergic agents (antipsychotics, antidepressants, antihistamines, antiparkinsonian agents, antiarrhythmics, antispasmodics, opiates, and antidiarrheals)
- α-adrenoceptor agonists and antagonists
- Calcium channel blockers
Psychological problems, including depression
Endocrine disorders (hypercalcemia, hyperglycemia)
Restricted mobility
Stool impaction

Ham RJ, Sloane PD: *Primary care geriatrics,* St Louis, 1997, Mosby.

Laboratory tests such as a fasting blood sugar (FBS) and a serum calcium might reveal hyperosmolar states that could contribute to a high urine volume and thus UI. A blood urea nitrogen (BUN) and creatinine would provide a rough indication of kidney function.

On physical examination the stress maneuver, which involves coughing or bearing down during the pelvic examination and then checking for urine leakage, could be used to look for stress incontinence.

THERAPEUTIC OPTIONS

Pharmacological

If a UTI is present, an appropriate medication could be chosen (probably a 3-day course of Bactrim DS).

There are pharmacological treatments for UI, including use of a sympathetic agonist such as pseudoephedrine for stress incontinence. A sympathetic agonist acts by increasing sphincter tone. Other drugs can be used to increase bladder tone (such as in overflow incontinence without outlet obstruction). An example would be bethanecol. Drugs may also be used to decrease bladder tone (anticholinergic) in a patient with an overactive detrusor. An example would be oxybutynin. These must be used with great caution, however, since urinary retention may be the result. Other drugs with anticholinergic effects may also contribute to urinary retention.

Educational and Other Nonpharmacological Options

Ms. Manjakhina can increase fluid intake to promote urinary output, although she will be hesitant to do so if she is still incontinent. Hygiene and sexuality issues can be discussed. She should avoid bladder irritants such as caffeine. Some patients anecdotally have indicated caffeine-free diet sodas as providing subjective symptoms.

She can attempt to plan her day based on her current voiding patterns. Urge control can be practiced by using deep breathing exercises. Kegel's exercises can be effective in decreasing UI, although the frequency with which they must be done and the fact that they must be kept up indefinitely limit the number of patients who benefit.

HEALTH PROMOTION/HEALTH MAINTENANCE

Immunization recommendations are similar in Russia to those in the United States. When Ms. Manjakhina was a child, immunizations were given on a routine schedule. She may need an update of her tetanus-diphtheria (Td) immunization, and as a smoker, a Pneumococcal vaccine would be recommended. An annual influenza vaccine should be given as well.

Ms. Manjakhina should have aggressive screening for cancers because of her age and possible previous environmental exposures. Her Pap smear was sent. Colon cancer screening should be considered and could begin with fecal occult blood testing (FOBT). This could wait for a later visit or begin now depending on your judgment. Clinical breast examination should be carried out, and a mammogram would also be recommended.

HRT is an issue that should be addressed in Ms. Manjakhina. It may protect her from cardiac disease and osteoporosis, although not all clinicians are convinced that the current evidence is compelling (US Preventive Services Task Force, 1996). It may also provide her with some subjective relief from her UI since it will increase estrogen effects in the vaginal area and thus make external sphincter closure more effective.

FOLLOW-UP

Ms. Manjakhina should be seen in about 2 weeks after laboratory testing is done and treatment of the UTI is completed.

References

Berkow R, editor: *Merck manual,* Rahway, NJ, 1992, Merck.

Ham RJ, Sloane PD: *Primary care geriatrics,* St Louis, 1997, Mosby.

Hutt E: The elderly patient. In Mladenovic J, editor: *Primary care secrets,* St Louis, 1995, Mosby.

US Preventive Services Task Force: *Clinical preventive services guidelines,* Baltimore, 1996, Williams & Wilkins.

CASE
38

2:30 PM
Justin Baker
Age 3 1/2 years

OPENING SCENARIO

Justin Baker is a 3 1/2-year-old male in your office with red, "weepy" eyes. His was last seen for an 18 month well child check (WCC).

HISTORY OF PRESENT ILLNESS

(Obtained from mother)

"This happens off and on. This is probably his third episode. I haven't really noticed a pattern. The other two episodes cleared up on their own. One episode was about 3 months ago, and the other one was about this same time last year. This episode started 3 days ago. I haven't done anything for it except some warm soaks with a wash cloth. He never had it this bad before, but his sister Jessie did, so I brought her in, got a cream, and it went away within a couple of days. Justin's right eye is now very red, and he feels like it has sand in it. It was just a little crusty this morning. The crust was yellowish. I just washed it off with a warm cloth. His left eye is red but less so, and it did not really have a crust on it this morning. He has had a runny nose this week as well but no other symptoms."

MEDICAL HISTORY

Normal spontaneous vaginal delivery. Apgar scores were 10 and 10. Ear infections at 2 months, 5 months, 9 months, and 18 months. Immunization record is shown in Table 38-1. Growth percentiles are consistent in the approximately 60th percentile for height and 80th for weight. Milestones all within normal limits on previous visits. Toilet trained but occasionally wakes up wet. Sleeps about 10 hours per night but really hates to go to bed. Likes to dress himself and likes to draw.

FAMILY MEDICAL HISTORY

MGM: 51 yr (diabetes mellitus [DM])
MGF: 53 yr (A&W)
PGM: 50 yr (A&W)
PGF: 53 yr (myocardial infarction [MI] 2 years ago)

Mother: 26 yr (A&W)
Father: 26 yr (A&W)
One sister: 20 mo (A&W)

SOCIAL HISTORY

Lives with both parents and younger sister (she is now 20 months old). Father works as a maintenance man at local factory (makes electrical parts for lamps, etc.). Mother works part time at local video store (Mondays, Wednesdays, and Fridays). Justin attends family daycare when his mother is working.

MEDICATIONS

None

ALLERGIES

None

REVIEW OF SYSTEMS

(Obtained from mother)
General: Good energy level
Skin: No itching or rashes

Table **38-1** *Immunization Record for Justin Baker*

VACCINE	DATE	INITIALS	NOTES
DPT	2 mo	MDO	Tetramune
DPT	4 mo	MDO	Tetramune
DPT	6 mo	MDO	Tetramune
DPT	18 mo	MDO	Acellular
Td			
Td			
IPV	2 mo	MDO	
IPV	4 mo	MDO	
OPV	18 mo	MDO	
OPV			
MMR	13 mo	MDO	
MMR			
HBV	2 mo	MDO	
HBV	4 mo	MDO	
HBV			
Hib	2 mo	MDO	Tetramune
Hib	4 mo	MDO	Tetramune
Hib	6 mo	MDO	Tetramune
Hib			

HEENT: No history of head injury; no corrective lenses; denies frequent colds, hay fever, or sinus problems; teeth present without gross defects

Neck: No lumps, goiters, or pain

Thorax: Denies shortness of breath

Heart: No chest pain; no shortness of breath with normal activity

Abdomen/Gastrointestinal: No nausea, vomiting, constipation, or diarrhea.

Genitourinary: No dysuria; no odor to urine

Extremities: No joint pain or swelling

Neurological: No seizures

Endocrine: No polyuria, polyphagia, polydipsia; temperature tolerances good

Hematological: No excessive bruising; no history of transfusions

Nutrition: Eats from all four food groups; frequent snacker and tends to like the same foods over and over again (scrambled eggs, pizza, fish sticks); drinks about 20 oz of milk per day

PHYSICAL EXAMINATION

Vital signs: Temperature: 98° F; *Pulse:* 76 beats/min; *Respirations:* 18 breaths/min

Weight: 39 lb

General: Well developed, well nourished; in no acute distress; appears stated age

HEENT: Normocephalic without masses or lesions; pupils equal, round, and reactive to light; extraocular movements intact; conjunctiva injected both palpebral and scleral; no ciliary flush; moderate amount of clear discharge present; nares patent and noninjected; throat without redness or lesions; tympanic membranes (TMs) noninjected; cone of light crisp; TMs mobile

Neck: Supple without thyromegaly or adenopathy

Thorax: Clear to auscultation and percussion

Heart: Regular rate and rhythm; no murmurs, rubs, or gallops

Abdomen/Gastrointestinal: No hepatosplenomegaly; abdomen soft, nontender; bowel sounds normoactive

Extremities: Range of motion functionally intact; no cyanosis, clubbing, or edema

Neurological: No Babinski signs present

ASSESSMENT   *Please indicate the problems or issues you have identified that will guide your care (preferably in list form):*

PLAN   *Please list your plans for addressing each of the problems or issues in your assessment:*

Community Clinic
Jeffrey A. Eaton, NP
Joyce D. Cappiello, NP

Name:_____ DOB_____
Address_____ Date_____

Rx

"label all unless indicated"
Refill:_____ times-- Do not refill ( )

Signed:_____
DO NOT TAKE THIS TO YOUR PHARMACIST

Community Clinic
Jeffrey A. Eaton, NP
Joyce D. Cappiello, NP

Name:_____ DOB_____
Address_____ Date_____

Rx

"label all unless indicated"
Refill:_____ times-- Do not refill ( )

Signed:_____
DO NOT TAKE THIS TO YOUR PHARMACIST

CASE
38 *Discussion*

LEARNING ISSUES

In order to resolve this patient's problem, you will need to consider and address the following issues (you may generate additional issues as well):

- **Causes for conjunctival injection**
- **Differential diagnosis of conjunctivitis**
- **Appropriate advice regarding problems with bedtime**
- **Immunizations and the episodic visit**
- **Health maintenance and the episodic visit in children**
- **Acellular pertussis vaccine**
- **Oral poliovirus (OPV) vaccine**
- ***Haemophilus influenzae* type b (Hib) vaccine**
- **Advice regarding occasional bedwetting in a 3 1/2 year old**
- **The varicella zoster virus (VZV) vaccine**

INITIAL IDEAS

Justin is a 3 1/2-year-old boy, and you have not seen him for 2 years. You do not know when you will see him again, so you want to do what you can in this 15-minute time slot. Based on the presenting history, you have probably created a problem list that looks something like this:

- Conjunctivitis (etiology)
- Problems with sleeping and/or bedtime
- Immunizations needed: Hepatitis B (HBV), VZV, Hib
- Health promotion/health maintenance

INTERPRETATION OF CUES, PATTERNS, AND INFORMATION (INCLUDING DIFFERENTIAL DIAGNOSIS)

Conjunctivitis

The first place you need to start is with the presenting problem. Your differential diagnosis for conjunctivitis will include the following:

1. Viral conjunctivitis
2. Bacterial conjunctivitis
3. Allergic conjunctivitis
4. Less common problems including trachoma (chlamydia), lyme disease, measles, and herpes simplex
5. Corneal abrasion or foreign body

Additional information about Justin's visual acuity would be helpful and might be obtainable using a Snellen E chart. He might not be able to cooperate, however, and you would have to proceed without this information. Many clinicians would not culture the eye drainage at this point but would if it recurs or does not get better.

The fact that it has happened "off and on" before makes it suspicious for an allergic conjunctivitis. He does not have many other allergic symptoms, however, so this makes it somewhat less probable, as does the fact that it occurred at different times of the year. If you were suspicious, questions about new pets, a seasonal pattern, or other questions appropriate to allergies could be asked.

The runny nose that he had earlier in the week could have been related to allergies, or it could represent a viral infection; thus a viral conjunctivitis is a possibility as well. Practically, it probably does not make much difference for today's visit because the key decision that you need to make is whether to start antibiotics. If a child has a crust in the morning, it supports a bacterial origin, and some clinicians use that as their criteria on whether to start antibiotics. The feeling of sand in the eye also makes some clinicians more apt to prescribe antibiotics since the child will get some subjective relief from the ointment as well as treatment for an infection that is either bacterial or soon will be. Many other clinicians will start antibiotics with any viral infection since the number that turn into a bacterial infection is quite high.

When would you suspect trachoma? If Justin was a Native American or living in the mountain areas of the southern United States, that might raise your level of suspicion. Trachoma is usually a chronic conjunctivitis with exacerbations and remissions, so Justin's presentation would not be entirely out of the question. Photophobia and eyelid edema might also raise the level of suspicion of trachoma as would granulations of the upper lid. If Justin's conjunctivitis recurred soon after a usual treatment approach, then consultation might be appropriate.

Herpes simplex virus (HSV) or VZV (although VZV would be quite unusual in this age group without coexisting chronic disease) might be suspected if there were vesicular lesions anywhere on the face with his conjunctivitis. Although most of children with HSV infection do well, referral to ophthalmology is usually done as a precaution.

Lyme disease or other noninfectious causes could also be suspected if Jake had other symptoms such as joint pain or a recurrence pattern.

A foreign body would be suspected based on history, but in a young child a complete history is difficult to obtain.

REVISED IDEAS

- Bacterial conjunctivitis
- Allergic or viral conjunctivitis with or without superimposed bacterial conjunctivitis
- Problems with sleeping and/or bedtime
- Immunizations needed: HBV, VZV, Hib
- Health promotion/health maintenance

DIAGNOSTIC OPTIONS

Most clinicians would do one of two things in this case, and the response of the parents to the options may be the deciding factor. Justin's problem could be treated as a viral or allergic conjunctivitis with supportive therapy and oral antihistamines. The other common approach would be a trial of therapy with antibiotics.

Another option would be a culture, but since the majority of children will respond to empiric therapy, it is probably not worth the cost at this point.

If there was suspicion of the more serious causes of conjunctivitis, then an optometrical or ophthalmological consultation as appropriate would be indicated. If Lyme disease was suspected, then antibody titers could be drawn.

Based on his history, you are probably not highly suspicious of a corneal abrasion or a foreign body. He did not have an abrupt onset, and his sister had something very similar recently. Based on this low probability and his being 3 years old, staining him with fluoroscein and using the Wood's lamp would not be a common practice.

THERAPEUTIC OPTIONS

Pharmacological

Ilotycin (Erythromycin) ointment is a reasonable choice since it does not burn, is relatively cheap, and has good coverage. A common prescription might be 1/4 to 1/2 inch to the affected eyes tid for 4 to 5 days. Textbooks often recommend 7- to 10-day treatment, but stopping at 4 to 5 days is reasonable if the child has been completely symptom free for a couple of days. Sodium Sulamyd 10% ointment (Bleph-10) is also a reasonable choice. The prescription might be similar at 1/4 to 1/2 inch qid for 5 to 7 days depending on the severity and reason for prescribing. Some clinicians prescribe it less frequently and some more. This case is relatively mild, so it probably is not necessary to be much more aggressive than this. Sulamyd drops are also used, but some complain of a mild burning sensation when they are instilled, and a few minutes of blurred vision caused by the ointment does not seem to be major problem for most 3 year olds. Bacitracin/polymixin ointment is also used.

Educational

Another issue that you will need to address is whether Justin should go to daycare tomorrow. Uphold and Graham (1996) say that eye secretions are infectious for 24 to 48 hours. One common practice is to suggest that he have at least three doses of antibiotic cream or drops before going back to daycare. This should not be a problem, so many clinicians would approve his going to daycare. Daycares are very (appropriately so) concerned about conjunctivitis. If Justin can stay home tomorrow, his mother will not run the risk of problems with the daycare.

Other instructions should include a call if no improvement in 2 to 3 days, careful handwashing, and disposal of the tube when completed (it is preferred that a separate tube be used for each eye, but this may not be agreeable to parents). Cool, moist compresses may decrease the discomfort.

Justin had other problems, and you may want to address them today or schedule him for a WCC. Either way you will need to think through those problems and possible solutions.

Problems with Sleeping and/or Bedtime You might explore the meaning of this problem to the mother to the extent time allows. Some reassurance that this is a common problem would be appropriate as well as some basic suggestions that she can use to try to address the problem. Limiting your advice to two or three suggestions may be best since you have only 15 minutes and several things with which to deal. Those suggestions would probably be to establish a routine at night and a special bed toy. Other suggestions may also be reasonable depending on further data collection. Try those two or three suggestions and a follow-up visit in 2 or 3 weeks.

You also may want to provide some reassurance that accidents are still quite common in boys this age who are toilet trained, and that they will gradually decrease over time.

Immunizations needed: HBV, VZV, Hib This level of illness is not a contraindication to giving immunizations, so the following could be given pending discussions with the mother and signature on appropriate informed consent forms:

1. *HBV:* HBV vaccine can be expensive, and 3 year olds are still not high risk. As with all vaccines, this choice is up to the parents. The strength of your recommendation will be based on a desire to provide herd immunity to this age cohort, an understanding of state funding and the direct cost to parents, and an understanding of the individual situation. If the parents are willing, HBV vaccine should be given today.

2. *VZV:* VZV vaccine is recommended for this age group but is still quite expensive ($45+ per dose), and availability is variable. (Adolescents need two doses, but this is not an issue for Justin). Many clinicians offer the vaccine and then let the parents decide. The vaccine does not have an extensive history, so the more long-term protective effects are not known. It is a live vaccine, so there is a remote risk to other family members. This of course would be covered in the informed consent process, but you could also check for people at risk to whom he could be exposed. There are also storage issues for the VZV vaccine, and the clinician may want to assure that the vaccine has been stored appropriately.

3. *Hib:* Because Justin was switched to the acellular diphtheria-pertussis-tetanus (DPT) vaccine, he seems to have missed a dose of Hib. Justin is still in the age group for epiglottitis risk. He had his first dose at age 2 months, and thus he should get a total of four doses of Hib vaccine. There is a combination vaccine available that combines Hib and HBV vaccine, so that would allow you to give Justin just one shot for these two vaccines.

HEALTH PROMOTION/HEALTH MAINTENANCE

You should base the amount of time spent on the following on whether you are running behind, whether there are any cancellations later in the afternoon, and how long the earlier components had taken. Depending on the parent, asking that Justin come back for immunizations and a check-up in about 1 month may be the appropriate intervention.

1. *Nutrition:* Like many toddlers, Justin is going through "food jags." Although you would like Justin to eat healthier, you also need to recognize that he is at an age that he is learning to make his own choices, and when possible you should try to respect that. Encouraging healthier foods by example as well as trying to prepare them in a way that he finds appetizing are probably reasonable approaches. Justin at about 3 1/2 years old is in the 50th percentile, so it looks like he is starting to slim down a little anyway. You would want to have the mother keep an eye on his weight to see where it goes. He is old enough to stand on a scale, and you should in fact get a reasonably accurate value. This also raises the issue of cholesterol in children. Justin's grandfather had an MI at age 51, which fits most definitions of early cardiovascular disease. Most clinicians would screen Justin for hyperlipidemia, although the benefit of doing so is somewhat controversial.

2. *Disease screening:* Looking for eye problems is reasonable, although sensitivity and specificity documentation of most tests is lacking. A cover test and visual acuity test are reasonable, although they may not be all that helpful. Tuberculosis (TB) testing could be considered in high-risk areas.

3. *Lead levels:* Lead levels should have been tested at 12 months. You should probably check to make sure these were done. Seeing whether he lives in an old home and whether his father's factory work puts him in contact with lead are useful. A lead questionnaire could also be used. Remember that screening for lead also has its own set of adverse effect (US Preventive Services Task Force, 1996).

4. *Bedwetting:* His occasional bedwetting is not unusual at this age, and his parents should be reassured about this. Some simple behavioral interventions such as having him void at bedtime and limiting fluids for a couple of hours before bedtime are worth a reminder.

General Anticipatory Guidance at this Age
- Some chores
- Brushing of his teeth (although some dentists recommend that an adult brush the teeth until age 5)
- Seat belts, smoke detectors, bike safety, water safety
- Ipecac may now be expiring; assure emergency numbers including poison control
- Sun screen
- Fluoride

FOLLOW-UP

Justin will need to be seen between ages 4 and 5 for his preschool immunizations. He should return if he worsens or if he is not improved in 24 to 48 hours.

References
US Preventive Services Task Force: *Guide to clinical preventive services,* Baltimore, 1996, Williams & Wilkins.

Uphold CR, Graham MV: *Guidelines in family practice,* Gainesville, Fla, 1996, Barramarrae.

CASE
39

OPENING SCENARIO

Curt Ozana is a 36-year-old male scheduled for an episodic visit. He is new to your practice.

HISTORY OF PRESENT ILLNESS

"Yesterday I began having pain in my right scrotum. The pain has been increasing. I don't remember any trauma to the area." The patient denies urethral discharge or burning. No history of prior urinary tract infections (UTIs), prostatitis, or renal calculi. New female sexual partner 2 months ago. Had vasectomy 2 years ago. Does not use condoms.

MEDICAL HISTORY

Denies any hospitalizations or major medical problems. Outpatient vasectomy 2 years ago.

Last physical examination was several years ago (does not remember exactly). Had all childhood immunizations, including measles-mumps-rubella (MMR) but not hepatitis.

FAMILY MEDICAL HISTORY

Mother: 70 (Parkinson's disease for 1 year)
Father: 72 (chronic obstructive pulmonary disease [COPD])
Sister: 40 yr (A&W)
Brother: 37 yr (A&W)

SOCIAL HISTORY

Divorced for 1 year. Has 2 children, ages 5 and 7. Works as a computer programmer. Nonsmoker.

MEDICATIONS

None

ALLERGIES

Penicillin

REVIEW OF SYSTEMS

General: States overall health is good
Cardiac: Denies any chest pain, dyspnea
Respiratory: Denies shortness of breath, asthma, enviromental allergies
Gastrointestinal: Denies hepatitis or liver problems; no abdominal or flank pain
Genitourinary: No history of undescended testicles; denies history of kidney or urinary tract problems; no recent instrumentation of urinary tract; no history of sexually transmitted diseases (STDs)

PHYSICAL EXAMINATION

Vital signs: Temperature: 98.4° F; *Pulse:* 74 beats/min; *Respirations:* 16 breaths/min; *BP:*110/74 mm Hg
Heart: Regular rate and rhythm, no murmurs, rubs, or gallops
Lungs: Clear to auscultation
Abdomen: No tenderness, guarding, or masses palpated; no hepatosplenomegaly, costovertebral angle (CVA) tenderness, or suprapubic tenderness noted; no inguinal masses or lymphadenopathy noted
Genitourinary: Right testis: red, swollen to twice the normal size, tender; raising testes decreases the pain; positive cremasteric reflex; transillumination negative; no hydrocele, spermatocele, varicocele, or epididymal cyst noted; Left testis: no redness, enlargement, or tenderness; no inguinal or femoral hernias noted; faint, dull red rash noted in right and left groin area; scaly plaques with distinct margins covering a small portion of groin area; when questioned, states this rash has been present for several months; states he has used some over-the-counter (OTC) cream when it is itchy and bothersome for a day or so, but then he forgets to use it once the itching improves; denies rashes elsewhere on body

ASSESSMENT   *Please indicate the problems or issues you have identified that will guide your care (preferably in list form):*

PLAN   *Please list your plans for addressing each of the problems or issues in your assessment:*

Community Clinic
Jeffrey A. Eaton, NP
Joyce D. Cappiello, NP

Name:_____ DOB_____
Address_____ Date_____

Rx

"label all unless indicated"
Refill:_____ times-- Do not refill ( )

Signed:_____
DO NOT TAKE THIS TO YOUR PHARMACIST

Community Clinic
Jeffrey A. Eaton, NP
Joyce D. Cappiello, NP

Name:_____ DOB_____
Address_____ Date_____

Rx

"label all unless indicated"
Refill:_____ times-- Do not refill ( )

Signed:_____
DO NOT TAKE THIS TO YOUR PHARMACIST

Community Clinic
Jeffrey A. Eaton, NP
Joyce D. Cappiello, NP

Name:_____ DOB_____
Address_____ Date_____

Rx

"label all unless indicated"
Refill:_____ times-- Do not refill ( )

Signed:_____
DO NOT TAKE THIS TO YOUR PHARMACIST

Community Clinic
Jeffrey A. Eaton, NP
Joyce D. Cappiello, NP

Name:_____ DOB_____
Address_____ Date_____

Rx

"label all unless indicated"
Refill:_____ times-- Do not refill ( )

Signed:_____
DO NOT TAKE THIS TO YOUR PHARMACIST

LEARNING ISSUES

In order to resolve this patient's problem, you will need to consider and address the following issues (you may generate additional issues as well):

- Genitourinary examination
- Surgical emergency with scrotal pain
- Role of STDs in causing epididymitis
- Useful physical examination techniques and diagnostic testing in making a diagnosis with complaint of scrotal pain

INITIAL IDEAS

Because of Mr. Ozana's history of a new sexual contact in the past 6 months, an STD is high on the differential list.

INTERPRETATION OF CUES, PATTERNS, AND INFORMATION

Torsion is a surgical emergency that should not be overlooked. How do you rule this out? Torsion is more commonly seen in young adolescent or prepubertal males rather than in a 36 year old. Physical examination findings are often helpful in distinguishing torsion from other conditions. Elevation of the scrotum often relieves the pain of epididymitis as with this patient but intensifies the discomfort in torsion. The cremasteric reflex is slow or absent in torsion but is present in other conditions that cause scrotal swelling. This reflex is present in Mr. Ozana. The urinalysis is normal in torsion but usually shows pyuria in epididymitis. If the diagnosis is still not clear or the diagnosis is torsion, immediate referral to a urologist is indicated.

A tumor would present as a firm, nontender or mildly tender mass rather than as an acutely painful problem. If this scrotal swelling does not clear with antibiotics in a few days, reconsider this diagnosis.

A hydrocele, a benign swelling of fluid in the scrotal sac, is usually easy to identify since it is painless, transilluminates, and often can be palpated as a separate structure from the testes. A spermatocele is a fluid-filled enlargement to the epididymis that usually cannot be palpated separately. It is also benign and painless. Epididymal cysts can be found anywhere along the course of the epididymis. They are often multiple and bilateral but are benign. They are not important in themselves but must be distinguished from a solid or inflammatory mass. A varicocele is a common variant made up of a convoluted mass of dilated veins in the spermatic cord. Its consistency has been called a "bag of worms." It will not transilluminate and rarely enlarges enough to cause discomfort. In severe cases, it may affect fertility. None of these were noted during the physical examination of Mr. Ozana.

Orchitis, an inflammation of the testes, can only be differentiated from epididymitis in the early stages since swelling will quickly spread to the entire scrotum, making differentiation impossible.

Fever, chills, and bladder irritability are common symptoms. Since orchitis can be an uncommon complication of mumps in adults, ask about his history of immunizations. If he has not had immunizations or the disease, check his parotid glands.

Epididymitis related to an STD remains high on the differential. The presence of a urethral discharge would certainly be suspicious. Chlamydia is the most common cause of epididymitis in men under 50, although gonorrhea may also be present. Sometimes no infectious organism is found.

The additional issue noted on the physical examination is the groin rash. It is not uncommon for individuals to forget to mention a problem that is not bothersome. The most common rash in this area is a superficial, intertriginous fungal infection called tinea cruris (jock itch). Predisposing factors include obesity, a warm, humid environment, and tight clothing. Groin infections are common since it is an area that is often warm and moist. Be sure to ask about a similar rash elsewhere. Tinea pedis (feet) thrives on the same conditions of a warm, humid environment.

REVISED IDEAS

- Torsion
- Orchitis
- Tumor
- STD
- Tinea cruris

HISTORY AND PHYSICAL EXAMINATION TECHNIQUES

Although the history will focus on his chief complaint of scrotal pain, a few quick questions about his overall health would identify any other major health problems that could influence your choice of medications, such as liver or kidney disease. Some clinicians listen to heart and lung sounds to obtain some basic data on any new patient regardless of the complaint.

DIAGNOSTIC OPTIONS

Laboratory Results

Epididymitis   The causative organism of epididymitis may be found with testing of the urethral area for chlamydia and gonorrhea. If your facility has the capability for Gram's staining, this can provide an immediate assessment of the likelihood of an STD. Otherwise, many providers use the Genprobe assay, which tests for both infections and would confirm a positive Gram's stain in a few days. The newer polymerase chain reaction (PCR) urine tests for chlamydia are more accurate and more user friendly in the male. PCR testing for both gonorrhea and chlamydia from a urine specimen will soon be commercially available. Urine PCR testing in the female is not accurate because of the variety of organisms present in the vagina, which may affect the urine testing. Gonorrhea testing currently will require a urethral specimen plated on a Thayer-Martin agar. If concerned about STD exposure, also consider screening for syphilis and human immunodeficiency virus (HIV).

A urinalysis will usually show pyuria, and a urine culture will be positive in a nonsexually transmitted epididymitis associated with UTIs caused by gram-negative enteric organisms. Empiric therapy is indicated before culture results are available.

Tinea cruris   Generally the diagnosis for tinea cruris is made by physical examination. If the diagnosis is unclear, a scraping can be taken from the edges of the rash with either another glass slide or with a #15 scalpel and then placed on a potassium hydroxide preparation on a glass slide, gently heated, and examined under a microscope for hyphae or spores.

THERAPEUTIC OPTIONS

Epididymitis

An antibiotic regimen of Ceftriaxone 250 mg IM in a single dose and doxycycline 100 mg po bid for 10 days is the recommended treatment (Centers for Disease Control and Prevention [CDC], 1993). The recommended treatment is unchanged in the 1997 guidelines that will soon be published. Scrotal support, rest, and sitz baths will usually control the infection and provide comfort within a few days. Failure to improve within 3 days would require reevaluation of both the diagnosis and therapy. Some edema may persist for several weeks after finishing therapy and is not a treatment failure.

What about Mr. Ozana's allergy to penicillin? The likelihood of cross-reactivity between penicillins and cephalosporins is not clear but is estimated to be approximately 3% to 7% in patients with a history of an accelerated reaction to penicillin (Koda-Kimble and Young, 1995). However, only approximately 10% of persons who report a history of severe allergic reactions to penicillin are still allergic (CDC, 1993). What does he mean by an allergy? Many patients will have an "amoxicillin rash" with no cross-reactivity with other penicillins (Koda-Kimble and Young, 1995). There is a recommended alternative regimen of Ofloxacin 300 mg orally bid for 10 days that Mr. Ozana could safely take since there is no cross-sensitivity with the quinolones.

Tinea cruris

Any number of topical antifungal agents are effective for the treatment of tinea cruris, many of which are over-the-counter. The imidazoles such as clotrimazole, miconazole, and ketoconazole are very effective if used regularly (Fitzpatrick et al, 1994). What happens with many patients, as has occurred with this individual, is that cream is used sporadically. The sporadic use decreased symptoms of this subacute infection but did not effectively treat the symptoms. Sustained use 2 to 3 times a day for 1 to 3 weeks until symptoms are cleared should clear the infection. Oral agents, such as fluconazole, are not recommended.

If there is any way he can decrease moisture in the groin, such as loose fitting boxers and cotton underwear, this may be helpful in clearing the infection and preventing its return.

Encourage condom use as a measure to reduce his risk of exposure to STDs.

Since Mr. Ozana is a new patient to your practice, encourage him to return for a more complete history and physical at some point. The yield on a physical of a healthy young man without major health problems is low, but it will give you a thorough database on him. This could very helpful in the future.

References

Centers for Disease Control and Prevention: Recommendations and reports: 1993 sexually transmitted disease treatment guidelines; *MMWR* 42:i-102, 1993.

Fitzpatrick T et al: *Color atlas and synopsis of clinical dermatology,* ed 2, New York, 1994, McGraw-Hill.

Koda-Kimble MA, Young L: *Applied therapeutics,* Vancouver, 1995, Applied Therapeutics.

3:00 PM
Melanie Roberge
Age 18 years

OPENING SCENARIO

Melanie Roberge is an 18-year-old female scheduled for an episodic visit. She is new to your practice.

HISTORY OF PRESENT ILLNESS

"I have a vaginal discharge that I want checked out. It is a yellow, smelly discharge. There is no itching, but it burns a little bit when I urinate. For the past 2 weeks I have had more cramping than usual. My last boyfriend was about 5 months ago. We used condoms most of the time, but I am scared that I might have a sexually transmitted disease (STD)."

MEDICAL HISTORY

No hospitalizations or surgery. Had all childhood immunizations when she was young except for hepatitis B. Unsure of last tetanus-diphtheria (Td) immunization.

FAMILY MEDICAL HISTORY

MGM: 61 yr (hypercholesterolemia)
MGF: 62 yr (lung problems, heavy smoker)
PGM: 65 yr (cirrhosis, alcoholic)
PGF: Deceased at 69 yr (colon cancer)
Mother: 40 yr (smoker)
Father: 42 yr (alcoholic)
Sister: 20 yr (A&W)

SOCIAL HISTORY

Lives at home with parents. Graduated from high school and now works cleaning houses. Nonsmoker. Admits to drinking alcohol (2 beers 2 to 3 times per week); smokes marijuana occasionally at parties on the weekends; when questioned about risk factors for an STD, admits to intravenous (IV) drug use. Has had a number of sexual partners in the past year, some of whom also used IV drugs. Has been using heroin over the past 6 months on a daily basis. States she does not share needles. States she would like some help with this problem.

MEDICATIONS

None

ALLERGIES

None

REVIEW OF SYMPTOMS

General: Appetite fair; no weight changes; denies fever, chills, night sweats; sleep 6 hours per night and fatigued during the day
HEENT: No history of frequent colds, sinusitis, rhinitis, environmental allergies, ear infections; hearing and vision normal; no dental problems, last saw a dentist 1 year ago
Cardiac: No chest pain, palpitations
Respiratory: No history of wheezing, asthma, shortness of breath, dyspnea
Gastrointestinal: No heartburn, nausea, vomiting, diarrhea; frequent constipation, no hemorrhoids; lower abdominal pain for 2 weeks
Genitourinary: G0P0; menarche at age 13; regular, 28-day menstrual cycles; mild cramping for 1 day premenstrually; last menstrual period (LMP) 3 weeks ago; last Pap smear 2 years ago within normal limits; contraception method is condoms 95% of the time; no history of STDs
Extremities: No history of fractures or sprains; occasional myalgias; no joint pain
Endocrine: Temperature tolerances good; no skin or hair changes; occasional fatigue
Neurological: Occasional headaches relieved by ibuprofen; no weakness, seizures; denies depression or history of psychiatric illness; denies current history of feeling sad, powerless

PHYSICAL EXAMINAITION

Vital signs: Temperature: 98.6° F; *Pulse:* 74 beats/min; *Respirations:* 20 breaths/min; *BP:* 130/76 mm Hg
Height: 5'1"; *Weight:* 135 lb, *BMI:* 26
General: Healthy appearing, slightly overweight young female; oriented to time and place
Skin: Ecchymotic area on right antecubital space
Gastrointestinal: Abdomen soft, no tenderness or masses; no hepatosplenomegaly
Genitourinary: Vulva: no lesions, redness; Vagina: moderate amount of gray discharge; Cervix: no lesions, negative cervical motion tenderness; Uterus: 14 to 16 week size; Adnexa: nontender, no enlargement bilaterally

ASSESSMENT   *Please indicate the problems or issues you have identified that will guide your care (preferably in list form):*

PLAN   *Please list your plans for addressing each of the problems or issues in your assessment:*

Community Clinic
Jeffrey A. Eaton, NP
Joyce D. Cappiello, NP

Name:_____ DOB_____
Address_____ Date_____

Rx

"label all unless indicated"
Refill:_____ times-- Do not refill ( )

Signed:_____

DO NOT TAKE THIS TO YOUR PHARMACIST

Community Clinic
Jeffrey A. Eaton, NP
Joyce D. Cappiello, NP

Name:_____ DOB_____
Address_____ Date_____

Rx

"label all unless indicated"
Refill:_____ times-- Do not refill ( )

Signed:_____

DO NOT TAKE THIS TO YOUR PHARMACIST

CASE
40 Discussion

LEARNING ISSUES

In order to resolve this patient's problem, you will need to consider and address the following issues (you may generate additional issues as well):

- Differential diagnosis of vaginal discharge
- Screening for drug use
- Criteria for identification of substance abuse
- Identifying readiness for behavior change
- STD screening
- Immunization needs
- Pap smear in the presence of vaginal discharge
- Human immunodeficiency virus (HIV) testing
- Evaluation of uterine enlargement

INITIAL IDEAS

Although her chief complaint is the vaginal discharge, further discussion revealed additional issues. She may not have wanted to acknowledge her drug use to the receptionist, and also, she may have wanted to establish a comfort level with you as her provider before divulging this information.

INTERPRETATION OF CLUES, PATTERNS, INFORMATION

1. Knowing about her history of drug use increases your concerns about exposure to hepatitis, HIV, syphilis, gonorrhea, and chlamydia. She needs thorough testing for all STDs plus specific evaluation of her vaginal discharge.

2. The *Healthy People 2000 Goals* identifies reducing the use of tobacco, alcohol, and other drugs as one of the priority areas for reducing risk factors and maintaining a healthy population. A goal has been set for 75% of primary care providers to screen for substance abuse by the year 2000.

How do you screen for drug use? There is little research data to determine whether the use of standardized screening questionnaires can increase the detection of potential drug problems among patients (US Preventive Services Task Force, 1996). The majority of the common standardized questionnaires deal with alcohol use rather than drug use. There is an Addiction Severity Index designed to evaluate treatment needs of patients with drug or alcohol problems, but it is too lengthy for use as a routine screening tool. The Drug Abuse Screening Test (DAST-10) is a drug use questionnaire that seems more appropriate for patients already identified as drug users.

The first DAST-10 question of, "Have you used drugs other than those required for medical purposes?" is a good screening question (Skinner, 1982). Some clinicians modify the CAGE by substituting the term "drug use" for alcohol use. It is easy to remember, especially if you are already used to using it as a screening tool for alcohol problems. The RAFFT screening questionnaire developed for use with adolescents may be the most useful with this patient:

- **R:** Do you drink or use drugs to RELAX, feel better about yourself, or fit in?
- **A:** Do you ever drink alcohol or use drugs while you are ALONE?
- **F:** Do you or any of your closest FRIENDS drink or use drugs?
- **F:** Does a close FAMILY member have a problem with alcohol or drug use?
- **T:** Have you ever gotten into TROUBLE from drinking or drug use (i.e., skipping school, bad grades, trouble with the law or parents)?

If there are any positive responses, then you can explore this further.

What behaviors meet the criteria for substance abuse? The symptoms of substance use disorders according to the Diagnostic and Statistical Manual of Mental Disorders (DSM-IV) (American Psychiatric Association, 1994) include the following:

1. Dependence criteria: three or more of the following symptoms:
    a. Dose increases or substance taken over longer time than was intended
    b. Desires to cut down but unable to
    c. More time taken up with thinking about, getting, using, or recovering from substances
    d. Important activities reduced or given up because of substance use
    e. Continues to use despite recognizing that the substances are contributing to psychological and/or physical problems
    f. Increased tolerance with diminished effect
    g. Experiences withdrawal symptoms
2. Abuse criteria: one or more of the following symptoms:
    a. Recurrent use of substance, which results in failure to fulfill major role obligations (e.g., work, school, parenting, etc.)
    b. Recurrent use of substance in situations that may cause potential physical harm (e.g., operating machinery, driving)
    c. Recurrent substance-related legal problems (e.g., arrests for disorderly conduct, driving while intoxicated [DWI])
    d. Continued substance use despite persistent or recurrent social problems caused or exacerbated by the effects of the substance (e.g., arguments with spouse about consequences of intoxication, physical fights)
    f. Symptoms persist for over 1 month and do not meet criteria for dependence

With Ms. Roberge, you just needed to ask the screening questions. It is unusual for someone with a substance abuse problem to be so forth coming. It appears she is wanting to address this issue but needs some encouragement. There is research by Prochaska, DiClemente, and Norcross (1992) that gives insight into a patient's readiness to change. Six stages of behavior change are identified:

- *Precontemplation:* There is no intention to change and there may be no awareness of a problem.
- *Contemplation:* There is an awareness of a problem, but there is ambivalence about making change. This stage can last for years.
- *Preparation:* There is an intent to quit, and small changes are starting to be made.
- *Action:* Changes are being made.
- *Maintenance:* Changes are stabilizing and relapses are prevented. This stage begins after 6 months of change and lasts about 5 years.
- *Relapse:* This is common and part of the process of behavior change for most individuals.

Ms. Roberge appears to be in the contemplation stage. She is aware of her problem and is willing to acknowledge it to a health provider. This is a major step in making behavior change.

What can health providers do at each stage? In the precontemplation stage, you can state your concern about the patient's substance abuse and provide reasons why they should consider changing their behavior to improve their health. Realistically, you will have little impact at this stage. In the contemplation stage, your information may be listened to and considered. In the preparation stage, you can assist patients in setting short-term goals for behavior change. Most of the brochures in office waiting rooms address this stage (e.g., tips on quitting smoking offer practical strategies for successful smoking cessation). At the maintenance stage, you can help patients predict risky situations where they may relapse and teach them problem solving strategies. In relapse, you need to encourage patients. Let them know that relapse is common, praise them for past accomplishments, and encourage further efforts.

3. Consider hepatitis A and B immunizations. The CDC recommend hepatitis A and B immunizations for users of IV drugs.

REVISED IDEAS
- Chlamydia
- Gonorrhea
- Vaginitis of non-STD origin.

DIAGNOSTIC OPTIONS

Routine screening for STDs will include a rapid plasma reagin (RPR) for syphilis, the highly accurate PCR chlamydia testing from a cervical specimen, and gonorrhea testing. A wet mount, pH of the vaginal discharge, and the whiff test will give information regarding non-STD causes of vaginitis such as bacterial vaginosis, monilia, or trichomonas.

A urine dipstick would rule out a urinary tract infection (UTI) as the cause of her mild dysuria.

A Pap smear may be less sensitive because of the presence of the discharge and the resulting inflammation. If you think you can convince her to return for a visit, then postpone the Pap smear until the discharge is treated; otherwise perform the test today.

Screening for condylomata, herpes, and the less common STDs is accomplished through the physical examination. If suspicious lesions are noted, then appropriate testing can be performed.

HIV testing is appropriate and necessary. The question is whether to order the test with results filled in the regular section of the chart or to refer the testing procedure to an anonymous testing site. There could be ramifications with insurance companies and subsequent coverage. Usually this is an issue with which your office will have previously wrestled and devised an appropriate system.

Do you test for hepatitis A or B before use of the vaccine? The decision to test patients before vaccination for prior infection is primarily a cost-effectiveness issue and should be based on whether the cost of testing balances the cost of the vaccine saved by not vaccinating individuals who have already been infected. Estimations of such cost-effectiveness depend on three variables: the cost of vaccination, the cost of testing for susceptibility, and the expected prevalence of immune individuals in the group. Testing in the groups with the highest risk is usually cost effective (e.g., IV drug users). IV drug use places the user in a high-risk group, so testing is cost effective. For routine testing of hepatitis B, only one antibody test is necessary, either antibody to the core (anti-HBc) or antibody to the surface antigen (anti-HBs). Anti-HBc identifies all previously infected persons, both carriers and those who are not carriers, but does not differentiate between members of each group. Anti-HBs identifies persons previously infected except for carriers. Neither test has a particular advantage for groups expected to have low carrier rates such as health care workers. Anti-HBc may be preferred for higher-risk groups to avoid unnecessary vaccination of carriers (US Department of Health and Human Services [USDHHS], 1990).

The discussion is similar for testing with anti-HAV (antibody to the hepatitis A virus) before use of the newer hepatitis A vaccine. In populations that have expected high rates of prior HAV infection, prevaccination testing may be considered to reduce costs by not vaccinating persons who have prior immunity. For adults the decision to test should be based on (1) the expected prevalence of immunity, (2) the cost of vaccination compared with the cost of serological testing (including the cost of an additional visit), and (3) the likelihood that testing will not interfere with initiating vaccination (USDHHS, 1996).

People for whom prevaccination testing will likely be more cost effective include adults who were either born or lived for extensive periods in geographic areas with a high incidence of HAV infection, older adolescents, adults in certain population groups (e.g., American Indians, Alaskan Natives, and Hispanics), and adults in certain groups that have a high prevalence of infection (e.g., men who have sex with men). In the late 1980s, 10% to 19% of people who had HAV reported a history of IV drug use. However, in recent years, less than 3% of infected persons are IV drug users. If Ms. Roberge were over 40 years of age, the estimated prevalence of HAV is generally greater than 33%, thus the cost of screening is one third the cost of the vaccination series. Prevaccination screening would then be cost effective (USDHHS, 1996). Since you as the provider know the risk in your community, you can decide according to prevalence. In the authors' area, the risk is low. Also, since the risk for IV drug users currently is less than 3%, it is probably not cost effective to screen Ms. Roberge before vaccination. Postvaccination testing is not recommended either.

Urine drug screening seems inappropriate for this woman. She admits to drug use and is seeking help. No further laboratory data is needed before referring her to a drug treatment program.

Even though this patient reports a history of regular menses with a normal bleeding 3 weeks ago, the clinician must consider pregnancy based on her enlarged uterus. She may be mistaken about the dates, or she may be having bleeding in pregnancy. The current office urine pregnancy tests have a sensitivity and a specificity of 98% to 99% along with offering immediate results. Serum levels are generally higher than urine levels for the first 2 weeks after conception and may offer some advantage during that time. An office urine test rather than a blood test is adequate since her uterus indicates an enlargement, if due to pregnancy, well beyond the first few weeks of pregnancy.

Laboratory Results

The following tests were performed in the office at the time of the visit:
- Whiff test: Positive
- pH: 5.5
- Wet prep: Clue cells, no trichomonas or hyphae
- Urine pregnancy test: Negative.
- Urine dipstick: Negative for leukocytes, nitrites

REVISED IDEAS

- Uterine mass of unknown origin
- Bacterial vaginosis
- At risk for STDs
- Substance abuse

THERAPEUTIC OPTIONS

1. The pelvic mass now takes priority in this workup. Since the urine tests have a high accuracy rate, especially in the 14- to 16-week stage of pregnancy, rather than repeat testing with a radioimmune assay blood pregnancy test, a pelvic ultrasound will be ordered.

2. Treat the bacterial vaginosis. The newer vaginal preparations are highly efficacious, have fewer interactions with alcohol than the past regimen of oral metronidazole, produce no gastrointestinal complaints, and are less teratogenic. Unfortunately, they are significantly more expensive than oral metronidazole. Although the diagnosis for bacterial vaginosis has been established using accepted criteria, an STD may be present concurrently.

3. Screen for STDs and evaluate risk and/or exposure to hepatitis A and B.

4. Give tetanus/diphtheria (Td) immunization.

5. Refer Ms. Roberge to a drug treatment program. If a program is unavailable, the primary care provider may need to provide medical care during the withdrawal process. It is most advantageous that the patient work with a counselor, even if a specific program is unavailable. Clonidine, nonsteroidal antiinflammatory drugs (NSAIDs) for the muscle spasms and aches, and antidepressants form the pharmacological cornerstone of treatment.

References

American Psychiatric Association: *Diagnostic and statistical manual of mental disorders,* ed 4, Washington, DC, 1994, American Psychiatric Association.

Prochaska JO, DiClemente CC, Norcross JC: In search of how people change: applications to addictive behaviors, *Amer Psychol* 47:1102, 1992.

Skinner HA: The Drug Abuse Screening Test, *Addict Behav* 7:363, 1982.

US Department of Health and Human Service: Prevention of hepatitis A through active or passive immunization: recommendations of the Immunization Practices Advisory Committee, *MMWR* 45, 1996.

US Department of Health and Human Services: Protection against viral hepatitis: recommendations of the Immunization Practices Advisory Committee, *MMWR* 39, 1990

US Preventive Services Task Force: *Guide to clinical preventive services,* ed 2, Baltimore, 1996, Williams & Wilkins..

3:15 PM
Renée Jones
Age 35 years

OPENING SCENARIO

Renée Jones is a 35-year-old female with a complaint of wrist pain near the base of her right thumb. This is her first visit to your office. Her provider over the past several years has been her certified nurse midwife (CNM). She is 16 weeks postpartum.

HISTORY OF PRESENT ILLNESS

"About 2 weeks ago I began to notice pain near the base of my right thumb. It is worse at the end of the day and after use. The pain is sharp at times but more often "achy" as the day goes on. Ice seems to ease the discomfort. Acetaminophen (2 tabs) has decreased the pain, but I am hesitant to use a large amount of any medication while nursing, even acetaminophen. I take a dose every 1 to 2 days. I am a physical therapist and do much writing and massaging in my work. I returned to work 4 weeks ago after an 12-week maternity leave. Other activities that aggravate my wrist include holding the baby while nursing and the usual household activities of cleaning and laundry. Currently I have no hobbies or specific exercise workout regimen other than walking. Also, I held off getting my second hepatitis B vaccine during pregnancy. I want to know if it is safe to have the immunization while breastfeeding. My first dose was 14 months ago."

She is right hand dominant. She has noticed a decreased range of motion of her right thumb, difficulty gripping, and catching and locking at the base of her thumb.

MEDICAL HISTORY

No surgeries. Three hospitalizations only for childbirth. Negative history of any major medical problems including arthritis. Had all usual childhood immunizations except hepatitis. Tetanus/diphtheria (Td) booster 3 years ago.

FAMILY MEDICAL HISTORY

Parents: A&W
One sibling: 30 yr (A&W)
Three children: newborn, 5, and 8 yr (A&W)

SOCIAL HISTORY

Married with three children. Nonsmoker. Alcohol: rarely, especially since pregnant and nursing. Sleep: interrupted, nurses infant twice per night. States that infant is gaining weight and thriving.

MEDICATIONS

Prenatal vitamins daily
Tylenol: 2 tabs every 1 to 2 days

ALLERGIES

None

REVIEW OF SYSTEMS

General: Feels her health is excellent
Genitourinary: No menses since delivery; lactating; uses diaphragm faithfully; had Pap smear, which was within normal limits at 6-week postpartum check
Extremities: No history of joint pain, arthralgias, myalgias; no history of sprains, fractures, or trauma; denies neck, shoulder, or elbow pain or injuries; low back discomfort during pregnancy, which resolved postpartum; aware of and uses appropriate body mechanics in her job

PHYSICAL EXAMINATION

Vital signs: Temperature: 97.8° F; *Pulse:* 90 beats/min; *Respirations:* 22 breaths/min; *BP:* 118/70 mm Hg
Height: 5' 7"; *Weight:* 172 lb; *BMI:* 27
Neck: Full active range of motion (AROM) without discomfort, no tenderness to palpation
Shoulder: Right: full AROM without discomfort, no tenderness to palpation
Elbow: Right: full AROM without discomfort, no tenderness to palpation
Wrist/hand: No redness, thenar atrophy, or dry skin; very mild soft tissue swelling; palpation reveals tenderness on the radial and ulnar borders of the anatomical snuff box; no tenderness on the floor of the snuffbox; pain with resisted movement of thumb and first extensor; ROM of thumb limited in the extremes by pain; some decrease in thumb abduction; strength and grip slightly less with right hand because of pain; mild crepitus with radial/ulnar movement; no neurosensory, neurovascular changes; full ROM of the wrist; Finkelstein test: positive; Phalen's test: negative; Tinel sign: negative

ASSESSMENT   *Please indicate the problems or issues you have identified that will guide your care (preferably in list form):*

PLAN   *Please list your plans for addressing each of the problems or issues in your assessment:*

Community Clinic

Jeffrey A. Eaton, NP
Joyce D. Cappiello, NP

Name:_____ DOB_____
Address_____ Date_____

Rx

"label all unless indicated"
Refill:_____ times-- Do not refill ( )

Signed:_____
DO NOT TAKE THIS TO YOUR PHARMACIST

Community Clinic

Jeffrey A. Eaton, NP
Joyce D. Cappiello, NP

Name:_____ DOB_____
Address_____ Date_____

Rx

"label all unless indicated"
Refill:_____ times-- Do not refill ( )

Signed:_____
DO NOT TAKE THIS TO YOUR PHARMACIST

LEARNING ISSUES

In order to resolve this patient's problem, you will need to consider and address the following issues (you may generate additional issues as well):

- Specific physical examination techniques with wrist and forearm pain
- Evaluating medication use in lactation
- Effective scheduling of hepatitis B immunizations, including during pregnancy and lactation
- Weight loss in a postpartum, lactating woman

INITIAL IDEAS

As often happens, other issues surface during the visit. The issues of the hepatitis B series and her slow postpartum weight loss need to be addressed. If the treatment plan for her wrist pain includes prescribing medications, care must be exercised with a lactating woman.

PROBLEM NUMBER ONE: WRIST PAIN

Interpretation of Cues, Patterns, and Information

Since the pain is most severe at the end of the day or after extended use, you can conclude that an activity performed frequently throughout the day is either causing or aggravating the condition. First, look at her daily work routine. As a physical therapist, she performs therapeutic massages on clients and is required to keep long notes and fill out many forms. Both of these involve wrist and thumb movements. After not working during a 12-week maternity leave, she has just returned to these activities 4 weeks ago.

Second, examine her activities at home, which may be aggravating factors. She states that she does the usual housework and laundry. She currently has no time for hobbies or any specific workout regimen other than walking. The obvious change in her home schedule is caring for the new baby including periods of time spent nursing. A review of how she holds the baby while nursing might be helpful to identify any malpositioning of her forearm.

Rheumatoid arthritis seems unlikely based on the absence of swollen, painful joints. Degenerative joint disease (DJD) could be considered if she had a history of trauma or long-standing repetitive motion injury. Carpal tunnel symptoms are common in pregnancy because of fluid changes, but these should not be an issue in this case.

Symptoms involving the hand can be referred from the elbow, the shoulder, and the cervical spine. The causes of referred pain to the wrist and hand include herniated cervical discs, osteoarthritis of the cervical spine and brachial plexus, thoracic outlet syndrome, and elbow and shoulder nerve entrapment. These related clinical areas should be evaluated.

Since Ms. Jones is a physical therapist, she may have a good sense of her own condition.

Revised Ideas

- Tenosynovitis (de Quervain's disease)
- Carpal tunnel syndrome
- Rheumatoid arthritis

Diagnostic Options

First of all, inspection is one of your most valuable diagnostic techniques. What you do not see can be as important as what you do see. The absence of redness, dryness, or atrophy of the thenar muscle are all encouraging signs.

Next, palpate over the anatomical snuffbox. The borders of the snuffbox are composed of the abductor pollicis longus and the extensor pollicis brevis tendons. These tendons become more prominent when the thumb is extended. They can be palpated near the site of insertion into one of the passageways of the dorsal part of the hand. This passageway is of clinical significance because it is the site for a tenosynovitis in which inflammation of the synovial lining of the tendon sheath narrows the tunnel opening and results in pain where the tendons move. Tenderness elicited in this area during palpation may be an indication of this condition. Any tenderness elicited on the floor of the snuffbox suggests a fracture.

To test specifically for this problem, use the Finkelstein test. Instruct the patient to make a fist with her thumb tucked inside of her other fingers. Then, as you stabilize her forearm with one hand, deviate her wrist to the ulnar side with the other hand. If she feels a sharp pain in the area of the tunnel, this is a positive Finkelstein test, which indicates strong evidence of stenosing tenosynovitis (Fig. 41-1).

Physical examination techniques used to test for carpal tunnel syndrome include the Tinel sign and Phalen's test. The Tinel sign is positive if you can elicit pain in the distribution of the medial nerve by tapping over the volar carpal ligament with the palm of the hand turned upward. The Phalen's test is positive if you can reproduce symptoms such as tingling of the fingers with flexion of the patient's wrist. Press the backs of each hand together with fingers pointing toward the floor. Both wrists are bent at a 90 degree angle (or maximum degree) and held for at least a minute; then record the onset of symptoms. For example, if Phalen's test is positive at 15 seconds, continue to test for the full minute to determine if symptoms increase. Numbness and tingling are present with a positive test. A negative Phalen's test and Tinel sign reduce the likelihood of carpel tunnel problems. If numbness is noted, check 2-point discrimination (Figs. 41-2 and 41-3).

X-ray examination is not usually helpful at this time.

There are many sites for tenosynovitis, but for the most part only the long tendons with sheaths, such as the dorsal extensor tendons of the wrist, are involved. Tenosynovitis most often occurs from excessive, repetitive hand motions as may occur with Ms. Jones' massage motions at work or some other nonrelated work activity.

Therapeutic Options

The initial therapy with the majority of musculoskeletal complaints is a trial of nonsteroidal anti-inflammatory drug (NSAID) therapy. There is a variety of prescription and over-the-counter (OTC) products from which to choose. Some have one-a-day or twice-a-day dosing to increase compliance, and others have an improved side-effect profile. In this case, choose an NSAID that has data regarding its safety profile in lactating women. Many resources that provide general information about medications do not give accurate information about the appearance of the drug in breast milk nor its risk to the infant. The book *Drugs in Pregnancy and Lactation* (Briggs, Freeman, and Yaffe, 1994) is a well referenced resource. It summarizes data that shows that ibuprofen can be used safely in lactating women since it does not enter human milk in significant quantities and is considered compatible with breastfeeding by the American Academy of Pediatrics.

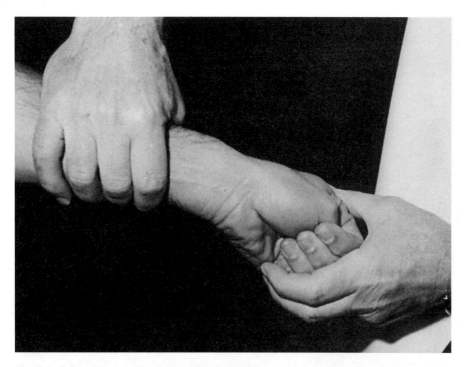

Fig. **41-1** Finkelstein's test suggests tendinitis of the thumb abductors and is performed by forcing the flexed and adducted thumb across the palm, stretching the tendons and causing pain. *(From Hawkins RJ: Musculoskeletal examination, St Louis, 1995, Mosby.)*

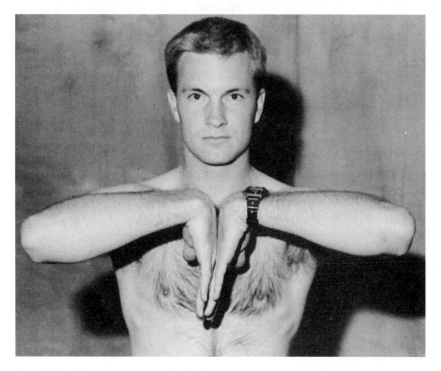

Fig. **41-2** Phalen's test has the patient forcibly flexing the wrists together, reproducing pain and paresthesias in the distribution of the median nerve, suggestive of a carpal tunnel syndrome. *(From Hawkins RJ: Musculoskeletal examination, St Louis, 1995, Mosby.)*

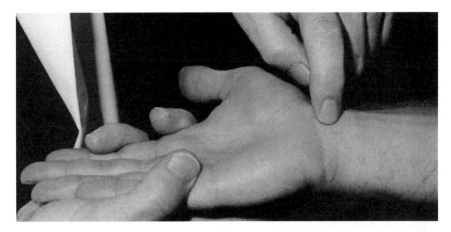

Fig. **41-3** Tinel's test, performed at the wrist, may produce paresthesias and pain in the distribution of the median nerve. *(From Hawkins RJ: Musculoskeletal examination, St Louis, 1995, Mosby.)*

A therapeutic dose is 600 mg tid, and improvement should be expected in several days. Therapy should be continued an additional 4 to 5 days to prevent relapses. This usually means 7 to 10 days of therapy. Because she has not yet resumed menstrual cycles, you cannot rely on the last menstrual period (LMP) to rule out a possible pregnancy. Fortunately, there are no published reports linking the use of ibuprofen with congenital defects (Briggs, Freeman, and Yaffe, 1994).

Ice is a mainstay of treatment, and since Ms. Jones has been applying ice and finds it helpful, encourage this four times per day if possible.

A thumb splint to help immobilize the thumb can be very helpful. Steroid injections are not usually first-line therapy but are more likely reserved for cases unresponsive to the above regimen. Hydrocortisone phonophoresis with ultrasound is also a helpful next step.

Ms. Jones may need to be out of work for this to heal. If this is necessary, the appropriate paperwork for worker's compensation will need to be completed.

Have Ms. Jones think through the position she uses to hold the baby during the day and with the nighttime feedings. If problematic, discuss modifying the position she is using to hold the baby for nursing. A "built-up" pen may decrease the discomfort of writing. She may be able to use her other hand or other parts of her hand for massage.

A follow-up appointment needs to be addressed. A return visit in 2 weeks seems reasonable or sooner if the pain does not improve.

PROBLEM NUMBER TWO: HEPATITIS B IMMUNIZATIONS

Ms. Jones held off getting her second hepatitis vaccine because she was pregnant. Is the vaccine contraindicated in pregnancy? Because the vaccine contains only noninfectious HBsAg (hepatitis B surface antigen) particles, there should be no risk to the fetus. In contrast, HBV infections of a pregnant woman may result in severe disease for the mother and chronic infections in the newborn. Therefore pregnancy or lactation should not be considered a contraindication to the use of this vaccine for persons who are otherwise eligible (US Department of Health and Human Services [USDHHS], 1990). It is likely that this patient chose not to immunize during pregnancy even with this information because she felt she was at low risk for exposure.

Now that she is in the office and inquiring about resuming the use of the vaccine, the vaccine can be given today. According to information provided by the Centers for Disease Control and Prevention, vaccine doses administered at longer intervals provide equally satisfactory protection, but optimal protection is not conferred until after the third dose. If the vaccine series is interrupted after the first dose, the second and third doses should be given separated by an interval of 3 to 5 months.

People who are late for the third dose should be given this dose when convenient. Postvaccination testing is not considered necessary in either situation (USDHHS, 1990).

Remember that 30% to 50% of people who developed antibodies with the vaccine will lose detectable antibody levels within 7 years, but protection against viremic infection and clinical disease appears to persist. The issue of booster doses is not completely settled since this vaccine has only been used for approximately 20 years, but given the current knowledge, it does not appear that boosters will be necessary (USDHHS, 1990).

Many times, providers and patients just assume that medications and vaccines cannot be given during pregnancy or lactation. However, there will be times that treatments are necessary and preferable in pregnancy. Again, the Briggs book can be helpful with medication decisions.

PROBLEM NUMBER THREE: POSTPARTUM WEIGHT LOSS

The fact that she is lactating is helpful for weight loss. Usually, women who are nursing lose more weight than women who do not breastfeed. Long-range studies suggest there is a lessened tendency for childbirth-associated obesity for those who breastfeed.

The nursing mother continues to need approximately 500 calories per day more than she did before the pregnancy. This can usually be met with four servings of calcium-rich foods such as low-fat milk. Generally, the focus should be on eating an assortment of fruits, vegetables, proteins, and calcium sources each day rather than on dieting. As the baby begins to eat solid foods and relies less on breast milk, the mother's appetite gradually decreases and the weight begins to return to prepregnancy levels more quickly.

An exercise program would be an appropriate step at this point as long as it did not involve upper body weights or activities that aggravate the wrist.

It can be difficult for many new mothers, and especially working mothers, to find the time to focus on exercise and meal preparation. This health professional may be well aware of what she wants to do but may need assistance in devising a plan to meet her current needs.

HEALTH PROMOTION/HEALTH MAINTENANCE

She had a recent Pap smear, is comfortable with her contraception method, is a nonsmoker, is up-to-date on her tetanus immunization, and will also be current with a hepatitis B immunization. Any additional issues can be addressed at subsequent visits.

References

Briggs GC, Freeman RK, Yaffe SJ: *Drugs in pregnancy and lactation,* ed 3, Baltimore, 1994, Williams & Wilkins.

US Department of Health and Human Services: Protection against viral hepatitis: recommendations of the Immunization Practices Advisory Committee, *MMWR* 39, 1990.

CASE
42

OPENING SCENARIO

Judy Marland is an 81-year-old female in your office for memory problems. She is accompanied by her daughter who lives 3 miles away. Her daughter tells you that she wanted somebody to look at her mother because she has been getting a lot more forgetful. She forgot to pay the phone bill for 2 months and the phone company was threatening to shut off her phone. She did not notice any major change; it just seems to have come on gradually. You have 30 minutes scheduled to obtain a history, do a physical examination, and review laboratory work that was done 2 months ago when Ms. Marland had cataract surgery. She is doing well postsurgery and says that her vision has improved significantly.

HISTORY OF PRESENT ILLNESS

"I have problems remembering sometimes, but who doesn't?" Based on history from her daughter, this 81-year-old woman has been becoming progressively more confused over the past 2 months. At times she is unable to find rooms in her own home and has forgotten to pay bills. Ms. Marland's history is limited by her memory and her daughter's lack of knowledge of events in the remote past.

MEDICAL HISTORY

Hysterectomy about 20 years ago. G3P2102. No other surgeries or hospitalizations. Had been followed by Dr. Breene who left the area about 1 year ago. Your practice assumed the care of Dr. Breene's patients, but no record can be found on Ms. Marland. Her complete blood count (CBC) (Table 42-1), chemistry profile, (Table 42-2), urinalysis (Table 42-3), and chest x-ray (CXR) examination (Box 42-1) are provided.

Table **42-1** *CBC for Judy Marland from 2 Months Ago*

CBC	RESULT	NORMAL
WBC	4.6	4.5-10.8
RBC	3.45 L	4.20-5.40
Hgb	10.1 L	12.0-16.0
Hct	33.2 L	37.0-47.0
MCV	78.3 L	81.0-99.0
MCH	28.2	27.0-32.0
MCHC	32.4	32.0-36.0
RDW	16.2 H	11.0-16.0
Platelets	221	150-450
Segs	66 H	50-65
Lymphocytes	21 L	25-45
Monocytes	8	0-10
Eosinophils	5 H	0-4

Table **42-2** *Chemistry Profile for Judy Marland from 2 Months Ago*

TEST	RESULT	NORMAL
FBS	130 H	60-110
BUN	27	8-28
Creatinine	1.0	0.5-1.5
Sodium	128 L	135-145
Potassium	5.3	3.5-5.5
Chloride	104	95-105
Albumin	3.8 L	4.0-6.0
Total protein	6.3 L	6.5-8.0
Alkaline phosphate	100	30-120
ALT	22	0-40
AST	28	0-40
LDH	134	50-150
Cholesterol	252 H	110-200
Calcium	8.4 L	8.8-10.2
GGT	29	0-30
Magnesium	2.1	1.6-2.4
Bilirubin	0.7	0.1-1.0
Conjugated bilirubin	0.1	0.0-0.2
Iron	17 L	60-160
Uric acid	6.3	2.0-7.0

Table 42-3 Urinalysis for Judy Marland from 2 Months Ago

Color	Yellow
Character	Clear
SG	1.025
Urine pH	5.0
Glucose	Negative
Nitrite	Negative
WBCs	0-2
RBCs	0-1
Epithelial cells	0-5
Crystals	None

Box 42-1 Chest X-ray Examination for Judy Marland from 2 Months Ago

The lung fields are clear of infiltrates. The pulmonary vasculature and markings are normal. The heart size is in the upper range of normal limits.
Impression: Normal chest x-ray examination
Boyd Bates, DO

FAMILY MEDICAL HISTORY

Mother: Died at 54 yr (breast cancer; had adult-onset diabetes mellitus [AODM])
Father: Died at 77 yr (stroke; also had AODM)
One child: Died 30 yr ago (automobile accident)
Daughter: 58 yr (A&W)
Son: 54 yr (high cholesterol)

SOCIAL HISTORY

Does not smoke or drink alcohol. She is a retired seamstress. Husband died 10+ years ago from myocardial infarction (MI) at age 74. Neighbor visits her at her home twice per week. Daughter lives 3 miles away and takes her to church on Sundays. Daughter is a school teacher, and son-in-law is an attorney. She has one son who lives about 1000 miles away.

MEDICATIONS

Triamterene/hydrochlorothiazide (Dyazide): 1 tab po qd
Digoxin: 0.125 mg po qd
Coumadin: 1 mg po qd
Benadryl: 25 mg at hs
Tums ii tabs tid
Multivitamin: 1 tab po qd

ALLERGIES

None

REVIEW OF SYSTEMS

General: Denies weight loss, night sweats
HEENT: Denies diplopia, blurring, hearing impairment, sore throats
Cardiac: Denies chest pain, shortness of breath, dyspnea on exertion, paroxysmal nocturnal dyspnea, or peripheral swelling
Abdomen/Gastrointestinal: Denies anorexia, nausea, vomiting, constipation, diarrhea, black or clay colored stools
Genitourinary: Denies dysuria, hematuria
Musculoskeletal: Denies joint or back pain
Hematological: Denies excessive bruising

PHYSICAL EXAMINATION

Vital signs: Temperature: 96.6° F; *Pulse:* 88 beats/min; *Respirations:* 24 breaths/min; *BP:* 108/44 mm Hg
Height: 5' 3"; *Weight:* 112 lb
Skin: Slightly pale without open areas
HEENT: Head is normocephalic, atraumatic; pupils equal, round, and reactive to light; extraocular movements intact; Snellen 20/40 using both eyes with glasses; tympanic membranes noninjected without excessive cerumen; whisper test 2/3 bilaterally; nares are patent without redness or exudate; throat is noninjected; tongue is midline; palate rises symmetrically; she is edentulous with well fitting dentures
Neck: Supple without thyromegaly, adenopathy, or carotid bruits
Heart: Regular rate and rhythm; no rubs, or gallops; Grade III/VI murmur heard at the fourth ICS LSB; peripheral pulses are 1+ at popliteal, dorsalis pedis, and posterior tibial; pulses 2+ at femoral, radial, and carotid
Lungs: Clear to auscultation and percussion except for fine bibasilar crackles, which clear with coughing.
Breasts: Without masses or discharge
Abdomen/Gastrointestinal: Soft, nontender; no hepatosplenomegaly; rectal is with brown stool, no masses; stool is guaiac negative
Genitourinary: Genitalia is without external lesions or rashes; pelvic examination not done
Extremities: Without cyanosis, clubbing, or edema; reflexes are 2+ at the biceps, triceps, brachioradialis, patellar, and Achilles; no Babinski signs present; strength and sensation in upper and lower extremities are symmetrical
Neurological: Cranial nerves 2 through 12 grossly intact

ASSESSMENT   *Please indicate the problems or issues you have identified that will guide your care (preferably in list form):*

PLAN   *Please list your plans for addressing each of the problems or issues in your assessment:*

Community Clinic
Jeffrey A. Eaton, NP
Joyce D. Cappiello, NP

Name:_____ DOB_____
Address_____ Date_____

Rx

"label all unless indicated"
Refill:_____ times-- Do not refill ( )

Signed:_____
DO NOT TAKE THIS TO YOUR PHARMACIST

Community Clinic
Jeffrey A. Eaton, NP
Joyce D. Cappiello, NP

Name:_____ DOB_____
Address_____ Date_____

Rx

"label all unless indicated"
Refill:_____ times-- Do not refill ( )

Signed:_____
DO NOT TAKE THIS TO YOUR PHARMACIST

Community Clinic
Jeffrey A. Eaton, NP
Joyce D. Cappiello, NP

Name:_____ DOB_____
Address_____ Date_____

Rx

"label all unless indicated"
Refill:_____ times-- Do not refill ( )

Signed:_____
DO NOT TAKE THIS TO YOUR PHARMACIST

Community Clinic
Jeffrey A. Eaton, NP
Joyce D. Cappiello, NP

Name:_____ DOB_____
Address_____ Date_____

Rx

"label all unless indicated"
Refill:_____ times-- Do not refill ( )

Signed:_____
DO NOT TAKE THIS TO YOUR PHARMACIST

LEARNING ISSUES

In order to resolve this patient's problem, you will need to consider and address the following issues (you may generate additional issues as well):

- **Causes of confusion**
- **Delirium**
- **Pseudodementia**
- **Dementia evaluation and diagnosis**
- **Safety concerns in confused elderly people**
- **Evaluation of heart murmur**
- **Digoxin in treatment of dysrhythmias**
- **Anticoagulation**
- **Causes of peripheral swelling**
- **Anemia as a cause of confusion**
- **Laboratory values in nutritional evaluation**
- **Hyponatremia**
- **Hyperlipidemias in the elderly**
- **Interpretation of the differential white blood cell (WBC) count**

INITIAL IDEAS

- Confusion: Review of dementia, delirium, depression
- Anemia (also possibly contributing to confusion)
- Hyponatremia (also possibly contributing to confusion)
- Possible nutritional deficiency (low albumin level)
- Heart murmur
- On anticoagulation for unknown reason
- Elevated serum cholesterol level
- Incomplete database; on Dyazide and digoxin for unknown reason

INTERPRETATION OF CUES, PATTERNS, AND INFORMATION

The first thing you must do is avoid being overwhelmed. Ms. Marland does not really have any conditions that would qualify as emergencies. Thus you have some time to think about her multiple problems and get help if you need it. (Sometimes the first thing you need to do is take your own pulse and wait for it to return to normal before you begin to address the patient's issues.)

The onset of Ms. Marland's confusion coinciding with her cataract surgery would make it very suspicious that her confusion is a delirium. She also has a hyponatremia that could be causing her confusion. A diagnosis of dementia requires that all reversible causes be ruled out. Therefore at this point, she clearly does not meet the criteria.

Depression, which presents as dementia, is also a possibility (so called pseudodementia). This is not as common as was once thought, and a fairly high percentage of these people progress to frank dementia within about 1 year; however, it still should be assessed.

Quantifying her confusion to the greatest extent possible will allow both an assessment of severity and a baseline by which to measure any changes. The Folstein Minimental Status Exam (MMSE) and clock drawing are good screens of cognitive function.

She has a microcytic anemia and thus probably an iron deficiency anemia (IDA). This could be confirmed with a serum ferritin and total iron binding capacity (TIBC). With her other laboratory tests indicating a nutritional deficiency, that is a reasonable probability for cause, but you also will need to rule out more serious causes such as an occult bleed. At a minimum, some stool guaiacs and other history collection looking for occult bleeding would be reasonable. Whenever a patient has IDA, you need to think both nutritional and bleeding. This is a relatively mild anemia, and you should have some time to work it up. Anemia can cause confusion, but in this case her anemia is relatively mild and she has several other more probable causes that should be explored.

Although Dyazide is a combination diuretic, it can still cause hyponatremia. Other causes of the syndrome of inappropriate antidiuretic hormone (SIADH) should be considered, however, and a common one is malignancy. Some clinicians would do a urine sodium and a serum osmolality, but alternatively a trial off Dyazide is probably reasonable. Her blood pressure (BP) looks like it can tolerate it, but if she does have any heart failure related to her valvular dysfunction, you would have to make sure that the increased volume would not exacerbate that problem. Her peripheral edema may be caused by heart failure or venous insufficiency, and you really do not have enough information at this point to decide which is the cause. Her serum protein levels are low but not low enough to result in osmotic edema.

In evaluation of her nutritional problems, her low albumin and total protein levels are of concern. Her serum cholesterol level may actually be reassuring because when people are profoundly nutritionally deficient, their cholesterol level will usually be low as well. Liver dysfunction can lower protein levels, but her transaminase levels are normal. Her hypocalcemia is almost definitely artifact related to her low albumin level since serum calcium is protein bound and serum levels will decrease whenever protein levels are low. Lymphocytes may also be decreased in a nutritional deficiency. The clinician must remember that the differential WBC count is expressed in terms of a percentage so that whenever one value changes it will affect the other values even though those absolute counts have not changed. Thus a low lymphocyte count can make the neutrophil and eosinophil counts appear elevated even when no increase in those counts exist.

Her murmur may represent an aortic sclerosis, possibly a mild stenosis, or even a mitral problem. If this is a new murmur or you are suspicious that her confusion is related, an echocardiogram is essential.

Most likely, her Coumadin medication is related to an inferred history of atrial fibrillation or prophylaxis of stroke. This is a finding, however, that is not really explained by your current data. Further questioning of the family and requests for old records may help. Most clinicians would leave her on the Coumadin until old records were obtained, but check a Pro-time in the interim.

Many clinicians would leave her elevated cholesterol level alone, at least until all of her other problems were addressed, but some would intervene sooner. Starting with a full lipid profile might be reasonable since this probably represents a cholesterol level on an already restricted diet. Consideration of the lack of data about older females and elevated cholesterol level not having a documented negative outcome versus the theoretic risks associated with hyperlipidemia would need to occur.

You suspect that Ms. Marland has hypertension, problems with peripheral edema, atrial fibrillation, congestive heart failure (CHF), or some combination of the above. As noted, changing the Dyazide may be reasonable but should be undertaken cautiously. A digoxin level should be checked since digitalis toxicity can cause delirium. Old records will also inform this decision.

Fine bibasilar crackles are common because of fibrotic changes and can be attributed as an age-related change especially when they clear with coughing. A high index of vigilance around CHF is still essential however, although lack of an S3 (no gallops) makes it somewhat less probable.

REVISED IDEAS

Your current working ideas have probably not changed much, although you may have new thoughts about how to approach them:

- Confusion: Review of dementia, delirium, depression
- Anemia (possibly contributing to confusion)
- Hyponatremia (also possibly contributing to confusion)
- Possible nutritional deficiency (low albumin level)
- Heart murmur
- On anticoagulation for unknown reason
- Elevated serum cholesterol level
- Incomplete database on Dyazide and digoxin for unknown reasons
- Digitalis toxicity

DIFFERENTIAL DIAGNOSIS

Each of the identified problems will have its own differential diagnosis. The overarching differential (and the one addressing the presenting problem) addresses the cause of her confusion. Dementia is primarily a diagnosis of exclusion since it requires that reversible causes of confusion be ruled out (American Psychiatric Association, 1994). Thus the first thing that must happen is a search for delirium. Differential diagnosis for delirium should include at least the following:

- **D:** Drugs
- **E:** Emotional disorders (including depression)
- **M:** Metabolic or endocrine disorders
- **E:** Eye and ear dysfunctions, environment
- **N:** Nutritional deficiencies, neurological problems
- **T:** Tumor and trauma
- **I:** Infections
- **A:** Arteriosclerotic complications (MI, CHF), alcohol, or anemia

DIAGNOSTIC OPTIONS

Since many causes of delirium are metabolic in origin, appropriate laboratory studies should be obtained. The chart shown in Box 42-2 is reproduced from Ham and Sloane (1997) and provides some guidance around choice of laboratories.

Some other thoughts regarding evaluation are as follows:

- Her fasting blood sugar (FBS) is not significantly elevated, but a 2-hour postprandial and/or some other capillary blood sugars could be considered. A glycosylated hemoglobin is not usually considered a diagnostic test, but some clinicians will order it.
- Obtain records from her cataract surgery.
- Her diphenhydramine (Benadryl) may be adding to her confusion, so it should probably be stopped.
- A key issue in this case is whether you are concerned about her safety. If so, explore whether she could stay with her daughter for a week or so until you know more about the cause of her confusion.

Box 42-2 Suggested Investigations in Dementia

ALL PATIENTS

- CBC
- TSH $\pm$ T_4 $\pm$ free T_4
- Vitamin B_{12} and folate
- Serological test for syphilis
- BUN and creatinine
- Calcium
- Glucose

MOST PATIENTS

- CT scan or MRI of brain (except in those severely demented with history over 3 years, nonabrupt onset, no history of head injury, and no early localized neurological symptoms or signs)
- Electrolytes
- Liver function
- ECG, CXR, urinalysis: often recommended baseline in all elders, not specific to dementia

SOME PATIENTS

- EEG
- SPECT
- Neuropsychological testing

From Ham RJ, Sloane PD: *Primary care geriatrics,* ed 3, St Louis, 1997, Mosby.

- Her blood urea nitrogen (BUN)/creatinine ratio was somewhat high, so chronic dehydration is also a consideration. Orthostatic BPs may be helpful. This is a mild elevation and would be unlikely to alter cognitive function.
- A geriatric depression scale or at least a fuller assessment of depression is reasonable. It is important to remember that depression in the elderly may present without sadness, so it becomes a greater diagnostic challenge.
- In the diagnosis of her anemia there are several options. It is apparently an IDA since it is microcytic. This could be caused by decreased intake, impaired absorption, or iron (blood) loss. You could order a test of serum ferritin levels. The most serious concern with Ms. Marland is an occult blood loss, so assessment should be carried out looking for a loss from the colon, urine, or a gynecological source. Simultaneous evaluation of her coagulation status related to her Coumadin should be carried out since it is possible that she has been over-anticoagulated and that this will explain her blood loss.
- To determine whether her hyponatremia is a drug effect, the Dyazide could be discontinued and the serum sodium rechecked in about 2 to 3 days. This is combination potassium sparing and thiazide diuretic, so potassium levels should also be watched. If an SIADH workup was needed, a urine sodium and a serum osmolality would be a place to start. This can be a difficult workup, and a curbside consult with an experienced clinician might be reasonable.
- In regard to the suspected nutritional deficiency, a diet history is probably a good place to start. This is another reason to explore whether she could stay with the daughter for a week or so since you may get a more objective evaluation of her dietary intake.
- She has a heart murmur of unknown etiology. An echocardiogram can be helpful, and if indicated, an ejection fraction will give an idea of cardiac function. An electrocardiogram (ECG) may not explain the murmur, but most clinicians would order it based on her medications and other symptoms.

- Why is she on anticoagulation? You will probably need old records to find out. In the meantime, a Pro-time and dosage change based on the international normalized ratio (INR) is the reasonable course. If there is no evidence of a prosthetic valve (thoracic cicatrix, heart sounds, or evidence on CXR), then the dosage can be adjusted to achieve an INR of 2.0 to 3.0 for the short term. Depending on the indications, other options could be evaluated.
- Some clinicians would get a lipid profile, but most would leave her elevated serum cholesterol alone for now. Later the decision can be made whether to work up further based on your review of the current literature around elevated cholesterol levels in elderly women and relative risks and benefits of treatment.
- You have an incomplete database. Why is Ms. Marland on Dyazide and digoxin? While waiting for her old records you can check a digoxin level. You would specifically request records from her cataract surgery and her previous primary care provider.

THERAPEUTIC OPTIONS

Therapeutic options will probably be deferred until evaluation is complete. Therapeutic changes described above are primarily trials to determine whether certain aspects of the current therapies are contributing to her confusion. Once a cause of her confusion has been determined, an appropriate plan for therapeutics will be developed. In the interim the only other therapeutic plan to be developed is to assure her safety.

HEALTH PROMOTION/HEALTH MAINTENANCE

With her confusion as the current problem, it is probably appropriate to hold these issues for a later visit. At that time, the following could be considered: mammogram, Pap smear, pneumococcal vaccine (if not given in the past 6 years), and an update of her tetanus-diphtheria (Td) vaccination.

An assessment of whether an advance directive exists should be done in this case, and appropriate suggestions and discussion carried out. It is worthwhile to have this discussion early. If it does not occur on this visit, a reminder to do it at a later visit is appropriate. The relative benefits of a living will, durable power of attorney (DPOA) for healthcare, and the combination of both should be described. You should not recommend these if the assessment indicates that Ms. Marland is not in an appropriate state to sign them at this time.

FOLLOW-UP

One option would be to see her about 1 to 2 weeks after the laboratory tests are back and old records are obtained. This would allow for planning for the next step. It may take several visits before you really have a sense of what is going on with Ms. Marland.

References

American Psychiatric Association: DSM IV (diagnostic and statitistical manual of mental disorders), ed 4, Washington, DC, 1994, American Psychiatric Association.

Ham RJ, Sloane PD: Primary care geriatrics, ed 3, St Louis, 1997, Mosby.

CASE
43

OPENING SCENARIO

Mr. Metcalf is a 64-year-old male on your schedule for difficulty starting his urine stream. His wife is a patient of yours, and she recommended that he come to see you. Mr. Metcalf had seen a physician about 5 years ago who had given him a prescription for nitroglycerin and did a workup for his chest pain. The cardiac workup was negative, and the physician told Mr. Metcalf that he thought his pain was probably gastrointestinal in origin.

HISTORY OF PRESENT ILLNESS

"I noticed about 1 year ago that my urine stream was decreasing slightly. Now I have to stand for a couple of minutes before I can urinate. I have to get up once or twice a night to urinate, disrupting my sleep." Mr. Metcalf denies hematuria and dysuria. He feels that his bladder does not empty completely. He urinates about every 2 or 3 hours during the day.

MEDICAL HISTORY

He has occasional "angina" (about once per month), but it is completely relieved by nitroglycerin. Has not tried antacids or H_2 blocker. Electrocardiogram (ECG) has been completely normal, and he has had an exercise tolerance test (ETT) without any evidence of ischemic changes (although it did not reproduce the pain). He had an appendectomy at age 19. He started taking Valium because he was feeling extremely stressed at work about 10 years ago. He felt that it makes it easier for him to get through the day, and he has no desire to change this medication.

FAMILY MEDICAL HISTORY

MGM: bilateral amputations from vascular disease
Mother: 85 yr (Type II diabetes mellitus)
Father: Deceased at 79 yr (cerebral infarct; partial gastrectomy at 38)
One brother: 60 yr (A&W)
Three children: 27, 29, 32 (A&W)

SOCIAL HISTORY

Bank loan officer. Drinks 2 to 3 beers per night. Has smoked 1 pack per day for 40 years. Married.

MEDICATIONS

Valium: 5 mg every morning
Nitroglycerin: 0.4 mg SL for chest pain as needed

ALLERGIES

None

REVIEW OF SYSTEMS

General: Denies night sweats, swelling
Skin: No excessive bruising
HEENT: Denies diplopia, blurring, hearing impairment, sore throats, chest pain, shortness of breath, dyspnea on exertion, paroxysmal nocturnal dyspnea
Gastrointestinal: Denies nausea, vomiting, constipation, diarrhea, anorexia, black or clay colored stools
Genitourinary: Denies dysuria, hematuria
Muscoluskeletal: Denies joint and back pain
Neurological: Denies fevers or chills

PHYSICAL EXAMINATION

Vital signs: Temperature: 98.9° F; *Pulse:* 82 beats/min; *Respirations:* 18 breaths/min; *BP:* 122/82 mm Hg
Height: 5' 11"; *Weight:* 220 lb
HEENT: Head is normocephalic, atraumatic; pupils equal, round, and reactive to light; extraocular movements intact; tympanic membranes are observable without excessive cerumen; nares are patent without redness or exudate; throat is noninjected; tongue is midline; palate rises symmetrically; teeth are in adequate repair
Neck: Supple; without thyromegaly, adenopathy, or carotid bruits
Heart: Regular rate and rhythm; no murmurs, rubs, or gallops
Lungs: Clear to auscultation and percussion
Abdomen: Soft, nontender; no hepatosplenomegaly
Gastrointestinal: Brown stool; no masses
Genitourinary: Prostate is firm, symmetrical, mildly enlarged (Grade I); genitalia is normal, circumcised male; testicles descended bilaterally; bladder not palpable; no urge to void on suprapubic palpation
Extremities: Without cyanosis, clubbing, or edema

Neurological: Reflexes are 2+ at the biceps, triceps, brachioradialis, patellar, and Achilles; no Babinski signs present; strength and sensation are symmetrical

LABORATORY RESULTS

Seen in emergency room about 6 months ago for a suspected pneumonia, but chest x-ray examination (CXR) was negative. He was treated for bronchitis and did well. He has a copy of his complete blood count (CBC) (Table 43-1), chemistry profile (Table 43-2), and urinalysis (Table 43-3). ECG is without evidence of ischemia or ectopy.

Table **43-1** *CBC for Wilson Metcalf from 6 Months Ago*

CBC	RESULT	NORMAL
WBC	9.9	4.5-10.8
RBC	5.1	4.2-5.4
Hgb	14.1	12.0-16.0
Hct	40.2	37.0-47.0
MCV	92.2	87.0-99.0
MCH	28.2	27.0-32.0
MCHC	32.8	32.0-36.0
RDW	13.7	11.0-16.0
Platelets	396	150-450
Segs	55	50-65
Lymphocytes	31	25-45
Monocytes	10	0-10
Eosinocytes	4	0-4

Table **43-3** *Urinalysis for Wilson Metcalf*

Color	Yellow
Character	Clear
SG	1.015
Urine pH	6.0
Glucose	Negative
Nitrite	Negative
Protein	Negative
Leukocytes	Negative
Blood	Negative

Table **43-2** *Chemistry Profile for Wilson Metcalf from 6 Months Ago*

TEST	RESULT	NORMAL
FBS	103	60-110
BUN	27	8-28
Creatinine	1.1	0.5-1.5
Sodium	138	135-145
Potassium	4.3	3.5-5.5
Chloride	101	95-105
Albumin	4.8	4.0-6.0
Total protein	7.3	6.5-8.0
Alkaline phosphate	100	30-120
ALT	22	0-40
AST	20	0-40
LDH	144	50-150
Cholesterol	200	110-200
GGT	26	0-30
Magnesium	2.2	1.6-2.4
Bilirubin	0.6	0.1-1.0
Conjugated bilirubin	0.1	0.0-0.2
Iron	80	60-160
Uric acid	6.4	2.0-7.0

ASSESSMENT   *Please indicate the problems or issues you have identified that will guide your care (preferably in list form):*

PLAN   *Please list your plans for addressing each of the problems or issues in your assessment:*

Community Clinic
Jeffrey A. Eaton, NP
Joyce D. Cappiello, NP

Name:_____ DOB_____
Address_____ Date_____

Rx

"label all unless indicated"
Refill:_____ times-- Do not refill ( )

Signed:_____
DO NOT TAKE THIS TO YOUR PHARMACIST

Community Clinic
Jeffrey A. Eaton, NP
Joyce D. Cappiello, NP

Name:_____ DOB_____
Address_____ Date_____

Rx

"label all unless indicated"
Refill:_____ times-- Do not refill ( )

Signed:_____
DO NOT TAKE THIS TO YOUR PHARMACIST

Community Clinic
Jeffrey A. Eaton, NP
Joyce D. Cappiello, NP

Name:_____ DOB_____
Address_____ Date_____

Rx

"label all unless indicated"
Refill:_____ times-- Do not refill ( )

Signed:_____
DO NOT TAKE THIS TO YOUR PHARMACIST

Community Clinic
Jeffrey A. Eaton, NP
Joyce D. Cappiello, NP

Name:_____ DOB_____
Address_____ Date_____

Rx

"label all unless indicated"
Refill:_____ times-- Do not refill ( )

Signed:_____
DO NOT TAKE THIS TO YOUR PHARMACIST

CASE
43 *Discussion*

LEARNING ISSUES

In order to resolve this patient's problem, you will need to consider and address the following issues (you may generate additional issues as well):

- **Benign prostatic hyperplasia (BPH)**
- **Prostate cancer screening**
- **Pharmacological options for BPH**
- **Evaluation of chest pain**

INITIAL IDEAS

Mr. Metcalf is having symptoms of what is commonly called prostatism. You must decide what factors are causing his symptoms. Possibilities include the following:

- BPH
- BPH with a urinary tract infection (UTI)
- BPH with urinary retention
- Prostate cancer located in an area of the prostate that causes an outlet obstruction

INTERPRETATION OF CUES, PATTERNS, AND INFORMATION

Based on the initial ideas, the most important thing that you must do is decide what is causing the resistance to urination and the degree to which the urine flow is being obstructed. Although there is a relatively low probability that the outlet obstruction is being caused by a prostatic cancer, the potential risks validate consideration. Mr. Metcalf is at an age where a prostatic cancer would not be unusual because it increases in frequency with age.

Mr. Metcalf has no symptoms of UTI, although the associated inflammatory changes of an infection can make a mild BPH much more severe. When the infection is treated in this case, the symptoms of prostatism will decrease.

There is nothing in Mr. Metcalf's history that will be problematic regarding treatment for his prostatism except possibly his chest pain. It does appear to be mild, and since the ETT was negative, it is possible that his angina is not cardiac in origin. His ECG is currently normal as well. One option would be to try another approach to his chest pain and suggest antacids or an H_2 blocker.

If a medication is chosen as the appropriate intervention for his BPH, his chest pain history will need to be considered in choice of medication. The decrease in blood pressure associated with the use of an alpha blocker may make this angina better or worse or have no effect.

Another issue of concern is whether the outlet obstruction is severe enough to have resulted in urinary retention. On physical examination, you found no real evidence of this, and it is probably not necessary to cathterize him for postvoid residual (PVR). If you were suspicious that he was experiencing incomplete emptying, then you would insert a Foley catheter or order an ultrasound to assure that he did not have a high PVR. Discussion with a urologist might be advisable at that point. If there was a very high PVR, a Foley catheter could be left in while you discuss it with the urologist and then left in for a few weeks if that is the urologist's suggestion.

Mr. Metcalf's intake of 2 to 3 beers per night might be worth further discussion. A CAGE questionnaire would give you a sense of whether this was causing his problems.

REVISED IDEAS

The ideas that you had going into the room are probably not significantly different than the ones you have now with the exception of your level of concern about urinary retention.
- BPH with or without urinary retention
- Prostatic cancer
- BPH complicated by a UTI
- Bladder dysfunction
- Prostatitis (although improbable with a relatively small, firm gland)

DIAGNOSTIC OPTIONS

One of the key issues in the case of Mr. Metcalf is if and/or how you are going to determine whether he has prostatic cancer. In a male with these symptoms, it would be unusual for these symptoms to be caused by a cancer, but whether that possibility needs to be ruled out should be considered. Many clinicians would order a prostate-specific antigen (PSA) and perform a digital rectal examination (DRE). If both are normal, then no further diagnostic testing is needed. If either is abnormal, then ultrasound examination of the prostate with a possible biopsy would be indicated. Goroll, May, and Mulley (1995) note that the prior probability of prostate cancer is not increased in a male with symptoms of prostatism. However, there is a 10% to 15% chance of the coincidence of the two problems, and if the decision is made to not screen, then the patient must understand and agree with that decision. In another practical consideration, all of the most common medications used for treatment of prostatism caused by BPH include a directive to rule out prostate cancer in their prescribing information.

An option that can be used to determine the severity of symptoms would be the American Urologic Association's Symptom Index, which can be found in the Agency for Health Care Policy and Research (AHCPR) Guidlines for BPH (1994).

If there was no evidence of cancer, then a trial of therapy for BPH would be appropriate. A UTI can worsen symptoms, so a urinalysis and culture are appropriate before considering a medication trial.

THERAPEUTIC OPTIONS

Pharmacological

If an infection was detected, then a 7-day course of Bactrim DS bid would be a reasonable approach. If there was not an infection, then there are essentially two medication options that are used in a general practice setting. The first would be finasteride, which causes the prostate to shrink. The second option would be an alpha blocker. The most commonly used alpha blockers are Cardura and Hytrin. These work by relaxing the area of the prostatic capsule, thus decreasing the amount of outflow obstruction. Alpha blockers can be given at half strength for a few days to allow the body to adjust and possibly decrease any orthostatic hypotension that may occur. Finasteride, a 5-alpha reductase inhibitor, blocks the conversion of testosterone to dihydrotestosterone and results in shrinkage of the prostate.

Educational

Mr. Metcalf will be taught about BPH, and the plan of diagnosis and treatment will be fully explained. He will also be instructed regarding the side effects of alpha blockers or finasteride if either of those options is chosen.

Nonpharmacological

It has only been in the past 10 years that medication has been a common approach to prostatism. Previously, the patients had the options of surgery or living with the symptoms and the increased risk of problems associate with the urinary outflow obstruction. When patients fail in a trial of medication therapy, then surgery is still an option.

HEALTH PROMOTION/HEALTH MAINTENANCE

These may be most appropriate to address at later visits, but plans should be made to ensure that these needs are addressed.

Mr. Metcalf clearly needs ongoing care. He has several lifestyle issues that should be evaluated. Is he having problems with alcohol? Should you try to taper and discontinue his Valium? Are there other things that should be done to help him deal with stress? These are all better dealt with in an annual physical time slot rather than in an episodic visit. At that time, other issues could be addressed:

- Updating his immunizations: Td, Pneumococcal vaccine, influenza vaccine, consideration of hepatitis B vaccine as indicated
- Cholesterol screening: His cholesterol was only 200. Would you want to check his high-density lipoproteins (HDLs)?
- Other disease screening that could be done, such as testing for colon cancer, assuring that his glaucoma testing is up-to-date, etc.
- Diet, exercise, and other general health-promotive behaviors

FOLLOW-UP

Follow-up depends on the relationship between the clinician and the patient. Many clinicians would instruct the patient to increase the alpha blocker at weekly intervals and return in about 1 month to see if it was effective. Finasteride may take several months to have any effect. If watchful waiting is chosen, then an invitation to return at any time is appropriate. As noted, scheduling for a general health-promotion and/or disease screening examination would be optimal.

References

Agency for Health Care Policy and Research: *Benign prostatic hyperplasia: diagnosis and treatment*, AHCPR Publication 94-0582, 1994.

Goroll AH, May LA, Mulley AG: *Primary care medicine*, Philadelphia, 1995, JB Lippincott.

CASE 44

PART 1

Opening Scenario

Kimberly Parsons is a 16-year-old female who is in your office for a 15-minute visit. Her mother is not present because she works and could not take the day off. Ms. Parsons says that her mother said to call her if there were any problems or questions. Kim has been coming to this practice for several years, but this is the first time you have seen her.

History Of Present Illness

"I go through periods when I cough a lot. I never cough up anything; it's just a dry, hacking cough. I have coughing episodes after I swim in the pool, and it seems like I just can't take a deep breath. I don't think I had this before last summer. It is actually better since I've been swimming in the pool, but I still cough when I get out. It was really bad last summer when I was at my grandmother's camp. I've never felt like I was wheezing." Ms. Parsons has four to five colds per year.

Medical History

Never hospitalized, no major accidents, no chronic illnesses. Her medical record shows previous visits for well child checks (WCCs), three episodes of otitis media all before age 18 months, and four upper respiratory infections (URIs) between the ages of 2 and 10. No surgery.

Social History

Does not smoke or drink alcohol. Lives with parents. She is an "A" student.

Medications

Occasional Dimetapp and Advil

Allergies

None

Review of Systems

Skin: Denies rashes or lesions; had eczema as a baby
HEENT: Denies frequent sore throats, headaches, ear pain, blurred or double vision
Cardiac: Denies chest pain, shortness of breath; good exercise tolerance except as noted above
Respiratory: See History of Present Illness
Gastrointestinal: Occasional diarrhea with high stress; gets gassy when she drinks milk
Genitourinary: No itching or discharge; never had a Pap smear; denies current sexual activity; no dysuria or hematuria
Hematological: No bruising

Physical Examination

Vital signs: Temperature: 98.4° F; *Pulse:* 70 beats/min; *Respirations:* 24 breaths/min; *BP:* 110/60 mm Hg
Height: 5' 5"; *Weight:* 120 lb
General: Appears stated age (or a little older); neatly dressed; cooperative; oriented to time and place
HEENT: Head is normocephalic, atraumatic; pupils equal, round, and reactive to light; extraocular movements intact; tympanic membranes observable without excessive cerumen; nares are patent without redness or exudate; nasal mucosa is a little pale; throat is noninjected; tongue is midline; palate rises symmetrically; teeth are in adequate repair
Neck: Supple without thyromegaly or adenopathy
Heart: Regular rate and rhythm; no murmurs, rubs, or gallops
Lungs: Clear to auscultation and percussion; peak expiratory flow rates (PEFRs): 290/310/320; her predicted is 453
Abdomen: Soft, nontender; no hepatosplenomegaly
Extremities: Without cyanosis, clubbing, or edema; reflexes are 2+ at the biceps, triceps, brachioradialis, patellar, and Achilles; no Babinski signs present; strength and sensation are symmetrical

ASSESSMENT   *Please indicate the problems or issues you have identified that will guide your care (preferably in list form):*

PLAN   *Please list your plans for addressing each of the problems or issues in your assessment:*

Community Clinic
Jeffrey A. Eaton, NP
Joyce D. Cappiello, NP

Name:_____ DOB_____
Address_____ Date_____

Rx

"label all unless indicated"
Refill:_____ times-- Do not refill ( )

Signed:_____
DO NOT TAKE THIS TO YOUR PHARMACIST

Community Clinic
Jeffrey A. Eaton, NP
Joyce D. Cappiello, NP

Name:_____ DOB_____
Address_____ Date_____

Rx

"label all unless indicated"
Refill:_____ times-- Do not refill ( )

Signed:_____
DO NOT TAKE THIS TO YOUR PHARMACIST

Community Clinic
Jeffrey A. Eaton, NP
Joyce D. Cappiello, NP

Name:_____ DOB_____
Address_____ Date_____

Rx

"label all unless indicated"
Refill:_____ times-- Do not refill ( )

Signed:_____
DO NOT TAKE THIS TO YOUR PHARMACIST

Community Clinic
Jeffrey A. Eaton, NP
Joyce D. Cappiello, NP

Name:_____ DOB_____
Address_____ Date_____

Rx

"label all unless indicated"
Refill:_____ times-- Do not refill ( )

Signed:_____
DO NOT TAKE THIS TO YOUR PHARMACIST

PART 2

"While I'm here, I was wondering if you could give me some birth control pills. I'm not having sex yet, but I think I'm going to soon." How will you respond to her request?

ASSESSMENT AND PLAN

Community Clinic
Jeffrey A. Eaton, NP
Joyce D. Cappiello, NP

Name:_____ DOB_____
Address_____ Date_____

Rx

"label all unless indicated"
Refill:_____ times-- Do not refill ( )

Signed:_____
DO NOT TAKE THIS TO YOUR PHARMACIST

Community Clinic
Jeffrey A. Eaton, NP
Joyce D. Cappiello, NP

Name:_____ DOB_____
Address_____ Date_____

Rx

"label all unless indicated"
Refill:_____ times-- Do not refill ( )

Signed:_____
DO NOT TAKE THIS TO YOUR PHARMACIST

LEARNING ISSUES

In order to resolve this patient's problem, you will need to consider and address the following issues (you may generate additional issues as well):

* **Differential diagnosis of cough**
* **Diagnostic criteria for asthma**
* **Types of asthma, including cough-variant asthma**
* **Treatment options in reactive airway disease**
* **Influenza vaccine in asthma**
* **Consents needed to treat a 16 year old**
* **Lactose intolerance**
* **Choice of contraceptive methods**
* **Need for evaluation before initiating contraceptive pills**

PART 1

Initial Ideas

* URI
* Asthma
* Nonrespiratory causes of cough such as gastroesophageal reflux disease (GERD)

Interpretation of Cues, Patterns, and Information

Ms. Parsons gives a history that is very suspicious of a reactive airway disease. It seems to worsen when she was at her grandmother's camp, which is in an area where she would be exposed to more outdoor allergens. Her symptoms also seem to increase when she is exercising, but it may be difficult to determine whether exercise actually exacerbates the problem or whether her symptoms are a result of a decreased baseline function, which limits her ability to respond to the increased oxygen needs of swimming. Her PEFRs tend to indicate that she may have some baseline decrease in her lung function since she is well below the predicted for her age and height.

Another issue that you should deal with at this point is whether you can or should be treating Ms. Parsons without specific consent from her parents. The laws vary somewhat from state to state, but for a nonemergent complaint such as this, most states would require consent. Some clinicians will go ahead and collect data but validate with parents before treating. A clinician should obviously know the law and make appropriate decisions in an individual case.

Although Ms. Parsons does not have a wheeze, she could still have asthma. Asthma, which has cough as the predominant symptom and does not include wheezing, is referred to as cough-variant asthma.

Ms. Parsons is a good example of a child who has had signs of allergies in the past, including apparent lactose intolerance, dermatitis, recurrent respiratory infections, and eczema as a baby. Prospectively this number of infections would not necessarily raise a red flag, but retrospectively it does add evidence to support the diagnosis of asthma.

Since Ms. Parsons' symptoms have been intermittent and associated with increased exercise, the probability of an infectious process at this point is remote.

Revised Ideas

- Exercise-induced asthma
- Cough-variant asthma (allergy mediated)

Differential Diagnosis

Ms. Parsons has essentially no gastrointestinal symptoms (her gassiness with milk probably represents a lactose intolerance), so cystic fibrosis (CF) is less probable. As always, if she failed to respond to the current treatment, a differential diagnosis would be regenerated that would probably include CF.

Mass lesions, cardiac problems, or GERD would also fall into the category of remote possibilities. Psychogenic cough also occurs, although Ms. Parsons' history is not typical.

It appears that you are dealing with asthma. Whether it is predominantly exercise or allergy induced seems to be the question as well as establishing a label for the severity of her asthma (Table 44-1).

One approach that may contribute to the differential diagnosis is to monitor her symptoms in relation to exercise and exposure to allergens to help decide whether her symptoms are caused or exacerbated by these factors. The response that she gets to different classes of pharmacological agents will also contribute evidence for the diagnosis.

Diagnostic Options

Pulmonary function tests (PFTs) would be helpful in quantifying the degree of reactive airway disease. Peak flow meters are not as accurate as PFTs, and thus many sources recommend validating findings with PFTs. Prebronchodilator and postbronchodilator PFTs also document the airway's response to beta agonists.

Some clinicians will go ahead on the current information with a trial of therapy. As a companion with this approach, PEFR monitoring at home may provide some important information, so Ms. Parsons should be encouraged to obtain a peak flow meter and instructed in its use. Peak flow meters can cost as much as $25, and insurance coverage is variable, so you should take this into

Table 44-1 *Determining Asthma Severity*

STEP	SYMPTOMS	LUNG FUNCTION
Step 1	Symptoms less than twice per week Normal PEFR between exacerbations Exacerbations often brief	PEFR over 80% of predicted
Step 2	Symptoms more than twice per week Exacerbations may affect activity	PEFR over 80% of predicted
Step 3	Daily use of short-acting beta agonist Exacerbations more than twice per week	PEFR between 60% and 80% of predicted
Step 4	Continual Limit activity Frequent exacerbations Frequent nighttime symptoms	PEFR less than 60% of predicted; may be quite variable

Modified from NHLBI: *Expert panel report 2: guidelines for the diagnosis and management of asthma*, Bethesda, Md, 1997, National Asthma Education and Prevention Program.

consideration. In this case, if PEFRs enter the normal range and symptoms abate, most clinicians would continue the current therapy and consider further diagnostics as needed.

Therapeutic Options

Pharmacological There are several options in Ms. Parsons' case, but some of the more common approaches would be as follows:

- Start Ms. Parsons on an inhaled beta agonist (such as albuterol, 2 puffs), cromolyn, or nedocromil before she swims. This may limit her symptoms enough that swimming is no longer problematic. Advantages to this approach are that it is of minimal cost and inconvenience.
- Start her on a longer-acting preventive regimen such as cromylyn, nedocromil, or inhaled steroids. These will be more effective in minimizing day-to-day effects. It is more expensive and commits Ms. Parsons three to four times a day to a metered dose inhaler (MDI). Some clinicians would choose this approach because of Ms. Parsons' apparent decreased PEFR even without exercise. An albuterol inhaler could be given in addition to this for exercise such as swimming.
- Since Ms. Parsons' PEFR is probably classified as at least Step 2, and if this PEFR is accurate Step 3 in the NHLBI guidelines, the case for an antiinflammatory such as nedocromil, cromylyn, or inhaled steroids is quite strong. Some clinicians would want to confirm this with PFTs. In Step 3 asthma (in someone over 12 years old), it is also reasonable to consider an oral medication such as zafirlukast (Accolate), but their position in therapy is not fully established (NHLBI, 1997).
- The issue of a spacer should be considered. Spacers will increase the amount of medication delivered, but if MDIs are being carried in pocketbooks or pockets, they add to inconvenience and make the process of taking an inhalation more obvious. In a teenager, a clinician needs to consider these social issues as well as the pharmacological ones.

Educational As noted, a peak flow meter and appropriate instructions will allow a monitoring of symptoms by Ms. Parsons and her family. Her parents should probably have instructions as well, and a follow-up appointment that included the parents would be desirable.

Although not all people with asthma are affected, some individuals are aspirin sensitive, and it will cause wheezing. This or any other medications (such as certain other nonsteroidal antiinflammatory drugs [NSAIDs]) that cause problems should be avoided.

Other Nonpharmacological Options Alteration of the environment may minimize the allergic symptoms. She may be able to avoid triggers to her asthma by covering her pillow and/or mattress. Minimizimg carpeting can also be helpful in some people. Allergy testing is also an option, but many clinicians will start with a simple approach first and progress to additional testing as needed.

Health Promotion/Health Maintenance

- Update tetanus-diphtheria (Td) immunization, consider hepatitis B vaccine, and consider varicella zoster virus (VZV) vaccine.
- HEADSS (Home, Education, Alcohol, Drugs, Sex, Suicide): You might ask questions as appropriate today and consider an annual examination for further follow-up.

Follow-Up

For her asthma, a few weeks to 1 month will be adequate to get a sense of whether the treatment is working. Both her PEFR readings and her subjective improvement of symptoms will be used as criteria in determining the relative success of the therapy.

PART 2

Should you go ahead and do a full evaluation regarding the appropriateness of oral contraceptives (OCs), including a pelvic examination? Should you ask a few essential questions and give her a supply for 1 or 2 months and then bring her back for the examination? Or should you tell her that she will have to come back for a family planning appointment before you can give her pills?

The decision will be based on many factors. Does your state, province, or country allow you to give her OCs without parental consent? Most do, but you must be aware of appropriate laws. Does your own value system allow you to give her OCs? If not, should you refer her elsewhere? Are you worried that she may become pregnant if you put her off? There is no real evidence that a couple of months of pills will do any harm, and there have actually been those who have advocated OCs as over-the-counter (OTC) medication. Should you let her know about emergency contraception?

Even if you decide to give Ms. Parsons OCs, the risk of sexually transmitted diseases (STDs) and the value of continuing to use condoms should be discussed. In fact, a brief discussion of sexuality may be appropriate. Beginning sexual activity should be her choice, and she may have questions or need information to help her make that choice.

The issue of whether to do a pelvic examination before beginning OCs deserves further discussion. The objective of doing a pelvic examination in a woman who is beginning OCs is to screen for gynecological cancers and STDs. In a girl this age who has not been sexually active, the probability of either is remote. Deferring the pelvic examination will probably not have any negative effects, and some clinicians believe that the pelvic examination will be easier and less uncomfortable if done after sexual activity has begun.

Deciding whether to give her OCs involves both evaluation of current research and personal philosophy. The clinician must be sure that the chosen approach will be reasonable, but this approach will vary.

References

National Heart, Lung, and Blood Institute: *Expert panel report 2: guidelines for the diagnosis and management of asthma,* Bethesda, Md, 1997, National Asthma Education and Prevention Program.

APPENDIX

Abbreviations

2f ↓ u	Two fingers below the umbilicus
A&W	Alive and well
AA	Alcoholics Anonymous
ACOG	American College of Obstetricians and Gynecologists
ACP	American College of Physicians
ADA	American Dietetic Association
AFP	Alpha fetoprotein
AG	Anticipatory guidance
AHCPR	Agency for Health Care Policy and Research
AIDS	Acquired immunodeficiency syndrome
ASA	Acetylsalicylic acid
ASCUS	Atypical cells of undetermined significance
AST	Aspartate aminotransferase
AUDIT	Alcohol Use Disorders Identification Test
AV/AF	Anteverted/anteflexed
bid	Twice a day
BM	Bowel movement
BMI	Body mass index
BP	Blood pressure
BPH	Benign prostatic hyperplasia
BUN	Blood urea nitrogen
CAD	Coronary artery disease
CAGE	Cut down, Annoyed, Guilty, Eye-opener
CARE	Cholesterol and Recurrent Events
CBC	Complete blood count
CCAIT	Canadian Atherosclerosis Intervention Trial
CDC	Centers for Disease Control and Prevention
CF	Cystic fibrosis

CFS	Chronic fatigue syndrome
CHD	Coronary heart disease
CHF	Congestive heart failure
CLIA	Clinical Laboratory Improvement Act
CNM	Certified nurse midwife
CMT	Cervical motion tenderness
COPD	Chronic obstructive pulmonary disease
CT	Computerized tomography
CVA	Costovertebral angle; cerebrovascular accident
CXR	Chest x-ray examination
DJD	Degenerative joint disease
DMPA	Depomedroxyprogesterone acetate
DM	Diabetes mellitus
DP	Dorsalis Pedis pulse
DPT	Diphtheria-pertussis-tetanus
DPOA	Durable power of attorney
ECG	Electrocardiogram
ECP	Emergency contraceptive pills
EDC	Estimated date of confinement
ER	Emergency room
ESR	Erythrocyte sedimentation rate
ETT	Exercise tolerance test
FBS	Fasting blood sugar
FDA	Food and Drug Administration
FHR	Fetal heart rate
FOBT	Fecal occult blood test
GABHS	Group A β-hemolytic streptococci
GC	Gonorrhea
GCPS	Guide to Clinical Preventive Services

GDS	Geriatric Depression Scale
GERD	Gastroesophageal reflux disease
GGT	γ-Glutamyl transferase
GTT	Glucose tolerance test
GxPxAbx	Gravida (#) Para (#) Abortions (#)
GxPxxxx	Gravida (#) Para (term, premature, abortions, living)
HBV	Hepatitis B virus
HCI	Hydrochloric acid
HCM	Hypertrophic cardiomyopathy
Hct	Hematocrit
HDL	High-density lipoproteins
HEENT	Head, eyes, ears, nose, throat
HELLP	Hypertension, Elevated Liver function, Low Platelets syndrome
Hgb	Hemoglobin
HGSIL	High-grade squamous intraepithelial lesions
Hib	*Haemophilus influenzae* type b
HIV	Human immunodeficiency virus
HMO	Health Maintenance Organization
HNP	Herniated nucleus pulposus
HPV	Human papillomavirus
HRT	Hormone replacement therapy
HSV	Herpes simplex virus
IBD	Inflammatory bowel disease
IBS	Irritable bowel syndrome
IBW	Ideal body weight
ICS	Intercostal space
ID	Intradermal
IDA	Iron deficiency anemia

IDDM	Insulin-dependent diabetes mellitus
IHSS	Idiopathic hypertrophic subaortic stenosis
INH	Isonicotinic acid hydrazide
INR	International normalized ratio
IPV	Inactivated poliovirus vaccine
IUD	Intrauterine device
IV	Intravenous
JVD	Jugular venous distention
LDH	Lactic dehydrogenase
LDL	Low-density lipoproteins
LE	Lower extremity
LFT	Liver function test
LGSIL	Low-grade squamous intraepithelial lesions
LMP	Last menstrual period
LRI	Lower respiratory infection
LSB	Left sternal border
MAO	Monoamine oxidase
MAST	Michigan Alcoholism Screening Test
MCH	Mean corpuscular hemoglobin
MCHC	Mean corpuscular hemoglobin concentration
MCV	Mean corpuscular volume
MDI	Metered dose inhaler
MGF	Maternal grandfather
MGM	Maternal grandmother
MI	Myocardial infarction
MMR	Measles-mumps-rubella
MMSE	Minimental Status Examination
MPV	Mean platelet volume
MRI	Magnetic resonance imaging
MVP	Mitral valve prolapse
NCEP	National Cholesterol Education Program
NSAID	Nonsteroidal antiinflammatory drug
OC	Oral contraceptive
OPV	Oral poliovirus vaccine
OTC	Over the counter
PCP	*Pneumocystis carinii* pneumonia
PCR	Polymerase chain reaction
PEFR	Peak expiratory flow rate
PFT	Pulmonary function test
PGF	Paternal grandfather
PGM	Paternal grandmother
PID	Pelvic inflammatory disease
PIH	Pregnancy-induced hypertension
PMS	Premenstrual syndrome
PND	Paroxysmal nocturnal dyspnea; postnasal drip
po	Per os (by mouth)
PPD	Purified protein derivative
pr	Per rectum
prn	As needed
PSA	Prostate-specific antigen
PT	Posterior tibial pulse; physical therapy
PVR	Postvoid residual
qd	Every day
qid	Four times a day
qxh	Every (#) hours
RBC	Red blood cell
RDA	Recommended Daily Allowance
RDW	Red cell distribution width
RPR	Rapid plasma reagin
4S	Scandinavian Simvastatin Survival Study
SC	Subcutaneously
SCOR	Specialized Center of Research
SD	Standard deviations
SEER	Surveillance, Epidemiology, and End Results
Segs	Segmented neutrophils
SG	Specific gravity
SGOT	Serum glutamic oxalocetic transaminase (also known as AST)
SHEP	Systolic Hypertension in the Elderly Project
SI	Sacroiliac
SIADH	Syndrome of inappropriate antidiuretic hormone
SL	Sublingual
SLR	Straight leg raise
s/p	Status post
SPECT	Single photon emission computed tomography
SSRI	Selective serotonin reuptake inhibitor
STD	Sexually transmitted disease
TAB	Therapeutic abortion
Tb	Tuberculosis
TCA	Tricyclic antidepressant
TCN	Tetracycline
Td	Tetanus-diphtheria
TIA	Transient ischemic attack
TIBC	Total iron binding capacity
tid	Three times a day
TMP/SMX	Trimethoprim sulfamethoxazole
TSH	Thyroid-stimulating hormone
UI	Urinary incontinence
URI	Upper respiratory infection
US	Ultrasound
UTI	Urinary tract infection
UV	Ultraviolet
VZIG	Varicella zoster immune globulin
VZV	Varicella zoster virus
WBC	White blood cell
WCC	Well child check
WHO	World Health Organization
WOSCOPS	West of Scotland Coronary Prevention Study

INDEX

Community Clinic
Jeffrey A. Eaton, NP
Joyce D. Cappiello, NP

Name:_____ DOB_____
Address_____ Date_____

Rx

"label all unless indicated"
Refill:_____ times-- Do not refill ( )

Signed:_____
DO NOT TAKE THIS TO YOUR PHARMACIST

Community Clinic
Jeffrey A. Eaton, NP
Joyce D. Cappiello, NP

Name:_____ DOB_____
Address_____ Date_____

Rx

"label all unless indicated"
Refill:_____ times-- Do not refill ( )

Signed:_____
DO NOT TAKE THIS TO YOUR PHARMACIST

Community Clinic
Jeffrey A. Eaton, NP
Joyce D. Cappiello, NP

Name:_____ DOB_____
Address_____ Date_____

Rx

"label all unless indicated"
Refill:_____ times-- Do not refill ( )

Signed:_____
DO NOT TAKE THIS TO YOUR PHARMACIST

Community Clinic
Jeffrey A. Eaton, NP
Joyce D. Cappiello, NP

Name:_____ DOB_____
Address_____ Date_____

Rx

"label all unless indicated"
Refill:_____ times-- Do not refill ( )

Signed:_____
DO NOT TAKE THIS TO YOUR PHARMACIST

Community Clinic

Jeffrey A. Eaton, NP

Joyce D. Cappiello, NP

Name:_____ DOB_____

Address_____ Date_____

Rx

"label all unless indicated"

Refill:_____ times-- Do not refill ( )

Signed:_____

DO NOT TAKE THIS TO YOUR PHARMACIST

Community Clinic

Jeffrey A. Eaton, NP

Joyce D. Cappiello, NP

Name:_____ DOB_____

Address_____ Date_____

Rx

"label all unless indicated"

Refill:_____ times-- Do not refill ( )

Signed:_____

DO NOT TAKE THIS TO YOUR PHARMACIST

Community Clinic

Jeffrey A. Eaton, NP

Joyce D. Cappiello, NP

Name:_____ DOB_____

Address_____ Date_____

Rx

"label all unless indicated"

Refill:_____ times-- Do not refill ( )

Signed:_____

DO NOT TAKE THIS TO YOUR PHARMACIST

Community Clinic

Jeffrey A. Eaton, NP

Joyce D. Cappiello, NP

Name:_____ DOB_____

Address_____ Date_____

Rx

"label all unless indicated"

Refill:_____ times-- Do not refill ( )

Signed:_____

DO NOT TAKE THIS TO YOUR PHARMACIST

Community Clinic
Jeffrey A. Eaton, NP
Joyce D. Cappiello, NP

Name:_____ DOB_____
Address_____ Date_____

Rx

"label all unless indicated"
Refill:_____ times-- Do not refill ( )

Signed:_____
DO NOT TAKE THIS TO YOUR PHARMACIST

Community Clinic
Jeffrey A. Eaton, NP
Joyce D. Cappiello, NP

Name:_____ DOB_____
Address_____ Date_____

Rx

"label all unless indicated"
Refill:_____ times-- Do not refill ( )

Signed:_____
DO NOT TAKE THIS TO YOUR PHARMACIST

Community Clinic
Jeffrey A. Eaton, NP
Joyce D. Cappiello, NP

Name:_____ DOB_____
Address_____ Date_____

Rx

"label all unless indicated"
Refill:_____ times-- Do not refill ( )

Signed:_____
DO NOT TAKE THIS TO YOUR PHARMACIST

Community Clinic
Jeffrey A. Eaton, NP
Joyce D. Cappiello, NP

Name:_____ DOB_____
Address_____ Date_____

Rx

"label all unless indicated"
Refill:_____ times-- Do not refill ( )

Signed:_____
DO NOT TAKE THIS TO YOUR PHARMACIST

Community Clinic
Jeffrey A. Eaton, NP
Joyce D. Cappiello, NP

Name:_____ DOB_____
Address_____ Date_____

Rx

"label all unless indicated"
Refill:_____ times-- Do not refill ( )

Signed:_____
DO NOT TAKE THIS TO YOUR PHARMACIST

Community Clinic
Jeffrey A. Eaton, NP
Joyce D. Cappiello, NP

Name:_____ DOB_____
Address_____ Date_____

Rx

"label all unless indicated"
Refill:_____ times-- Do not refill ( )

Signed:_____
DO NOT TAKE THIS TO YOUR PHARMACIST

Community Clinic
Jeffrey A. Eaton, NP
Joyce D. Cappiello, NP

Name:_____ DOB_____
Address_____ Date_____

Rx

"label all unless indicated"
Refill:_____ times-- Do not refill ( )

Signed:_____
DO NOT TAKE THIS TO YOUR PHARMACIST

Community Clinic
Jeffrey A. Eaton, NP
Joyce D. Cappiello, NP

Name:_____ DOB_____
Address_____ Date_____

Rx

"label all unless indicated"
Refill:_____ times-- Do not refill ( )

Signed:_____
DO NOT TAKE THIS TO YOUR PHARMACIST

Community Clinic
Jeffrey A. Eaton, NP
Joyce D. Cappiello, NP

Name:_____ DOB_____
Address_____ Date_____

Rx

"label all unless indicated"
Refill:_____ times-- Do not refill ( )

Signed:_____
DO NOT TAKE THIS TO YOUR PHARMACIST

Community Clinic
Jeffrey A. Eaton, NP
Joyce D. Cappiello, NP

Name:_____ DOB_____
Address_____ Date_____

Rx

"label all unless indicated"
Refill:_____ times-- Do not refill ( )

Signed:_____
DO NOT TAKE THIS TO YOUR PHARMACIST

Community Clinic
Jeffrey A. Eaton, NP
Joyce D. Cappiello, NP

Name:_____ DOB_____
Address_____ Date_____

Rx

"label all unless indicated"
Refill:_____ times-- Do not refill ( )

Signed:_____
DO NOT TAKE THIS TO YOUR PHARMACIST

Community Clinic
Jeffrey A. Eaton, NP
Joyce D. Cappiello, NP

Name:_____ DOB_____
Address_____ Date_____

Rx

"label all unless indicated"
Refill:_____ times-- Do not refill ( )

Signed:_____
DO NOT TAKE THIS TO YOUR PHARMACIST

Community Clinic
Jeffrey A. Eaton, NP
Joyce D. Cappiello, NP

Name:_____ DOB_____
Address_____ Date_____

Rx

"label all unless indicated"
Refill:_____ times-- Do not refill ( )

Signed:_____
DO NOT TAKE THIS TO YOUR PHARMACIST

Community Clinic
Jeffrey A. Eaton, NP
Joyce D. Cappiello, NP

Name:_____ DOB_____
Address_____ Date_____

Rx

"label all unless indicated"
Refill:_____ times-- Do not refill ( )

Signed:_____
DO NOT TAKE THIS TO YOUR PHARMACIST

Community Clinic
Jeffrey A. Eaton, NP
Joyce D. Cappiello, NP

Name:_____ DOB_____
Address_____ Date_____

Rx

"label all unless indicated"
Refill:_____ times-- Do not refill ( )

Signed:_____
DO NOT TAKE THIS TO YOUR PHARMACIST

Community Clinic
Jeffrey A. Eaton, NP
Joyce D. Cappiello, NP

Name:_____ DOB_____
Address_____ Date_____

Rx

"label all unless indicated"
Refill:_____ times-- Do not refill ( )

Signed:_____
DO NOT TAKE THIS TO YOUR PHARMACIST

Community Clinic
Jeffrey A. Eaton, NP
Joyce D. Cappiello, NP

Name:_____ DOB_____
Address_____ Date_____

Rx

"label all unless indicated"
Refill:_____ times-- Do not refill ( )

Signed:_____
DO NOT TAKE THIS TO YOUR PHARMACIST

Community Clinic
Jeffrey A. Eaton, NP
Joyce D. Cappiello, NP

Name:_____ DOB_____
Address_____ Date_____

Rx

"label all unless indicated"
Refill:_____ times-- Do not refill ( )

Signed:_____
DO NOT TAKE THIS TO YOUR PHARMACIST

Community Clinic
Jeffrey A. Eaton, NP
Joyce D. Cappiello, NP

Name:_____ DOB_____
Address_____ Date_____

Rx

"label all unless indicated"
Refill:_____ times-- Do not refill ( )

Signed:_____
DO NOT TAKE THIS TO YOUR PHARMACIST

Community Clinic
Jeffrey A. Eaton, NP
Joyce D. Cappiello, NP

Name:_____ DOB_____
Address_____ Date_____

Rx

"label all unless indicated"
Refill:_____ times-- Do not refill ( )

Signed:_____
DO NOT TAKE THIS TO YOUR PHARMACIST

Community Clinic
Jeffrey A. Eaton, NP
Joyce D. Cappiello, NP

Name:_____ DOB_____
Address_____ Date_____

Rx

"label all unless indicated"
Refill:_____ times-- Do not refill ( )

Signed:_____
DO NOT TAKE THIS TO YOUR PHARMACIST

Community Clinic
Jeffrey A. Eaton, NP
Joyce D. Cappiello, NP

Name:_____ DOB_____
Address_____ Date_____

Rx

"label all unless indicated"
Refill:_____ times-- Do not refill ( )

Signed:_____
DO NOT TAKE THIS TO YOUR PHARMACIST

Community Clinic
Jeffrey A. Eaton, NP
Joyce D. Cappiello, NP

Name:_____ DOB_____
Address_____ Date_____

Rx

"label all unless indicated"
Refill:_____ times-- Do not refill ( )

Signed:_____
DO NOT TAKE THIS TO YOUR PHARMACIST

Community Clinic
Jeffrey A. Eaton, NP
Joyce D. Cappiello, NP

Name:_____ DOB_____
Address_____ Date_____

Rx

"label all unless indicated"
Refill:_____ times-- Do not refill ( )

Signed:_____
DO NOT TAKE THIS TO YOUR PHARMACIST

Community Clinic
Jeffrey A. Eaton, NP
Joyce D. Cappiello, NP

Name:_____ DOB_____
Address_____ Date_____

Rx

"label all unless indicated"
Refill:_____ times-- Do not refill ( )

Signed:_____
DO NOT TAKE THIS TO YOUR PHARMACIST

Community Clinic
Jeffrey A. Eaton, NP
Joyce D. Cappiello, NP

Name:_____ DOB_____
Address_____ Date_____

Rx

"label all unless indicated"
Refill:_____ times-- Do not refill ( )

Signed:_____
DO NOT TAKE THIS TO YOUR PHARMACIST

Community Clinic
Jeffrey A. Eaton, NP
Joyce D. Cappiello, NP

Name:_____ DOB_____
Address_____ Date_____

Rx

"label all unless indicated"
Refill:_____ times-- Do not refill ( )

Signed:_____
DO NOT TAKE THIS TO YOUR PHARMACIST

Community Clinic
Jeffrey A. Eaton, NP
Joyce D. Cappiello, NP

Name:_____ DOB_____
Address_____ Date_____

Rx

"label all unless indicated"
Refill:_____ times-- Do not refill ( )

Signed:_____
DO NOT TAKE THIS TO YOUR PHARMACIST

Community Clinic
Jeffrey A. Eaton, NP
Joyce D. Cappiello, NP

Name:_____ DOB_____
Address_____ Date_____

Rx

"label all unless indicated"
Refill:_____ times-- Do not refill ( )

Signed:_____
DO NOT TAKE THIS TO YOUR PHARMACIST

Community Clinic
Jeffrey A. Eaton, NP
Joyce D. Cappiello, NP

Name:_____ DOB_____
Address_____ Date_____

Rx

"label all unless indicated"
Refill:_____ times-- Do not refill ( )

Signed:_____
DO NOT TAKE THIS TO YOUR PHARMACIST

Community Clinic
Jeffrey A. Eaton, NP
Joyce D. Cappiello, NP

Name:_____ DOB_____
Address_____ Date_____

Rx

"label all unless indicated"
Refill:_____ times-- Do not refill ( )

Signed:_____
DO NOT TAKE THIS TO YOUR PHARMACIST

Community Clinic
Jeffrey A. Eaton, NP
Joyce D. Cappiello, NP

Name:_____ DOB_____
Address_____ Date_____

Rx

"label all unless indicated"
Refill:_____ times-- Do not refill ( )

Signed:_____
DO NOT TAKE THIS TO YOUR PHARMACIST

Community Clinic
Jeffrey A. Eaton, NP
Joyce D. Cappiello, NP

Name:_____ DOB_____
Address_____ Date_____

Rx

"label all unless indicated"
Refill:_____ times-- Do not refill ( )

Signed:_____
DO NOT TAKE THIS TO YOUR PHARMACIST

Community Clinic
Jeffrey A. Eaton, NP
Joyce D. Cappiello, NP

Name:_____ DOB_____
Address_____ Date_____

Rx

"label all unless indicated"
Refill:_____ times-- Do not refill ( )

Signed:_____
DO NOT TAKE THIS TO YOUR PHARMACIST

Community Clinic
Jeffrey A. Eaton, NP
Joyce D. Cappiello, NP

Name:_____ DOB_____
Address_____ Date_____

Rx

"label all unless indicated"
Refill:_____ times-- Do not refill ( )

Signed:_____
DO NOT TAKE THIS TO YOUR PHARMACIST

Community Clinic
Jeffrey A. Eaton, NP
Joyce D. Cappiello, NP

Name:_____ DOB_____
Address_____ Date_____

Rx

"label all unless indicated"
Refill:_____ times-- Do not refill ( )

Signed:_____
DO NOT TAKE THIS TO YOUR PHARMACIST

Community Clinic
Jeffrey A. Eaton, NP
Joyce D. Cappiello, NP

Name:_____ DOB_____
Address_____ Date_____

Rx

"label all unless indicated"
Refill:_____ times-- Do not refill ( )

Signed:_____
DO NOT TAKE THIS TO YOUR PHARMACIST

Community Clinic
Jeffrey A. Eaton, NP
Joyce D. Cappiello, NP

Name:_____ DOB_____
Address_____ Date_____

Rx

"label all unless indicated"
Refill:_____ times-- Do not refill ( )

Signed:_____
DO NOT TAKE THIS TO YOUR PHARMACIST

Community Clinic
Jeffrey A. Eaton, NP
Joyce D. Cappiello, NP

Name:_____ DOB_____
Address_____ Date_____

Rx

"label all unless indicated"
Refill:_____ times-- Do not refill ( )

Signed:_____
DO NOT TAKE THIS TO YOUR PHARMACIST

Community Clinic
Jeffrey A. Eaton, NP
Joyce D. Cappiello, NP

Name:_____ DOB_____
Address_____ Date_____

Rx

"label all unless indicated"
Refill:_____ times-- Do not refill ( )

Signed:_____
DO NOT TAKE THIS TO YOUR PHARMACIST

Community Clinic
Jeffrey A. Eaton, NP
Joyce D. Cappiello, NP

Name:_____ DOB_____
Address_____ Date_____

Rx

"label all unless indicated"
Refill:_____ times-- Do not refill ( )

Signed:_____
DO NOT TAKE THIS TO YOUR PHARMACIST

Community Clinic
Jeffrey A. Eaton, NP
Joyce D. Cappiello, NP

Name:_____ DOB_____
Address_____ Date_____

Rx

"label all unless indicated"
Refill:_____ times-- Do not refill ( )

Signed:_____
DO NOT TAKE THIS TO YOUR PHARMACIST

Community Clinic
Jeffrey A. Eaton, NP
Joyce D. Cappiello, NP

Name:_____ DOB_____
Address_____ Date_____

Rx

"label all unless indicated"
Refill:_____ times-- Do not refill ( )

Signed:_____
DO NOT TAKE THIS TO YOUR PHARMACIST

Community Clinic
Jeffrey A. Eaton, NP
Joyce D. Cappiello, NP

Name:_____ DOB_____
Address_____ Date_____

Rx

"label all unless indicated"
Refill:_____ times-- Do not refill ( )

Signed:_____
DO NOT TAKE THIS TO YOUR PHARMACIST

Community Clinic
Jeffrey A. Eaton, NP
Joyce D. Cappiello, NP

Name:_____ DOB_____
Address_____ Date_____

Rx

"label all unless indicated"
Refill:_____ times-- Do not refill ( )

Signed:_____
DO NOT TAKE THIS TO YOUR PHARMACIST

Community Clinic
Jeffrey A. Eaton, NP
Joyce D. Cappiello, NP

Name:_____ DOB_____
Address_____ Date_____

Rx

"label all unless indicated"
Refill:_____ times-- Do not refill ( )

Signed:_____
DO NOT TAKE THIS TO YOUR PHARMACIST

Community Clinic
Jeffrey A. Eaton, NP
Joyce D. Cappiello, NP

Name:_____ DOB_____
Address_____ Date_____

Rx

"label all unless indicated"
Refill:_____ times-- Do not refill ( )

Signed:_____
DO NOT TAKE THIS TO YOUR PHARMACIST

Community Clinic
Jeffrey A. Eaton, NP
Joyce D. Cappiello, NP

Name:_____ DOB_____
Address_____ Date_____

Rx

"label all unless indicated"
Refill:_____ times-- Do not refill ( )

Signed:_____
DO NOT TAKE THIS TO YOUR PHARMACIST

Community Clinic
Jeffrey A. Eaton, NP
Joyce D. Cappiello, NP

Name:_____ DOB_____
Address_____ Date_____

Rx

"label all unless indicated"
Refill:_____ times-- Do not refill ( )

Signed:_____
DO NOT TAKE THIS TO YOUR PHARMACIST

Community Clinic
Jeffrey A. Eaton, NP
Joyce D. Cappiello, NP

Name:_____ DOB_____
Address_____ Date_____

Rx

"label all unless indicated"
Refill:_____ times-- Do not refill ( )

Signed:_____
DO NOT TAKE THIS TO YOUR PHARMACIST

Community Clinic
Jeffrey A. Eaton, NP
Joyce D. Cappiello, NP

Name:_____ DOB_____
Address_____ Date_____

Rx

"label all unless indicated"
Refill:_____ times-- Do not refill ( )

Signed:_____
DO NOT TAKE THIS TO YOUR PHARMACIST

Community Clinic
Jeffrey A. Eaton, NP
Joyce D. Cappiello, NP

Name:_____ DOB_____
Address_____ Date_____

Rx

"label all unless indicated"
Refill:_____ times-- Do not refill ( )

Signed:_____
DO NOT TAKE THIS TO YOUR PHARMACIST

Community Clinic
Jeffrey A. Eaton, NP
Joyce D. Cappiello, NP

Name:_____ DOB_____
Address_____ Date_____

Rx

"label all unless indicated"
Refill:_____ times-- Do not refill ( )

Signed:_____
DO NOT TAKE THIS TO YOUR PHARMACIST

Community Clinic
Jeffrey A. Eaton, NP
Joyce D. Cappiello, NP

Name:_____ DOB_____
Address_____ Date_____

Rx

"label all unless indicated"
Refill:_____ times-- Do not refill ( )

Signed:_____
DO NOT TAKE THIS TO YOUR PHARMACIST

Community Clinic
Jeffrey A. Eaton, NP
Joyce D. Cappiello, NP

Name:_____ DOB_____
Address_____ Date_____

Rx

"label all unless indicated"
Refill:_____ times-- Do not refill ( )

Signed:_____
DO NOT TAKE THIS TO YOUR PHARMACIST

Community Clinic
Jeffrey A. Eaton, NP
Joyce D. Cappiello, NP

Name:_____ DOB_____
Address_____ Date_____

Rx

"label all unless indicated"
Refill:_____ times-- Do not refill ( )

Signed:_____
DO NOT TAKE THIS TO YOUR PHARMACIST

Community Clinic
Jeffrey A. Eaton, NP
Joyce D. Cappiello, NP

Name:_____ DOB_____
Address_____ Date_____

Rx

"label all unless indicated"
Refill:_____ times-- Do not refill ( )

Signed:_____
DO NOT TAKE THIS TO YOUR PHARMACIST

Community Clinic
Jeffrey A. Eaton, NP
Joyce D. Cappiello, NP

Name:_____ DOB_____
Address_____ Date_____

Rx

"label all unless indicated"
Refill:_____ times-- Do not refill ( )

Signed:_____
DO NOT TAKE THIS TO YOUR PHARMACIST

Community Clinic
Jeffrey A. Eaton, NP
Joyce D. Cappiello, NP

Name:_____ DOB_____
Address_____ Date_____

Rx

"label all unless indicated"
Refill:_____ times-- Do not refill ( )

Signed:_____
DO NOT TAKE THIS TO YOUR PHARMACIST

Community Clinic
Jeffrey A. Eaton, NP
Joyce D. Cappiello, NP

Name:_____ DOB_____
Address_____ Date_____

Rx

"label all unless indicated"
Refill:_____ times-- Do not refill ( )

Signed:_____
DO NOT TAKE THIS TO YOUR PHARMACIST

Community Clinic
Jeffrey A. Eaton, NP
Joyce D. Cappiello, NP

Name:_____ DOB_____
Address_____ Date_____

Rx

"label all unless indicated"
Refill:_____ times-- Do not refill ( )

Signed:_____
DO NOT TAKE THIS TO YOUR PHARMACIST

Community Clinic
Jeffrey A. Eaton, NP
Joyce D. Cappiello, NP

Name:_____ DOB_____
Address_____ Date_____

Rx

"label all unless indicated"
Refill:_____ times-- Do not refill ( )

Signed:_____
DO NOT TAKE THIS TO YOUR PHARMACIST

Community Clinic
Jeffrey A. Eaton, NP
Joyce D. Cappiello, NP

Name:_____ DOB_____
Address_____ Date_____

Rx

"label all unless indicated"
Refill:_____ times-- Do not refill ( )

Signed:_____
DO NOT TAKE THIS TO YOUR PHARMACIST

Community Clinic
Jeffrey A. Eaton, NP
Joyce D. Cappiello, NP

Name:_____ DOB_____
Address_____ Date_____

Rx

"label all unless indicated"
Refill:_____ times-- Do not refill ( )

Signed:_____
DO NOT TAKE THIS TO YOUR PHARMACIST

Community Clinic
Jeffrey A. Eaton, NP
Joyce D. Cappiello, NP

Name:_____ DOB_____
Address_____ Date_____

Rx

"label all unless indicated"
Refill:_____ times-- Do not refill ( )

Signed:_____
DO NOT TAKE THIS TO YOUR PHARMACIST

Community Clinic
Jeffrey A. Eaton, NP
Joyce D. Cappiello, NP

Name:_____ DOB_____
Address_____ Date_____

Rx

"label all unless indicated"
Refill:_____ times-- Do not refill ( )

Signed:_____
DO NOT TAKE THIS TO YOUR PHARMACIST

Community Clinic
Jeffrey A. Eaton, NP
Joyce D. Cappiello, NP

Name:_____ DOB_____
Address_____ Date_____

Rx

"label all unless indicated"
Refill:_____ times-- Do not refill ( )

Signed:_____
DO NOT TAKE THIS TO YOUR PHARMACIST

Community Clinic
Jeffrey A. Eaton, NP
Joyce D. Cappiello, NP

Name:_____ DOB_____
Address_____ Date_____

Rx

"label all unless indicated"
Refill:_____ times-- Do not refill ( )

Signed:_____
DO NOT TAKE THIS TO YOUR PHARMACIST

Community Clinic
Jeffrey A. Eaton, NP
Joyce D. Cappiello, NP

Name:_____ DOB_____
Address_____ Date_____

Rx

"label all unless indicated"
Refill:_____ times-- Do not refill ( )

Signed:_____
DO NOT TAKE THIS TO YOUR PHARMACIST

Community Clinic
Jeffrey A. Eaton, NP
Joyce D. Cappiello, NP

Name:_____ DOB_____
Address_____ Date_____

Rx

"label all unless indicated"
Refill:_____ times-- Do not refill ( )

Signed:_____
DO NOT TAKE THIS TO YOUR PHARMACIST

Community Clinic
Jeffrey A. Eaton, NP
Joyce D. Cappiello, NP

Name:_____ DOB_____
Address_____ Date_____

Rx

"label all unless indicated"
Refill:_____ times-- Do not refill ( )

Signed:_____
DO NOT TAKE THIS TO YOUR PHARMACIST

Community Clinic
Jeffrey A. Eaton, NP
Joyce D. Cappiello, NP

Name:_____ DOB_____
Address_____ Date_____

Rx

"label all unless indicated"
Refill:_____ times-- Do not refill ( )

Signed:_____
DO NOT TAKE THIS TO YOUR PHARMACIST

Community Clinic
Jeffrey A. Eaton, NP
Joyce D. Cappiello, NP

Name:_____ DOB_____
Address_____ Date_____

Rx

"label all unless indicated"
Refill:_____ times-- Do not refill ( )

Signed:_____
DO NOT TAKE THIS TO YOUR PHARMACIST

Community Clinic
Jeffrey A. Eaton, NP
Joyce D. Cappiello, NP

Name:_____ DOB_____
Address_____ Date_____

Rx

"label all unless indicated"
Refill:_____ times-- Do not refill ( )

Signed:_____
DO NOT TAKE THIS TO YOUR PHARMACIST

Community Clinic
Jeffrey A. Eaton, NP
Joyce D. Cappiello, NP

Name:_____ DOB_____
Address_____ Date_____

Rx

"label all unless indicated"
Refill:_____ times-- Do not refill ( )

Signed:_____
DO NOT TAKE THIS TO YOUR PHARMACIST

Community Clinic
Jeffrey A. Eaton, NP
Joyce D. Cappiello, NP

Name:_____ DOB_____
Address_____ Date_____

Rx

"label all unless indicated"
Refill:_____ times-- Do not refill ( )

Signed:_____
DO NOT TAKE THIS TO YOUR PHARMACIST

Community Clinic
Jeffrey A. Eaton, NP
Joyce D. Cappiello, NP

Name:_____ DOB_____
Address_____ Date_____

Rx

"label all unless indicated"
Refill:_____ times-- Do not refill ( )

Signed:_____
DO NOT TAKE THIS TO YOUR PHARMACIST

Community Clinic
Jeffrey A. Eaton, NP
Joyce D. Cappiello, NP

Name:_____ DOB_____
Address_____ Date_____

Rx

"label all unless indicated"
Refill:_____ times-- Do not refill ( )

Signed:_____
DO NOT TAKE THIS TO YOUR PHARMACIST

Community Clinic
Jeffrey A. Eaton, NP
Joyce D. Cappiello, NP

Name:_____ DOB_____
Address_____ Date_____

Rx

"label all unless indicated"
Refill:_____ times-- Do not refill ( )

Signed:_____
DO NOT TAKE THIS TO YOUR PHARMACIST

Community Clinic
Jeffrey A. Eaton, NP
Joyce D. Cappiello, NP

Name:_____ DOB_____
Address_____ Date_____

Rx

"label all unless indicated"
Refill:_____ times-- Do not refill ( )

Signed:_____
DO NOT TAKE THIS TO YOUR PHARMACIST

Community Clinic
Jeffrey A. Eaton, NP
Joyce D. Cappiello, NP

Name:_____ DOB_____
Address_____ Date_____

Rx

"label all unless indicated"
Refill:_____ times-- Do not refill ( )

Signed:_____
DO NOT TAKE THIS TO YOUR PHARMACIST

Community Clinic
Jeffrey A. Eaton, NP
Joyce D. Cappiello, NP

Name:_____ DOB_____
Address_____ Date_____

Rx

"label all unless indicated"
Refill:_____ times-- Do not refill ( )

Signed:_____
DO NOT TAKE THIS TO YOUR PHARMACIST

Community Clinic
Jeffrey A. Eaton, NP
Joyce D. Cappiello, NP

Name:_____ DOB_____
Address_____ Date_____

Rx

"label all unless indicated"
Refill:_____ times-- Do not refill ( )

Signed:_____
DO NOT TAKE THIS TO YOUR PHARMACIST

Community Clinic
Jeffrey A. Eaton, NP
Joyce D. Cappiello, NP

Name:_____ DOB_____
Address_____ Date_____

Rx

"label all unless indicated"
Refill:_____ times-- Do not refill ( )

Signed:_____
DO NOT TAKE THIS TO YOUR PHARMACIST

Community Clinic
Jeffrey A. Eaton, NP
Joyce D. Cappiello, NP

Name:_____ DOB_____
Address_____ Date_____

Rx

"label all unless indicated"
Refill:_____ times-- Do not refill ( )

Signed:_____
DO NOT TAKE THIS TO YOUR PHARMACIST

Community Clinic
Jeffrey A. Eaton, NP
Joyce D. Cappiello, NP

Name:_____ DOB_____
Address_____ Date_____

Rx

"label all unless indicated"
Refill:_____ times-- Do not refill ( )

Signed:_____
DO NOT TAKE THIS TO YOUR PHARMACIST

Community Clinic
Jeffrey A. Eaton, NP
Joyce D. Cappiello, NP

Name:_____ DOB_____
Address_____ Date_____

Rx

"label all unless indicated"
Refill:_____ times-- Do not refill ( )

Signed:_____
DO NOT TAKE THIS TO YOUR PHARMACIST

Community Clinic
Jeffrey A. Eaton, NP
Joyce D. Cappiello, NP

Name:_____ DOB_____
Address_____ Date_____

Rx

"label all unless indicated"
Refill:_____ times-- Do not refill ( )

Signed:_____
DO NOT TAKE THIS TO YOUR PHARMACIST

Community Clinic
Jeffrey A. Eaton, NP
Joyce D. Cappiello, NP

Name:_____ DOB_____
Address_____ Date_____

Rx

"label all unless indicated"
Refill:_____ times-- Do not refill ( )

Signed:_____
DO NOT TAKE THIS TO YOUR PHARMACIST

Community Clinic
Jeffrey A. Eaton, NP
Joyce D. Cappiello, NP

Name:_____ DOB_____
Address_____ Date_____

Rx

"label all unless indicated"
Refill:_____ times-- Do not refill ( )

Signed:_____
DO NOT TAKE THIS TO YOUR PHARMACIST

Community Clinic
Jeffrey A. Eaton, NP
Joyce D. Cappiello, NP

Name:_____ DOB_____
Address_____ Date_____

Rx

"label all unless indicated"
Refill:_____ times-- Do not refill ( )

Signed:_____
DO NOT TAKE THIS TO YOUR PHARMACIST

Community Clinic
Jeffrey A. Eaton, NP
Joyce D. Cappiello, NP

Name:_____ DOB_____
Address_____ Date_____

Rx

"label all unless indicated"
Refill:_____ times-- Do not refill ( )

Signed:_____
DO NOT TAKE THIS TO YOUR PHARMACIST

Community Clinic
Jeffrey A. Eaton, NP
Joyce D. Cappiello, NP

Name:_____ DOB_____
Address_____ Date_____

Rx

"label all unless indicated"
Refill:_____ times-- Do not refill ( )

Signed:_____
DO NOT TAKE THIS TO YOUR PHARMACIST

Community Clinic
Jeffrey A. Eaton, NP
Joyce D. Cappiello, NP

Name:_____ DOB_____
Address_____ Date_____

Rx

"label all unless indicated"
Refill:_____ times-- Do not refill ( )

Signed:_____
DO NOT TAKE THIS TO YOUR PHARMACIST

Community Clinic
Jeffrey A. Eaton, NP
Joyce D. Cappiello, NP

Name:_____ DOB_____
Address_____ Date_____

Rx

"label all unless indicated"
Refill:_____ times-- Do not refill ( )

Signed:_____
DO NOT TAKE THIS TO YOUR PHARMACIST

Community Clinic
Jeffrey A. Eaton, NP
Joyce D. Cappiello, NP

Name:_____ DOB_____
Address_____ Date_____

Rx

"label all unless indicated"
Refill:_____ times-- Do not refill ( )

Signed:_____
DO NOT TAKE THIS TO YOUR PHARMACIST

Community Clinic
Jeffrey A. Eaton, NP
Joyce D. Cappiello, NP

Name:_____ DOB_____
Address_____ Date_____

Rx

"label all unless indicated"
Refill:_____ times-- Do not refill ( )

Signed:_____
DO NOT TAKE THIS TO YOUR PHARMACIST

Community Clinic
Jeffrey A. Eaton, NP
Joyce D. Cappiello, NP

Name:_____ DOB_____
Address_____ Date_____

Rx

"label all unless indicated"
Refill:_____ times-- Do not refill ( )

Signed:_____
DO NOT TAKE THIS TO YOUR PHARMACIST

Community Clinic
Jeffrey A. Eaton, NP
Joyce D. Cappiello, NP

Name:_____ DOB_____
Address_____ Date_____

Rx

"label all unless indicated"
Refill:_____ times-- Do not refill ( )

Signed:_____
DO NOT TAKE THIS TO YOUR PHARMACIST

Community Clinic
Jeffrey A. Eaton, NP
Joyce D. Cappiello, NP

Name:_____ DOB_____
Address_____ Date_____

Rx

"label all unless indicated"
Refill:_____ times-- Do not refill ( )

Signed:_____
DO NOT TAKE THIS TO YOUR PHARMACIST

Community Clinic
Jeffrey A. Eaton, NP
Joyce D. Cappiello, NP

Name:_____ DOB_____
Address_____ Date_____

Rx

"label all unless indicated"
Refill:_____ times-- Do not refill ( )

Signed:_____
DO NOT TAKE THIS TO YOUR PHARMACIST

Community Clinic
Jeffrey A. Eaton, NP
Joyce D. Cappiello, NP

Name:_____ DOB_____
Address_____ Date_____

Rx

"label all unless indicated"
Refill:_____ times-- Do not refill ( )

Signed:_____
DO NOT TAKE THIS TO YOUR PHARMACIST

Community Clinic
Jeffrey A. Eaton, NP
Joyce D. Cappiello, NP

Name:_____ DOB_____
Address_____ Date_____

Rx

"label all unless indicated"
Refill:_____ times-- Do not refill ( )

Signed:_____
DO NOT TAKE THIS TO YOUR PHARMACIST

Community Clinic
Jeffrey A. Eaton, NP
Joyce D. Cappiello, NP

Name:_____ DOB_____
Address_____ Date_____

Rx

"label all unless indicated"
Refill:_____ times-- Do not refill ( )

Signed:_____
DO NOT TAKE THIS TO YOUR PHARMACIST